Recognizing and Correcting Developing Malocclusions

A Problem-Oriented Approach to Orthodontics

Second Edition

Edited by

Eustáquio A. Araújo, DDS, MDS
Professor Emeritus – Saint Louis University
Clinical Professor – University of Pittsburgh
Professor – Faculdade de Ciências Médicas de Minas Gerais

Peter H. Buschang, MA, PhD
Regents Professor and Director of Orthodontic Research
Department of Orthodontics
Texas A&M University Baylor College of Dentistry
Dallas, TX, USA

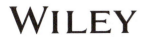

Copyright © 2025 John Wiley & Sons, Inc. All rights reserved, including rights for text and data mining and training of artificial technologies or similar technologies.

Published by John Wiley & Sons, Inc., Hoboken, New Jersey.
Published simultaneously in Canada.

No part of this publication may be reproduced, stored in a retrieval system, or transmitted in any form or by any means, electronic, mechanical, photocopying, recording, scanning, or otherwise, except as permitted under Section 107 or 108 of the 1976 United States Copyright Act, without either the prior written permission of the Publisher, or authorization through payment of the appropriate per-copy fee to the Copyright Clearance Center, Inc., 222 Rosewood Drive, Danvers, MA 01923, (978) 750-8400, fax (978) 750-4470, or on the web at www.copyright.com. Requests to the Publisher for permission should be addressed to the Permissions Department, John Wiley & Sons, Inc., 111 River Street, Hoboken, NJ 07030, (201) 748-6011, fax (201) 748-6008, or online at http://www.wiley.com/go/permission.

Trademarks: Wiley and the Wiley logo are trademarks or registered trademarks of John Wiley & Sons, Inc. and/or its affiliates in the United States and other countries and may not be used without written permission. All other trademarks are the property of their respective owners. John Wiley & Sons, Inc. is not associated with any product or vendor mentioned in this book.

Limit of Liability/Disclaimer of Warranty: While the publisher and author have used their best efforts in preparing this book, they make no representations or warranties with respect to the accuracy or completeness of the contents of this book and specifically disclaim any implied warranties of merchantability or fitness for a particular purpose. No warranty may be created or extended by sales representatives or written sales materials. The advice and strategies contained herein may not be suitable for your situation. You should consult with a professional where appropriate. Further, readers should be aware that websites listed in this work may have changed or disappeared between when this work was written and when it is read. Neither the publisher nor authors shall be liable for any loss of profit or any other commercial damages, including but not limited to special, incidental, consequential, or other damages.

For general information on our other products and services or for technical support, please contact our Customer Care Department within the United States at (800) 762-2974, outside the United States at (317) 572-3993 or fax (317) 572-4002.

Wiley also publishes its books in a variety of electronic formats. Some content that appears in print may not be available in electronic formats. For more information about Wiley products, visit our web site at www.wiley.com.

Library of Congress Cataloging-in-Publication Data Applied for:
Paperback ISBN: 9781119912545

Cover Design: Wiley
Cover Images: © Eustáquio A. Araújo

Set in 9.5/12.5pt STIXTwoText by Straive, Pondicherry, India

Printed in Singapore

M122685_171224

Dedications

To my family, particularly my wife Teresa, my daughter Kika, my son Chico, his wife Veronica, and my grandchildren Julia and Davi for the support and constant inspiration. To my parents, especially my father who, through his example, led me into dentistry. To each of my mentors, alumni from PUCMinas, Ciências Médicas de Minas Gerais and Saint Louis University, present residents, colleagues, and to each one of my patients who helped me to become a better clinician and professor. In addition, a special thanks to Drs. Orlando Tanaka, Jose Mauricio Vieira, Roberto Vieira, Júnia Lucia Vieira, and Gabriel Miranda for their help and friendship.

Eustáquio A. Araújo

Also to my family, particularly my wife Joyce, whose support and wisdom has sustained me. And to the orthodontic faculty, alumni, and residents that I have been privileged to work with – they have helped me to see the way. Together, they have made it all worthwhile.

Peter H. Buschang

Contents

List of Contributors *xiii*
Foreword *xv*
Preface *xvii*

1 **A guide for timing orthodontic treatment** *1*
Eustáquio A. Araújo, DDS, MDS and Bernardo Q. Souki, DDS, MSD, PhD
1.1 Occlusal deviations with indications for interceptive orthodontic treatment *3*
1.2 Ideal timing for early treatment *5*
1.2.1 Psychological aspects *5*
1.2.2 Severity of the malocclusion *5*
1.2.3 Effectiveness and efficiency concepts *6*
1.2.4 Maturational stage of development *7*
References *7*

2 **Development of the occlusion: what to do and when to do it** *9*
Bernardo Q. Souki, DDS, MSD, PhD
2.1 Stage 1—eruption of deciduous teeth *9*
2.1.1 Biogenesis of the deciduous dentition *9*
2.1.2 Dimensional changes of the dental arches at stage 1 *11*
2.1.3 Management of occlusal development at stage 1 *11*
2.2 Stage 2—completion of the deciduous dentition *11*
2.2.1 Dimensional changes in the dental arches at stage 2 *13*
2.2.2 Management of occlusion development at stage 2 *14*
2.3 Stage 3—eruption of first permanent molars *16*
2.3.1 Management of occlusion development at this stage *17*
2.4 Stage 4—eruption of permanent incisors *18*
2.4.1 Dimensional changes in the dental arches at this stage *18*
2.4.2 Management of occlusal development at this stage *19*
2.5 Stage 5—eruption of mandibular canines and first premolars *20*
2.5.1 Management of occlusal development at this stage *21*
2.6 Stage 6—eruption of second premolars *21*
2.6.1 Management of occlusal development at this stage *23*
2.7 Stage 7—eruption of maxillary canines and second molars *23*
2.7.1 Management of occlusal development at this stage *23*
2.8 Conclusions *24*
References *24*

3 Mixed dentition diagnosis: assessing the degree of severity of a developing malocclusion 27
Eustáquio A. Araújo, DDS, MDS
3.1   Assessing treatment need, complexity, and outcome 27
3.1.1 Summers' Occlusal Index 28
3.1.2 Dental Aesthetic Index (DAI) 28
3.1.3 Peer Assessment Rating (PAR) 28
3.1.4 Index of Orthodontic Treatment Need (IOTN) 28
3.1.5 Index of Complexity, Outcome, and Need (ICON) 29
3.1.6 The American Board of Orthodontics complexity index and outcome assessment 29
3.2   Assessing interceptive treatment outcome 31
3.2.1 Class I 31
3.2.2 Class II 31
3.2.3 Class III 32
        References 33

4 The genetics of the dental occlusion and malocclusion 35
Robyn Silberstein, DDS, PhD and Mary MacDougall, PhD
4.1   Introduction 35
4.1.1 Personalized medicine 35
4.1.2 Clinical examination 35
4.1.3 Principles of dysmorphology: variable expressivity and etiologic heterogeneity 36
4.2   Chromosomal abnormalities 37
4.3   Single gene defects 38
4.4   Multifactorial inheritance 38
4.5   Genetics of nonsyndromic malocclusion 40
4.6   Altered tooth number 42
4.7   Altered tooth structure 43
4.8   Altered eruption 43
4.9   Radiographic deviations associated with genetic conditions 45
4.10   Conclusion 47
        References 47

5 Class I: Recognizing and correcting intraarch deviations 51
5.1 Section I: The development and etiology of a Class I malocclusion 51
Peter H. Buschang, MA, PhD
5.1   Introduction 51
5.2   Prevalence of Class I malocclusion and changes in arch form 52
5.3   Class I malocclusion and the dental compensatory mechanism 58
5.4   What is anterior mandibular malalignment is related to? 60
5.4.1 Predisposing factors 60
5.4.2 Eruption problems associated with space loss 61
5.4.3 Contact displacements associated with relapse and tooth movements 62
        References 63

5.2	**Section II: Intercepting developing Class I problems** *67*	
	Eustáquio A. Araújo, DDS, MDS	
5.5	Tooth size arch length discrepancy (TSALD) *67*	
5.6	The assessment of crowding in the mixed dentition *68*	
5.6.1	Zero to minor TSALD *68*	
5.6.2	Small to moderate TSALD *69*	
5.6.2.1	Taking advantage of the transitional dentition *69*	
5.6.3	Gaining spaces in the dental arches *71*	
5.6.3.1	The importance of the leeway space/E space *71*	
5.6.3.2	Etiology of maxillary transverse deficiency *72*	
5.6.3.3	Maxillary expansion and headgear *73*	
5.6.3.4	Gaining space in the mandibular arch *83*	
5.6.3.5	Arch dimensions changes *84*	
5.6.3.6	Arch length and mandibular molar/MP *84*	
5.6.3.7	Arch length and mandibular incisors/MP *84*	
5.6.3.8	Transverse changes *84*	
5.6.3.9	Incisor irregularity changes *84*	
5.6.3.10	The Schwarz appliance *86*	
5.6.3.11	Two-by-four fixed therapy *86*	
5.6.4	Severe TSALD: fundamentals of serial extraction *92*	
5.6.5	Indications and contraindications for serial extraction (SE) *93*	
5.6.5.1	Additional important fundamentals in serial extraction *94*	
5.6.5.2	Sequence and timing of extractions *95*	
5.6.5.3	Alternative extraction sequences *95*	
	References *102*	
6	**Recognizing and correcting Class II malocclusions** *107*	
6.1	**Section I: The development, phenotypic characteristics, and etiology of Class II malocclusion** *107*	
	Peter H. Buschang, MA, PhD	
6.1	Introduction *107*	
6.1.1	Prevalence *109*	
6.2	Characterization of the Class II, division 2 phenotype *110*	
6.3	Characterization of the Class II division 1 phenotype *111*	
6.3.1	Hyperdivergent vs. hypodivergent Class II division 1 malocclusion *114*	
6.4	Developmental changes of Class IIs *115*	
6.5	Class II developmental changes *118*	
6.6	Etiology *119*	
	References *123*	
6.2	**Section II: Class II treatment: problems and solutions** *131*	
	Eustáquio A. Araújo, DDS, MDS	
6.7	Early Class II adjustment *132*	
6.8	Treatment *136*	
	References *158*	

7	**Recognizing and correcting Class III malocclusions** *161*
7.1	**Section I: The development, phenotypic characteristics, and etiology of Class III malocclusion** *161*
	Peter H. Buschang, MA, PhD
7.1	Introduction *161*
7.2	Characterization of the Class III phenotype *163*
7.3	Class III development *168*
7.4	Etiology *170*
	References *175*
7.2	**Section II: Class III treatment: problems and solutions** *179*
	Eustáquio A. Araújo, DDS, MDS
7.5	Diagnosis *183*
7.5.1	Facial diagnosis *183*
7.5.2	Cephalometric diagnosis *183*
7.5.3	Dental diagnosis *183*
7.5.4	Functional diagnosis *184*
7.5.5	Hereditary diagnosis *185*
7.6	Communication *187*
7.7	Early intervention *188*
7.8	Orthopedic maxillary expansion *188*
7.9	Face mask and/or chincup orthopedics *191*
7.9.1	The face mask *191*
7.9.2	The chincup *193*
7.10	Leeway space control *194*
7.11	Orthodontic mechanics *194*
7.12	Finishing *194*
7.13	Retention *194*
7.14	Growth reevaluation *195*
	References *221*
8	**Special topics** *225*
8.1	**Section I: Habit control: the role of function in open-bite treatment** *225*
	Ildeu Andrade, Jr., DDS, MS, PhD and Eustáquio A. Araújo, DDS, MDS
8.1	Nutritive vs. nonnutritive sucking habits *225*
8.2	Tongue physiology *226*
8.3	Tongue thrusting and forward resting posture of the tongue *227*
8.4	Breaking the habit *227*
8.4.1	How and when should a clinician intervene? *227*
8.4.2	The Araújo approach *227*
8.5	Treatment *229*
	References *235*

8.2	**Section II: Eruption deviations** *239*	
	Bernardo Q. Souki, DDS, MSD, PhD and Eustáquio A. Araújo, DDS, MDS	
8.6	Eruption deviations *239*	
8.7	Eruption deviation and PIOM: what are the most frequent eruption disturbances in each stage of dental development? *241*	
8.7.1	Stage 2 – Completion of deciduous dentition *241*	
8.7.2	Stage 3 – Eruption of the first permanent molars *241*	
8.7.3	Stage 4 – Eruption of the permanent incisors *241*	
8.7.4	Stage 5 – Eruption of the mandibular canines and the first premolars *242*	
8.7.5	Stage 6 – Eruption of the second premolars *247*	
8.7.6	Stage 7 – Eruption of maxillary canines and second molars *247*	
	References *253*	
8.3	**Section III: Strategies for managing missing second premolar teeth in the young patient** *255*	
	David B. Kennedy, BDS, LDS (RCSEng), MSD, FRCD(C)	
8.8	General concepts *255*	
8.9	Longevity of the second deciduous molar, resorption, and infraocclusion *256*	
8.9.1	Resorption *256*	
8.9.2	Infraocclusion *257*	
8.10	The alveolar ridge in extracted deciduous molars *257*	
8.11	Overall dental health and cost *258*	
8.12	Case histories *258*	
8.13	Summary *270*	
	References *270*	
8.4	**Section IV: Principles and techniques of premolar autotransplantation** *273*	
	Ewa M. Czochrowska, DDS, PhD and Paweł Plakwicz, DDS, PhD	
8.14	Class II malocclusion with congenitally missing lower second premolars *274*	
8.15	Traumatic loss of upper incisor/s *274*	
8.16	Uneven tooth distribution with multiple agenesis *274*	
8.17	Surgery *277*	
8.18	Selection of anesthesia (local vs. general) *277*	
8.19	Premolar to premolar transplantation *277*	
8.20	Premolar to anterior maxilla transplantation *279*	
8.21	Postoperative instructions *279*	
8.22	Follow-up *279*	
8.23	Pulp healing *280*	
8.24	Periodontal healing *281*	
8.25	Root growth *281*	
8.26	Reshaping to incisor morphology *281*	
8.27	Alveolar bone after autotransplantation *281*	
	References *282*	

8.5	**Section V: Dental trauma: revisiting posttrauma protocols and long-term follow-ups** *285*	
	Eustaquio A. Araújo, DDS, MDS and Gabriel Miranda, DDS, MS	
8.28	An overview of dental trauma *285*	
8.29	Orthodontic treatment and dental trauma *286*	
8.30	Managing traumatized teeth and preserving bone width – The decoronation approach *288*	
8.31	Final considerations *295*	
	References *297*	
8.6	**Section VI: Sleep-disordered breathing (SDB) in the growing child** *299*	
	Juan Martin Palomo, DDS, MDS and Luciane M. de Menezes, PhD	
8.32	The need for sleep *299*	
8.33	Diagnosis and management of sleep-disordered breathing (SDB) and obstructive sleep apnea (OSA) in children *300*	
8.34	Risk factors for OSA in children *302*	
8.34.1	Enlarged tonsils and adenoids *302*	
8.34.2	Obesity *304*	
8.34.3	Allergies and respiratory infections *304*	
8.34.4	Structural abnormalities and craniofacial anomalies *305*	
8.35	Consequences of SDB in children *305*	
8.36	Treatment options for the dental and skeletal consequences of SDB in children *309*	
8.37	New technologies: the use of apps and devices for SDB and OSA in children *310*	
8.38	Conclusion *310*	
	References *311*	
8.7	**Section VII: Mixed dentition orthodontic mechanics** *313*	
	Gerald S. Samson, DDS	
8.39	Definitions and terminology *314*	
8.39.1	Center of mass and center of resistance *315*	
8.39.2	Orders of tooth movements and orthodontic terminology *316*	
8.39.3	Force systems *316*	
8.39.4	Single-point force and moment of force *316*	
8.39.5	Additive and subtractive couples *316*	
8.39.6	Equilibrium and tooth movement – Newton's third law *317*	
8.39.7	Force systems and tooth movements *318*	
8.39.8	Mixed dentition example of one tube (bracket) and one couple system *319*	
8.39.9	Mixed dentition: maxillary anterior root convergence *320*	
8.39.10	Orthodontic treatment of teeth with open apices *320*	
8.39.11	Two brackets – two equal and oppositely directed couples *320*	
8.39.12	Two brackets – two unequal oppositely directed couples *321*	
8.39.13	Two brackets – two "same direction, additive" couples including increased anterior incisor root torque *322*	
8.39.14	Clinical application – mixed dentition openbite, two "same direction, additive" couples including increased anterior incisor root torque *324*	
	References *326*	

Index *327*

List of Contributors

Ildeu Andrade Jr., DDS, MS, PhD
Department of Orthodontics, School of Dental Medicine
University of Pittsburgh
Pittsburgh, PA
USA

Eustáquio A. Araújo, DDS, MDS
Department of Orthodontics, Center for Advanced Dental Education
Saint Louis University
St. Louis, MO
USA

Peter H. Buschang, MA, PhD
Department of Orthodontics
Texas A&M University School of Dentistry
Dallas, TX
USA

Ewa M. Czochrowska, DDS, PhD
Department of Orthodontics
Medical University of Warsaw
Warsaw
Poland

David B. Kennedy, BDS, LDS (RCSEng), MSD, FRCD(C)
Faculty of Dentistry
University of British Columbia
Vancouver, BC
Canada

Mary MacDougall, PhD
Faculty of Dentistry
University of British Columbia
Canada

Luciane M. de Menezes, PhD
Department of Orthodontics
Case Western Reserve University
Cleveland, OH
USA

Pontifical Catholic University of Rio Grande do Sul
Porto Alegre/RS
Brazil

Gabriel Miranda, DDS, MS
Department of Orthodontics
Saint Louis University
St. Louis, MO
USA

Juan Martin Palomo, DDS, MDS
Department of Orthodontics
Case Western Reserve University
Cleveland, OH
USA

Paweł Plakwicz, DDS, PhD
Department of Periodontology
Medical University of Warsaw
Poland

Gerald S. Samson, DDS
Department of Orthodontics, Center of
Advanced Dental Education
Saint Louis University
St. Louis, MO
USA

Robyn Silberstein, DDS, PhD
Department of Orthodontics, College of
Dentistry (retired)
University of Illinois at Chicago
Chicago, IL
USA

Bernardo Q. Souki, DDS, MSD, PhD
Department of Dentistry
Pontifical Catholic University of Minas Gerais
Belo Horizonte
Brazil

Foreword

Orthodontic educators are often confronted by loaded questions where the questioners really just want to know if their biases are shared by the educator. One of the most common questions is: "Do you teach early treatment to your students?" From experience, I know that the answer either lines up with the questioner's bias and a conversation of great agreement will follow, or the answer does not line up with their bias and a conversation of great disagreement will follow, so I prefer to provide neither expected answer, but instead aim to stimulate thought. So my answer might well be "Yes, we teach early treatment and late treatment and also very early and very late treatment. We also perform 1-phase treatment, 2-phase treatment, 3-phase, 4-, 5-, 6-, 7-, 8-, and even 9-phase treatment ... or more, if need be."

Of course, this answer is very perplexing and I am asked to explain what I mean – which I am happy to do. To provide support to my answer, I provide several examples. For one of these, I talk about a study that was performed long ago by a former graduate student named Greg Dyer [1]. He took a sample of treated adolescent females and a similar sample of treated adult females and compared the outcomes of the treatments performed. Importantly, in the adolescent group he found that growth provided 70% of the correction (i.e. the mandible outgrew the maxilla) while only 30% of the correction was due to tooth movement. In the adult sample, the growth was nil, or in some cases the maxilla outgrew the mandible and the amount of tooth movement that was necessary to correct the malocclusion was 119% – that is, the practitioner had to do all the work, and more, to make up for the poor growth, in order to correct the problem. For me, this is ample evidence that it is better to treat early (as an adolescent) as opposed to late (as an adult) in this particular situation. This example points to the meaning of my response to the question posed initially. It is not whether I am biased so that I believe only in early treatment or only in late treatment as a single choice that must be made, but rather it is that the question can only be answered in the context of the situation that is presented. In this example, my answer would be to treat early (in this case, adolescence) when you are confronted by a Class II female adolescent; don't wait till they become adults.

In the case of treatment performed in multiple phases, again it is the context of the patient's situation that dictates what to do. There is plenty of research and clinical experience available that suggests that a cleft palate patient is best treated early and often over many years, according to the many types of treatments that are arranged across many phases. There are also questions as to how many phases of treatment should be involved in an orthognathic surgery case.

So, the point that I am trying to make is that it matters little whether a practitioner "believes" in early treatment or not, and it makes little difference whether the practitioner "believes" in single-phase treatments or some other number of phases. What really matters is that the practitioner evaluates the condition that the patient presents and then applies the best available evidence to the situation in deciding if, when, and how the treatment should be rendered. To believe otherwise suggests that the doctor can decide the approach before even seeing the patient. But adopting a prefabricated approach is seldom the best choice because patients are all custom-made.

What follows in the pages to come is blended (some old, but mostly new) information concerning genetics, normal, and abnormal growth of the craniofacial skeleton, and the development of the occlusion. Such information will form the basis for understanding and determining the timing of treatment.

You will also find important information on the construction of a diagnosis, treatment plan, and estimation of prognosis, all based on available diagnostic records produced by both old and new technologies. All three types of Angle classes will be considered in terms of development, etiology, and treatment; that is the meat of this book.

Finally, information will be provided with regard to certain overriding topics such as biomechanics, and what might be considered "orphan topics" including problems attendant to abnormal eruption, function, aesthetics, congenitally missing teeth, autotransplantation, and habits.

So, how is this book different from previous books on the topic of early and preventive orthodontic treatment? Considering the comments made earlier in this preface, this book is based on available evidence, not bias, passion, or faith; it is meant to make you think and then apply what is proven. This book is also different in that the authors are very knowledgeable each in their own areas, and each is cognizant of the value of current science and the knowledge that science generates.

Those readers who are open to the development of new information and new ideas should enjoy and embrace the knowledge and direction contained within. For those who are very biased in their thoughts and actions do not be afraid to read this book; it will open your mind and help you adjust your thoughts and actions in a positive way.

Have a good read; I think you will find it worth the effort in terms of thought and then reasoned actions that will prove beneficial to your patients.

Rolf G. Behrents

Reference

1 Dyer, GS. Age effects of orthodontic treatment: adolescents contrasted with adults. MS Thesis, The University of Tennessee, 1989.

Preface

Recognizing and Correcting Development Malocclusions: A Problem-Oriented Approach to Orthodontics, in its second edition, continues to provide evidence-based approach to early age orthodontics, an often controversial topic. Based on decades of experience in clinical practice and education, Drs. Araujo and Buschang with the support of an outstanding team of contributors, present treatment protocols for early age orthodontics treatment with various malocclusions and other problems.

Class I, Class II, and Class III malocclusions are extensively covered, along with eruption deviations and developing hyperdivergence growth and open bites. This second edition brings new topics such as Trauma and Sleep Apnea in children. The literature is comprehensively reviewed to ensure that the reader thoroughly understands the development, phenoptic characteristics, and etiology of each type of malocclusion.

Taking a problem-oriented approach, the editors and contributors provide detailed information for each case, develop comprehensive problem lists, and then provide evidence-based treatment solutions.

The clinical focus of the text is ideally suited for the private practice clinician, with numerous references and academic underpinnings to ensure its suitability for orthodontic and pediatric dentistry residents.

Eustáquio A. Araújo
Center for Advanced Dental Education
Saint Louis University, St. Louis, MO, USA
19 September 2024

Peter H. Buschang
Regents Professor and Director
of Orthodontic Research
Department of Orthodontics
Texas A&M University Baylor
College of Dentistry
Dallas, TX, USA
19 September 2024

1

A guide for timing orthodontic treatment

Eustáquio A. Araújo, DDS, MDS[1] and Bernardo Q. Souki, DDS, MSD, PhD[2]

[1] *Department of Orthodontics, Center for Advanced Dental Education, Saint Louis University, St. Louis, MO, USA*
[2] *Department of Dentistry, Pontifical Catholic University of Minas Gerais, Belo Horizonte, Brazil*

When the decision was made to work on this book, the heavy responsibility of embracing the topic without bias or radicalism increased. Clinicians and academicians were initially consulted and asked to provide questions that would help establish priorities for early interventions. The responses came rapidly and contained all the sorts of questions one would imagine. ***Recognizing and Correcting Developing Malocclusions*** will try to address the collected questions and themes.

The term "early treatment" has been used for a long time, and it seems now to be fixed. Although "early" could suggest "too soon," for the sake of practicality it will be used in this book. The text will eventually also refer to timely or interceptive treatment.

Initiating orthodontic treatment during the growth spurt was often used to be considered the "gold standard" for treatment timing. The pendulum that regulates the initiation of orthodontic treatment has been swinging in different directions for many years. At present, this balance seems to have been shifting, as the pendulum appears to be swinging toward an earlier start, preferably at the late mixed dentition. The possibility of successfully managing the E-space has dramatically influenced the decision-making on the timing of orthodontic treatment [1].

At the beginning of the 20th century, some consideration was given to early treatment. A quote from Lischer [2] in 1912 says,

> Recent experiences of many practitioners have led us to a keener appreciation of the "golden age of treatment" by which we mean that time in an individual's life when a change from the temporary to the permanent dentition takes place. This covers the period from the sixth to the fourteenth year.

Soon after, in 1921, a publication [3] titled "The diagnosis of malocclusion with reference to early treatment," discusses the concepts of function and form and gives notable consideration to the role of heredity in diagnosis—so the topic with its controversies is an old one.

"The emancipation of dentofacial orthopedics," an editorial by Hamilton [4] supports early treatment. In summary, he states that:

a) healthcare professionals must do everything possible to help their patients, including early treatment;
b) it is irresponsible and unethical to prescribe treatment for financial betterment and for the sake of efficiency;
c) if the orthodontist is not willing to treat patients at a young age, others in the dental

---

Recognizing and Correcting Developing Malocclusions: A Problem-Oriented Approach to Orthodontics,
Second Edition. Edited by Eustáquio A. Araújo and Peter H. Buschang.
© 2025 John Wiley & Sons, Inc. Published 2025 by John Wiley & Sons, Inc.

profession will, and it is in the patients' best interest that we, as specialists, treat these patients. After all, our flagship journal includes "Dentofacial Orthopedics" in its title;

d) it is the highest calling of healthcare professionals to incorporate prevention as a primary means of treatment, and therefore early treatment is important;
e) pediatric dentists and other health professionals are incorporating early treatment in their practice because orthodontists are waiting too long to initiate treatment;
f) orthodontic programs have the responsibility to educate orthodontists about early treatment.

On the other hand, Johnston [5] indicates in "Answers in search of questioners" that:

a) little evidence exists that two-phase early treatment has a significantly greater overall treatment effect compared with treating in one phase and considering E-space preservation;
b) treatment aimed at the mandible typically has an effect on the maxilla;
c) early treatment is not efficient for the patient or doctor and results in an increased burden of treatment;
d) functional appliances do not eliminate the need for premolar extraction, as bone cannot grow interstitially and arch perimeter is not gained with their use;
e) patients occasionally endure psychological trauma due to dental deformity, but these isolated instances are not enough to "support what amounts to an orthodontic growth industry."

In an effort to establish grounds to initiate treatment earlier or later, we must try to answer two key questions:

1) Should developing problems be intercepted and treated in two phases?
2) Which malocclusions should receive consideration for treatment at an early age?

Undoubtedly, there is much agreement on what to treat, but there is still great disagreement on when to intervene.

What are achievable objectives for early treatment? Some of the most relevant ones are using growth potential appropriately, taking advantage of the transitional dentition, improving skeletal imbalances, eliminating functional deviations, managing arch development, improving self-esteem, minimizing trauma, and preventing periodontal problems.

Early orthodontic treatment offers several potential advantages, including better patient compliance, emotional satisfaction, and the ability to harness growth potential. It may also simplify the second phase of treatment and reduce the need for extractions. Additionally, early treatment can benefit practice management. However, there are also disadvantages, such as inefficiency, prolonged treatment time, patient immaturity, challenges with maintaining oral hygiene, difficulty in caring for appliances, and higher costs. It is crucial for orthodontists to carefully weigh these benefits and risks, providing evidence-based and well-reasoned recommendations on whether or not to initiate treatment. This chapter offers guidance on the optimal timing for orthodontic interventions.

The ideal timing for treating malocclusions in growing patients has been a controversial and widely discussed topic throughout the history of orthodontics [1, 6–10]. One of the most important debates in our field is whether to interrupt the development of problems with early treatment or to postpone therapy until later [1, 9]. Such controversies are likely due to the lack of a scientific basis for therapeutic clinical decisions [8]. Historically, dentistry has been an empirical science. Even today, most dentists choose to employ solutions and techniques that were first learned in dental school or those that they believe will work [1, 9]. In such cases, there is a high probability of treatment failure or a low-quality treatment outcome.

During the search for excellence in orthodontics, the concepts of effectiveness and efficiency have been emphasized [1]. Orthodontic clinical decisions should be scientifically based. Accordingly, treatment must be postponed until strong arguments in favor of beginning the therapy are present [9].

A follow-up protocol in which patients are re-examined periodically during growth and the development of occlusion allows the clinician to decide whether the cost/benefit of early treatment is justifiable. At this time, the program "preventive and interceptive orthodontic monitoring," or simply PIOM, as devised by Souki [11] is introduced.

Conceptually, PIOM is a program of sequential attention that aims to monitor the development of "normal" occlusion and seeks to diagnose any factors that may compromise the quality or quantity of orthodontic treatment and the establishment of an appropriate occlusion. Seven objectives govern PIOM:

1) Provide prospective monitoring with a minimal intervention philosophy;
2) Provide comprehensive orthodontic care with functional and esthetically harmonious adult occlusion as the ultimate goal;
3) Establish parameters so that orthodontists are not in a hurry to start treatment but are able to have a deadline to complete treatment;
4) Establish scientific parameters as guidelines for beginning therapy at each stage of maturation;
5) Respect the normal range of occlusal development;
6) Reduce dependence on patient compliance;
7) Delay phase II, if possible, until the time when second permanent molars can be included in the final occlusion.

During the years that separate the eruption of the first deciduous tooth and the full intercuspation of the second permanent molars, many morphogenetic influences and environmental factors act on the maturation of the dental arches and the occlusal pattern. Therefore, human occlusion should be viewed dynamically.

Clinicians must understand that during occlusal development, there is not just one line of ideal characteristics but a wide range of normal characteristics. In the mixed dentition, a larger variety of normal characteristics compared to the deciduous and permanent dentitions is encountered. Knowledge of normal features of occlusal maturation is important for the practice of orthodontics within PIOM. Throughout the history of medicine/dentistry, identifying signs or symptoms of a deviation from normal has been viewed as a situation requiring interceptive action. In lay terms, it has been thought that allowing a disease to evolve naturally (without therapy) may possibly make the disease more difficult to treat or even make it incurable [7]. This belief, when applied to orthodontics, may produce unnecessary interventions for occlusal characteristics that are totally within the range of normal (Figure 1.1), treatment of transitional deviations for which interceptive treatment (phase I) is not needed (Figure 1.2), and interceptive treatment before the appropriate time (Figure 1.3).

As mentioned earlier, the orthodontist should focus on two key questions: the first deals with the ideal timing for interceptive orthodontics, incorporating the decision between one- and two-phase treatments and the second hinges on identifying malocclusions that would benefit from an early intervention.

1.1 Occlusal deviations with indications for interceptive orthodontic treatment

Interceptive problems are those that, if not stopped during the course of their maturation, may become sufficiently severe to increase the complexity and difficulty of definitive treatment, compromise the final quality, or expose

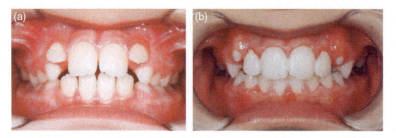

Figure 1.1 (a) A 8-year-old boy during "ugly duckling" phase presenting labial-distal displacement of maxillary lateral incisors and a diastema between the central incisors. (b) Same patient 3 years later without any orthodontic treatment. The incisors' alignment and leveling were naturally achieved.

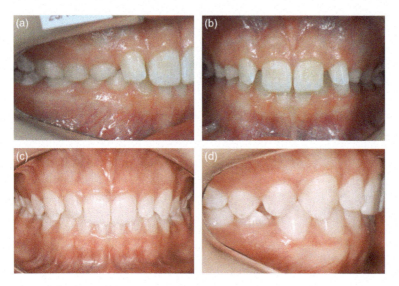

Figure 1.2 (a, b) A 9-year-old girl presenting deep bite and positive space discrepancy. Such transitional deviations (deep bite and positive space discrepancy) have no indication of interceptive orthodontics unless palatal soft tissue impingement is observed or aesthetics is a major concern. (c, d) Same girl 5 years later presenting significant natural improvements in the deep bite and space discrepancy with no phase I treatment.

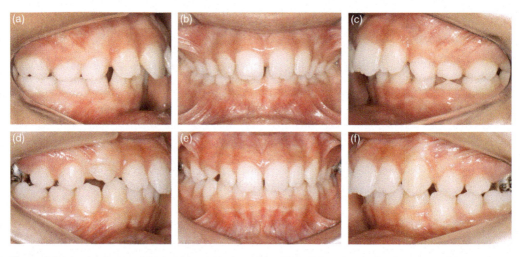

Figure 1.3 (a–c) A 9-year-old mixed dentition boy with a Class II/1 malocclusion but no psychosomatic concerns. The evaluation of a low/moderate risk of traumatic injuries in the maxillary front teeth indicated postponing to a single-phase orthodontic treatment. (d–f) Patient at 12 years old, during early permanent dentition. No interceptive orthodontic treatment was performed. After 5 months of headgear appliance, the patient is now going into the 12–18 months multibrackets comprehensive orthodontic treatment. Efficiency was achieved by postponing the Class II correction to a single-phase approach.

the individual to psychosocial conditions while waiting for a final corrective solution. Disagreements certainly exist among scholars regarding the clinical situations with indications for early orthodontic treatment. The list of issues presented by the American Association of Pediatric Dentistry [12] may serve as the starting point for this guideline. Based on their list, the following situations are suggested as candidates for early treatment: 1) prevention and interception of oral habits; 2) space management; 3) interception of deviations in eruption; 4) anterior crossbite; 5) posterior crossbite; 6) excessive overjet; 7) Class II malocclusion, when associated with psychological problems, increased risk of traumatic injury and hyperdivergence; 8) Class III malocclusion.

1.2 Ideal timing for early treatment

Several aspects must be considered by the clinician when deciding on the ideal timing for early treatment. Four basic considerations are: 1) psychosocial aspects; 2) the severity and etiology of the malocclusion; 3) the concepts of effectiveness and efficiency; 4) the patient's stage of the development.

1.2.1 Psychological aspects

Psychological aspects are often neglected by orthodontists and unfortunately have not been routinely considered during the early treatment decision-making process [13, 14].

At a time when bullying has been extensively discussed [15] and has been widely studied by psychopedagogues, clinicians must be constantly aware of the fact that, as providers, they can in many instances improve the self-esteem and quality of life (QoL) of their patients [16].

For many, the relationship between a patient's well-being and his/her malocclusion, along with possible associated sequelae has been thought to be of only minor importance [17]. Consideration must be given to each patient's QoL and the associated impact that postponement or avoidance of treatment may carry. Although somewhat vague and abstract, the concept of QoL is current and should be emphasized in orthodontics [18].

The literature provides evidence of an association between QoL and malocclusions. The methodologies of QoL studies, however, have not been homogeneous, and the samples are often constructed based on convenience, making it difficult to offer a reliable analysis. The lack of randomized samples hinders the interpretation of the evidence [18, 19].

Young people are motivated to seek orthodontic treatment because of their esthetic dissatisfaction [13], referrals from dentists [20], parental concerns [13], and the influence of peers [21]. Orthodontic treatment does improve QoL [19], but over time, the gain in QoL may be lost. When a malocclusion causes discomfort to a patient with the potential for generating a psychological imbalance [20], there is certainly an indication for early treatment [13], despite the fact that efficiency may be adversely affected [1].

1.2.2 Severity of the malocclusion

Malocclusions differ among patients presenting a wide range of severity. Therefore, it seems reasonable to think that, in infancy and adolescence, a mild malocclusion has a lower interceptive priority than a more severe one. For example, a posterior crossbite with mandibular shift (Figure 1.4a) should have treatment priority as compared to malocclusions with minor shift or not associated with functional deviations (Figure 1.4b). In the first scenario, the deviation can lead to asymmetric facial growth, making future therapy more complex [22]. There is less urgency for treatment of a single lateral incisor crossbite than a two-central-incisor crossbite (Figure 1.5), although there is a lack of evidence in the current literature about postponing interceptive approach of crossbites. It must be understood that the

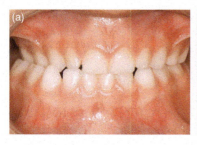 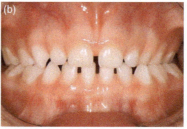

Figure 1.4 (a) Posterior crossbite with mandibular shift. (b) Posterior crossbite with no mandibular shift.

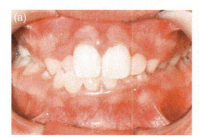 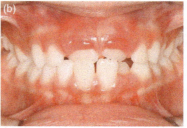

Figure 1.5 (a) A 8-year-old boy, Class I dental-skeletal pattern, presenting a single lateral incisor crossbite. (b) A 7-year-old girl, Class I dental-skeletal pattern, presenting two central incisors crossbite. Because periodontal and dentofacial growth impairments are more likely to happen in "b," it is reasonable to infer that interceptive approach should be addressed urgently.

severity of the malocclusion is not the only criterion for deciding on interceptive treatment. For example, if a Class III malocclusion is very severe in childhood, with skeletal components indicating that surgical correction may be required in the future, it is reasonable to consider delaying treatment until the end of growth to reduce extensive interceptive treatment [23, 24]. In other words, in some situations, it is advisable to postpone the correction of the malocclusion until a single-phase orthodontic-surgical treatment can be undertaken. On the other hand, many other Class III malocclusions in children may benefit greatly from an interceptive approach [24, 25].

1.2.3 Effectiveness and efficiency concepts

The decision on the best time for orthodontic treatment must also consider the aspects of effectiveness and efficiency [10]. Effectiveness is a concept that expresses the ability to effectively solve a problem. Will it work at all? How much improvement will be produced? This concept is important in the search for excellence in orthodontics. Orthodontic interceptive actions should be considered if there is evidence that the problem to be treated will, in fact, be solved by early treatment. If the problem is not intercepted, will it lead to a less acceptable final result or cause greater difficulty in obtaining a good result?

Efficiency is a formula that correlates result with time. How much time will be needed to achieve the goals? Will the financial, biological, and interpersonal burden be worth the outcome? In the contemporary world, the concept of efficiency has been an important criterion in deciding implementations of actions and services. If the cost–benefit of a phase I is unfavorable, should one consider the benefits of early orthodontic treatment?

In summary, the treatment of malocclusions in children should be considered an acceptable option if there is evidence that the outcome will add quality (effectiveness) and will be obtained with less effort (efficiency). Be sure to get the best result in the shortest amount of time possible.

1.2.4 Maturational stage of development

The orthodontist should consider several maturational aspects [26–28]. The presence of a minimal emotional maturity is essential for beginning any orthodontic procedure, even in patients with low-complexity malocclusions [29]. These considerations are essential to improve patient comfort [30] and to reduce the risk of accidents in young children. Thus, the cooperation of the child in the clinical examination becomes the first parameter used by orthodontists in judging the potential for early treatment. Depending on the child's behavior and compliance, the clinician will decide if orthodontic records should be taken.

Psychosocial maturity is normally associated with chronological age. The American Association of Orthodontists (AAO) in its brochure *Your Child's First Check-up* recommends that children have a check-up with an orthodontic specialist no later than age 7. However, decisions about early treatment should be undertaken on an individual basis. Other parameters of maturity should also be considered. Assessment of the dental age should be made when intra-arch problems suggest early treatment. On the other hand, skeletal age should be used as a guide for the best time to intercept sagittal and vertical interarch problems [26, 27].

In conclusion, it seems clear that a thorough consideration of all the factors described here will serve two purposes: 1) to determine whether or not early treatment is necessary and 2) to provide guidelines for determining when treatment should be initiated.

References

1 Proffit WR. The timing of early treatment: an overview. *Am J Orthod Dentofacial Orthop* 2006;**129**(4 Suppl):S47–9.

2 Lischer BE. *Principles and methods of orthodontics: An introductory study of the art for students and practitioners of dentistry.* Philadelphia, PA and New York: Lea & Febinger, 1912.

3 Johnson LR. The diagnosis of malocclusion with reference to early treatment. *J Dent Res* 1921;**3**(1):v–xx.

4 Hamilton DC. The emancipation of dentofacial orthopedics. *Am J Orthod Dentofacial Orthop* 1998;**113**(1):7–10.

5 Johnston L Jr. Answers in search of questioners. *Am J Orthod Dentofacial Orthop* 2002;**121**(6):552–95.

6 Freeman JD. Preventive and interceptive orthodontics: a critical review and the results of a clinical study. *J Prev Dent* 1977;**4**(5):7–14, 20–3.

7 Ackerman JL, Proffit WR. Preventive and interceptive orthodontics: a strong theory proves weak in practice. *Angle Orthod* 1980;**50**(2):75–87.

8 Livieratos FA, Johnston LE. A comparison of one-stage and two-stage non-extraction alternatives in matched Class II samples. *Am J Orthod Dentofacial Orthop* 1995;**108**(2):118–31.

9 Bowman SJ. One-stage versus two-stage treatment: are two really necessary? *Am J Orthod Dentofacial Orthop* 1998;**113**(1):111–6.

10 Arvystas MG. The rationale for early orthodontic treatment. *Am J Orthod Dentofacial Orthop* 1998;**113**(1):15–8.

11 Souki BQ. Desenvolvimento da oclusão. In: Toledo OA (ed), *Odontopediatria: fundamentos para a prática clínica.* 4th edn. Rio de Janeiro: Medbook, 2012. p. 307–27.

12 American Academy on Pediatric Dentistry. Management of the developing dentition and occlusion in pediatric dentistry. In: *The reference manual of pediatric dentistry*. Chicago, IL: American Academy of Pediatric Dentistry, 2022. p. 424–41.

13 Kiyak HA. Patients' and parents' expectations from early treatment. *Am J Orthod Dentofacial Orthop* 2006;**129**(4 Suppl):S50–4.

14 Tung AW, Kiyak HA. Psychological influences on the timing of orthodontic treatment. *Am J Orthod Dentofacial Orthop* 1998;**113**(1):29–39.

15 Takizawa R, Maughan B, Arseneault L. Adult health outcomes of childhood bullying victimization: evidence from a five-decade longitudinal British birth cohort. *Am J Psychiatry* 2014;**171**(7):777–84.

16 Bogart LM, Elliott MN, Klein DJ, et al. Peer victimization in fifth grade and health in tenth grade. *Pediatrics* 2014;**133**(3):440–7.

17 Carvalho AC, Paiva SM, Viegas CM, et al. Impact of malocclusion on oral health-related quality of life among Brazilian preschool children: a population-based study. *Braz Dent J* 2013;**24**(6):655–61.

18 Zhou Y, Wang Y, Wang X, et al. The impact of orthodontic treatment on the quality of life a systematic review. *BMC Oral Health* 2014;**14**:66 http://www.ncbi.nlm.nih.gov/pmc/articles/PMC4060859/.

19 Perillo L, Esposito M, Caprioglio A, et al. Orthodontic treatment need for adolescents in the Campania region: the malocclusion impact on self-concept. *Patient Prefer Adherence* 2014;**8**:353–9 Available from PubMed: http://www.ncbi.nlm.nih.gov/pmc/articles/PMC3964173/.

20 Miguel JAM, Sales HX, Quintão CC, et al. Factors associated with orthodontic treatment seeking by 12–15-year-old children at a state university-funded clinic. *J Orthod* 2010;**37**(2):100–6.

21 Burden DJ. The influence of social class, gender, and peers on the uptake of orthodontic treatment. *Eur J Orthod* 1995;**17**(3):199–203.

22 Lippold C, Stamm T, Meyer U, et al. Early treatment of posterior crossbite – a randomised clinical trial. *Trials* [Internet]. 2013 Jan 22]; 14:20. Available from PubMed: http://www.ncbi.nlm.nih.gov/pmc/articles/PMC3560255/

23 Fudalej P, Dragan M, Wedrychowska-Szulc B. Prediction of the outcome of orthodontic treatment of Class III malocclusions – a systematic review. *Eur J Orthod* 2011;**33**(2):190–7.

24 Mandall N, DiBiase A, Littlewood S, et al. Is early Class III protraction facemask treatment effective? A multicentre, randomized, controlled trial: 15-month follow-up. *J Orthod* 2010;**37**(3):149–61.

25 Masucci C, Franchi L, Defraia E, et al. Stability of rapid maxillary expansion and facemask therapy: a long-term controlled study. *Am J Orthod Dentofacial Orthop* 2011;**140**(4):493–500.

26 McNamara JA, Franchi L. The cervical vertebral maturation method: a user's guide. *Angle Orthod* 2018;**88**(2):133–43.

27 Gu Y, McNamara JA. Mandibular growth changes and cervical vertebral maturation. A cephalometric implant study. *Angle Orthod* 2007;**77**(6):947–53.

28 Mohlin B, Kurol J. To what extent do deviations from an ideal occlusion constitute a health risk? *Swed Dent J* 2003;**27**(1):1–10.

29 DiBiase A. The timing of orthodontic treatment. *Dent Update* 2002;**29**(9):434–41.

30 Gecgelen M, Aksoy A, Kirdemir P, et al. Evaluation of stress and pain during rapid maxillary expansion treatments. *J Oral Rehabil* 2012;**39**(10):767–75.

2

Development of the occlusion: what to do and when to do it

Bernardo Q. Souki, DDS, MSD, PhD

Department of Dentistry, Pontifical Catholic University of Minas Gerais, Belo Horizonte, Brazil

This chapter presents the rationale for preventive and interceptive orthodontic monitoring (PIOM) in relation to the seven stages of dental occlusal development. If occlusal development from the deciduous dentition until the end of the eruption of permanent cuspids and permanent second molars is correctly classified into stages, and if irregularities in each stage are identified, proper treatment decisions can be made in a timely manner. By the time that the permanent dentition is completed, deviations would have been adequately managed, respecting the contemporary concepts of effectiveness and efficiency. These stages (Table 2.1), if well understood and identified, represent a unique opportunity for rendering high-quality orthodontic care. While the chronological ages and developmental sequences may vary considerably among individuals, the anatomic entities are the foundations of occlusal management.

2.1 Stage 1 – eruption of deciduous teeth

Dental eruption is a biological process subject that is highly variable, both in sequence and in chronology [1]. The eruption of deciduous teeth into the oral cavity begins most often by the sixth month of postnatal life with the emergence of the mandibular central incisors (Table 2.1). At 30 months, all deciduous teeth will have erupted in approximately 70% of children, but a high degree of variation is likely to occur. At 14 months, both a child who has had no teeth erupted and a child who has all of their deciduous teeth in the oral cavity may be considered normal [2]. If a child has had no deciduous teeth erupted by 16 months, a radiographic investigation should then be performed.

An early eruption pattern of the deciduous dentition may indicate a tendency for an early transition between deciduous and mixed dentition [3]. Variations in the eruption sequence are very common but do not appear to cause significant disturbance in the development of the deciduous dentition and are usually not important unless teeth erupt in an ectopic position and block the eruption of other teeth. This is rare at this stage of occlusal development. The most prevalent eruption sequences for the deciduous dentition are A, B, D, C, and E [2].

2.1.1 Biogenesis of the deciduous dentition

The biogenesis of the deciduous dentition can be divided into four phases:

Phase 1 comprises the eruption of the maxillary and mandibular deciduous incisors

---

Recognizing and Correcting Developing Malocclusions: A Problem-Oriented Approach to Orthodontics, Second Edition. Edited by Eustáquio A. Araújo and Peter H. Buschang.
© 2025 John Wiley & Sons, Inc. Published 2025 by John Wiley & Sons, Inc.

Table 2.1 Clinical stages of occlusal development.

Stage	Description
1	Eruption of deciduous teeth
2	Completion of the deciduous dentition
3	Eruption of the first permanent molars
4	Eruption of the permanent incisors
5	Eruption of the mandibular canines and of the first premolars
6	Eruption of the second premolars
7	Eruption of maxillary canines and second molars

(Figures 2.1a and 2.1b). Due to the absence of posterior primary teeth, there is an excessive overbite, and the mandibular excursions are large. The immature anatomy of the temporomandibular joint (TMJ) favors this type of movement [4]. At this stage, the condyles are incipient, and the articular fossae are flat.

Phase 2 begins with the eruption of primary molars and their intercuspation (Figures 2.1c and 2.1d). This phenomenon promotes the first gain of the occlusal vertical dimension. Thanks to this uprising of the bite, there is a reduction in the excessive overbite. The occlusal morphology of the deciduous molars promotes the first occlusal reference and stimulates the morphological maturation of the TMJ [5].

Phase 3 starts with the eruption of the deciduous canines (Figure 2.1e). This phase is important for the establishment and maintenance of the primate spaces. In the maxillary arch, the primate space is located between the lateral incisors and the canines. In the mandible, it is located between the canines and first deciduous molars [6].

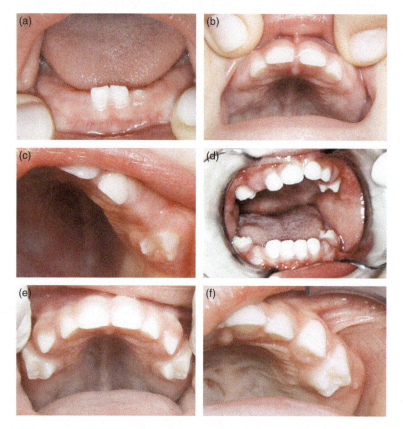

Figure 2.1 Stage 1: eruption of deciduous teeth.

The size of the primate spacing varies from less than 1 to 5 mm.

Phase 4 is marked by the eruption of the deciduous second molars (Figure 2.1f). This phase includes the consolidation of the primary occlusion and of the vertical dimension, initiated with the eruption of the first deciduous molar. This period ends with the intercuspation of all deciduous teeth, between the 30th and 36th months of life.

2.1.2 Dimensional changes of the dental arches at stage 1

There is an evidence [7] that significant gains in arch perimeter happen during the first 2 years of life (i.e., during the eruption of the deciduous dentition).

2.1.3 Management of occlusal development at stage 1

The incidence of a malocclusion at this stage is very low; however, clinicians should provide guidance to parents about the wide range of normality in regard to the chronology and sequence of tooth eruption. During the eruption of the deciduous dentition, interceptive orthodontic treatment is not indicated. Even when there is an early diagnosis of abnormalities in occlusal development, such as crossbites or space problems, it is recommended to wait until the deciduous dentition matures to decide on the best therapeutic approach. Radical attempts to encourage the abandonment of thumb sucking are not needed currently. The use of a pacifier is acceptable during most of this stage in the vast majority of children, since there is no permanent damage to the occlusion [8]. There is evidence that suppressing the pacifier at the end of this stage (approximately 2–3 years of age) will permit self-correction of dentoalveolar sequelae [9]. When dealing with late pacifier use, a closer evaluation of the patient's skeletal pattern should be implemented. A pacifier in a hypodivergent subject may be much less harmful than in a hyperdivergent one [10].

During Stage 1, clinicians should also be able to detect mouth breathing. Upper airway obstruction by adenotonsillar hyperplasia may disrupt the harmony of facial development in this age group. There is evidence that breathing patterns should be normalized during the first 4 years of life, when 60% of facial growth is attained.

2.2 Stage 2 – completion of the deciduous dentition

Although it is sometimes overlooked because only the deciduous teeth are present, occlusal normality during this stage favors the development of a good permanent dentition. However, even in Stage 2, a child with a normal occlusion has a significant chance that irregularities in the following stages of development may still occur. Figure 2.2 shows a panoramic radiograph and Figure 2.3 shows an intraoral view of a child with a normal occlusal relationship at this stage.

Most frequently, this stage includes children from 3 to 6 years of age. At the earliest part of Stage 2, immediately after the eruption of the deciduous second molars, diastemas are usually present between the crowns of these teeth and the adjacent deciduous first molars (Figure 2.4a). However, over the coming months, this physiological spacing tends to disappear, depending on the natural mesial migration of the maxillary and mandibular deciduous second molars, which drift as a response to the development of the adjacent first permanent molars (Figure 2.4b). The child at the end of the deciduous dentition (approximately 6 years of age) has no more spacing between the deciduous teeth except for the incisors in a Baume Type I occlusion (Figure 2.4c). There is a marked reduction of the arch perimeter. Generally, there is no crowding in the late deciduous dentition [11]. Spacing in the anterior region during this stage, however,

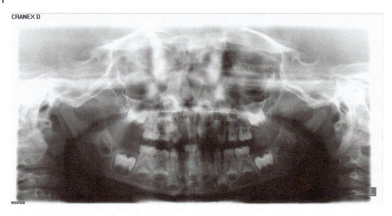

Figure 2.2 Panoramic radiograph of 3-year-old child.

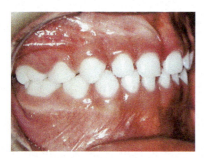

Figure 2.3 Normal characteristics of the deciduous dentition.

is highly desirable considering that the succedaneous permanent incisors have a greater mesiodistal diameter and need room to be aligned [12]. Table 2.2, based on charts from white North American boys [13], provides the average diameter of the deciduous and permanent incisors and provides a comparison between the average values for each dental unit and for the entire incisor region. The negative sign indicates a negative balance resulting from the larger size of the permanent teeth.

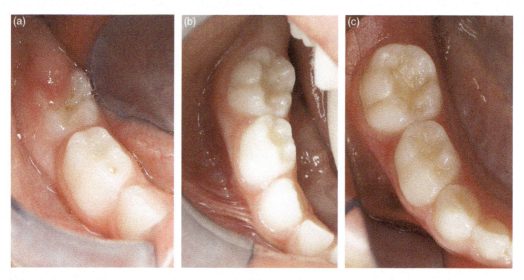

Figure 2.4 Interdental spacing closure in the deciduous dentition.

2.2 Stage 2–completion of the deciduous dentition

Table 2.2 Mesiodistal measurements of deciduous and permanent incisors, discrepancy of the size of deciduous vs. permanent incisors, and anterior segment discrepancy.

Arch	Incisor	Deciduous mean size (mm)	Permanent mean size (mm)	Deciduous vs. permanent tooth discrepancy (mm)	Anterior segment discrepancy (mm)
Maxillary	Central	6.41 ± 0.43	8.91 ± 0.59	−2.50	−8.24
	Lateral	5.26 ± 0.37	6.88 ± 0.64	−1.62	
Mandibular	Central	4.06 ± 0.35	5.54 ± 0.32	−1.48	−5.36
	Lateral	4.64 ± 0.43	6.04 ± 0.37	−1.40	

Based on charts of white North America boys, Moyers' Handbook of Orthodontics [13].

According to Baume [14], deciduous arches may or may not have generalized interdental spacing. Both forms are considered normal [6]. However, in dental arches with physiological or developmental spacing, known as Type I, a transition to mixed dentition with a lower risk of space deficiency is more likely to occur [12].

Deciduous teeth roots in their bony bases are nearly perpendicular, and the dental crowns are vertically positioned with no buccal-lingual angulation. Therefore, during deciduous dentition, the interincisal angle is close to 180°. In the posterior region, the curve of Wilson does not exist, and the curve of Spee is flat to mild [11]. Light to moderate abrasion wear on the incisors is considered normal in deciduous dentition [15].

The relationship of the maxillary cuspids with the mandibular dental arch is the major reference for sagittal classification during deciduous stage [6, 16]. The occlusion is considered normal when the long axis of the deciduous maxillary cuspid is in the direction of the interproximal surface of the lower deciduous first molar and lower deciduous cuspid (Figure 2.3). This relationship is called normo-occlusion. Analogous to the classification suggested by Angle for the permanent dentition, this occlusal pattern is clinically known as a "Class I canine relationship." The prevalence of a normal sagittal relationship, characterized by the key deciduous canines, is approximately 80% [8]. Also in the sagittal perspective, 0–3 mm overjet during Stage 2 is considered normal [6].

A normal transverse relationship is characterized by a positive overjet of the buccal cusps of the deciduous molars relative to the same cusps of the lower arch and the palatal cusps of the deciduous molars resting in the pits of their antagonist lower molars. The palatal surfaces of the upper deciduous canines maintain occlusal contact with the buccal surface of the deciduous canines and the first deciduous molars.

There is a wide range of normality for overbite in Stage 2. Overbites of ⅔ the incisal coverage as well as an edge-to-edge bite are considered normal. In this period, due to the high prevalence of nonnutritive sucking habits, the prevalence of an anterior open bite tends to be higher [17].

2.2.1 Dimensional changes in the dental arches at stage 2

Evidence indicates that, in most children, the deciduous maxillary and mandibular arch length and perimeter undergo a small reduction between 3 and 6 years of age [18]. Conversely, some investigators have found that the arch length of the deciduous dentition does not decrease, whereas Baume [14] reported an 89% and an 83% rate of maxillary and mandibular change or sagittal decrease, respectively. No increase in the length of the arch during

Table 2.3 Orthodontic interceptive procedures and their indication in each of the seven stages of occlusal development, according to color-coded convention.

Procedures	Stages of occlusal development						
	1	2	3	4	5	6	7
Manage oral habits	Maybe	Yes	Yes	Yes	Maybe	Yes	Maybe
Space maintenance	No	Yes	Yes	Yes	Maybe	Yes	Yes
Space regaining	No	Maybe	Yes	Yes	Yes	Yes	Yes
Space creation	No	No	No	Maybe	Maybe	No	No
Anterior crossbite	No	Yes	Yes	Yes	Yes	Maybe	Maybe
Posterior crossbite	Yes	Yes	Yes	Yes	Yes	Maybe	Maybe
Class II malocclusion	No	No	No	Maybe	Maybe	Yes	Yes
Class III malocclusion	No	Yes	Yes	Yes	Maybe	Yes	Yes

- Yes
- Maybe
- No

this developmental stage of occlusion was observed.

The deciduous dental arch width, measured at the intercanine and intermolar distances, is reported to be stable during Stage 2 [18, 19], but transverse changes from the ages of 4–6 were found in other studies [13].

2.2.2 Management of occlusion development at stage 2

During this period, several factors may contribute to malocclusion exposing children to the risk of developing occlusal abnormalities. Table 2.3 presents a synthesis of the preventive and interceptive orthodontic procedures recommended for each of the seven stages of occlusal development.

- **Oral habits:** Mouth breathing habits should be evaluated, and a referral to an ear, nose, and throat (ENT) should be provided. Figure 2.5 illustrates a 3-year-old girl immediately before adenotonsillectomy and 48 hours after surgical airway clearance. There was a marked improvement in the muscular facial balance with the normalization of the breathing pattern.

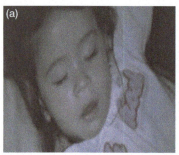
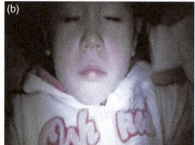

Figure 2.5 A 3-year-old mouth-breathing girl. (a) Night before adenotonsillectomy, (b) 48 hours after airway normalization.

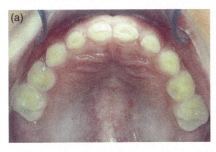 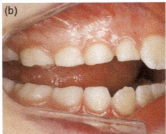

Figure 2.6 Bruxism in the deciduous and early mixed dentition. (a) Severe abrasion. (b) Moderate abrasion.

As with other controversial issues, any extreme decision on sucking habits is not correct [9, 10]. Clinicians should recognize the individual variations among children and their sucking habits and should be aware that some children do, in fact, rely on digit sucking for emotional support and security, whereas others find it a meaningless and empty habit that can be discontinued without psychological trauma [20].

Bruxism in this stage is also frequently noted and should be a problem only if excessive tooth abrasion is identified (Figure 2.6a). A small amount of occlusal wear on the deciduous teeth may be considered physiologic (Figure 2.6b).

- **Space maintenance:** When only the first deciduous molar is lost, space maintenance can be accomplished with simple fixed or removable devices. However, when early loss of a second deciduous molar occurs before the eruption of the adjacent first permanent molars, therapeutic options are limited, and the prognosis is less favorable. In the anterior region, from the perspective of space maintenance, there is no need to install removable or fixed devices if the loss of one or more incisors occurred after the eruption of the primary canines [21]. The early loss of deciduous canines at this stage is rare; in the event that it occurs, any intervention, if considered, has to be carefully planned.
- **Space regaining:** Premature loss of a deciduous first molar most likely allows the mesial drifting of the adjacent deciduous second molar, resulting in loss of the dental arch perimeter. Space regaining with fixed or removable appliances should be considered.
- **Space creation:** Permanent incisors require more space than their deciduous predecessors (Table 2.2). In the absence of interdental spacing of the deciduous incisors, a significant arch development may be necessary to avoid crowding in the anterior region during the transitional stage. However, there is no scientific evidence to prove the effectiveness of deciduous arch development with orthodontic or orthopedic techniques.
- **Anterior crossbite:** Anterior crossbites may interfere with normal skeletal growth, as well causing tooth abrasion and gingival recession. Early treatment is usually indicated [22] with the objectives of reestablishing a normal development and preventing dentofacial growth impairments (Figure 2.7). The determination of the appropriate timing for intercepting an anterior crossbite hinges upon several crucial factors, namely the degree of difficulty it creates to physiological growth, patient maturity, and compliance.
- **Posterior crossbite:** It is recommended to eliminate occlusal interferences (prematurities) that lead to mandibular anterior and lateral shifts (Figure 2.7). The literature indicates that, as a rule, posterior crossbites should be treated, if possible, as soon as detected, taking advantage of the immaturity of the midpalatal suture.
- **Class II malocclusion:** At this stage, in general, an interceptive treatment for a Class II malocclusion is not recommended.

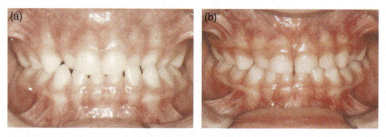

Figure 2.7 Deciduous dentition: anterior and posterior crossbite. (a) Pretreatment. (b) Posttreatment.

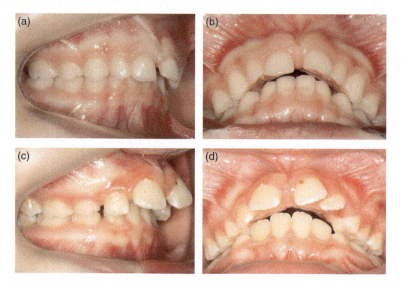

Figure 2.8 Untreated Class II malocclusion. (a) Age 4, deciduous dentition. (b) Mixed dentition. Note the dramatic detrimental changes in the dental relationship without early therapeutic actions in the sagittal relationship.

But the assistant orthodontist might recommend early treatment for severe Class II malocclusion during deciduous dentition if there is a predicted deterioration of the dental relationship during the transition of dentitions (Figure 2.8). In selected cases of severe mandibular micrognathia with a medical recommendation for mandibular advancement, the orthodontist may be part of the team responsible for performing a therapeutic intervention, particularly when there is evidence of sleep apnea (obstructive sleep apnea [OSA]). The efficiency of Class II therapy during this particular phase of skeletal maturation is often low. Therefore, it is critical to have a prior assessment indicating a high likelihood of success before considering early treatment during this stage of dental development.

- **Class III malocclusion:** Depending on the emotional maturity of the patient, there are strong indications for early treatment of Class III malocclusions at this stage (Figure 2.9). Chapter 7 describes procedures that may be implemented.

2.3 Stage 3 – eruption of first permanent molars

Generally, the mixed dentition begins with the eruption of the mandibular central permanent incisors. The mandibular first permanent molars erupt at about the same time, followed

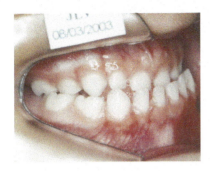

Figure 2.9 Skeletal Class III malocclusion in the deciduous dentition.

The eruption of the first permanent molars coincides with the juvenile growth spurt [23] and with the second physiological gain in the vertical dimension of the occlusion.

Normal occlusion during Stage 3 most often has the following characteristics: a Class I relationship or a cusp-to-cusp sagittal relationship of the first permanent molars; a Class I relationship of the deciduous canines; an overjet of 0–3 mm; an overbite ranging from edge-to-edge to 3/4 incisal coverage; and a normal transverse interarch relationship.

2.3.1 Management of occlusion development at this stage

- **Oral habits:** Same as Stage 2.
- **Space maintenance:** After the first permanent molar eruption, it is easier to install fixed space maintainers supported by these teeth.
- **Space regaining:** Ectopic eruption of the maxillary first permanent molars is quite common. A detailed description on the management of this deviation is given in Chapter 8.
- **Space creation:** Not indicated in this stage.
- **Anterior crossbite:** Same indications as in Stage 2.
- **Posterior crossbite:** Same indications as in Stage 2. However, after the eruption of the first permanent molars, regardless of whether the permanent incisors have erupted or not, a critical appraisal of the posterior crossbite should be performed to determine whether or not maxillary permanent first molars need to be incorporated in the appliance (Figure 2.10a). If no functional deflection is observed, or no transverse growth restriction is detected in the deciduous canines area, the crossbite correction limited to the first molar can be postponed (Figure 2.10b).
- **Class II malocclusion:** No treatment may be indicated at this stage as the effectiveness will not be greater than if done at a later time, and the efficiency is less. Treatment is indicated only when there

by their maxillary counterparts, although it is common to observe the first permanent molars erupt before the lower central incisors. These sequences do not seem to convey clinically significant differences. The eruption of the permanent incisors and first molars is known as the first transitional period. For didactic reasons, this chapter will presume that the first permanent molars erupt first. Although the average age for the eruption of the first permanent molars is 6 years, the normal range is ages 4–8.

The first permanent molars are added to the deciduous dentition utilizing the space created by appositional growth distally to the second deciduous molars. At birth, the lower first permanent molar is located near the junction of the mandibular corpus and ramus, with the crown mesially inclined. In very young children, the upper first permanent molars are located in the maxillary tuberosity, with the crown distally tipped. During the process of eruption, the maxillary first permanent molars gradually incline mesially and are guided by the distal surfaces of the second deciduous molars to their final occlusion.

Thus, it is generally agreed that the pattern of the terminal plan of the deciduous second molars is of paramount importance in the early intercuspation of the first permanent molars. However, as mentioned in Stage 2, the analysis of the terminal planes of the deciduous molars should be evaluated along with the deciduous canines' relationship.

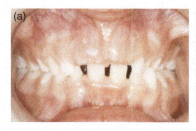 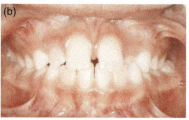

Figure 2.10 Posterior crossbite after the eruption of the first permanent molars. (a) Maxillary left deciduous teeth in crossbite. Minor functional shift of the mandible. (b) Only left first permanent molars are in crossbite. No functional deflection.

are psychosocial concerns or a high risk of trauma to the incisors.
- **Class III malocclusion:** Same indications as in Stage 2.

2.4 Stage 4—eruption of permanent incisors

During the first transitional period, there is the exchange of the deciduous for the permanent incisors. The first transitional period lasts approximately 2 years (6–8 years of age). Then, an intermediate rest period occurs, lasting approximately 2 years. Some children experience a longer intermediate period.

While in the previous three stages, deviations from an "ideal" position of the teeth were less frequent, during Stage 4, the incidence of deviations from the "ideal" is very high. It is important to note that although the term "normal" development means "naturally occurring," during this stage some malpositioning of the incisors may be considered normal, and "ideal" occlusion would be difficult to find. Understanding the mechanisms that lead to these deviations from ideal tooth positioning is essential for appropriate clinical management favoring observation rather than intervention.

The mandibular permanent incisors develop in a lingual position in relation to the predecessor deciduous teeth. During eruption, these teeth often emerge in a lingual position in the oral cavity. Due to this lingual eruption pattern, the roots of the deciduous incisors often may not be naturally resorbed, and natural exfoliation can be impaired.

During the eruption of the maxillary permanent incisors, they often participate in the root resorption of deciduous incisors and emerge with acceptable alignment in the oral cavity. But the maxillary lateral incisors may sometimes erupt palatally, particularly in patients with space deficiency.

During this stage, the maxillary incisors may have a distal crown angulation with the lateral incisors in particular more angulated. Earlier literature describes this positioning of the upper incisors as the "ugly duckling phase" (see Chapter 1, Figure 1.1). This dental compensation is a natural mechanism of the permanent incisors root structure protection from traumatic contact with the enamel of the adjacent erupting permanent canines. The closure of the diastema between the incisors, as well as a change in the inclination of the lateral incisors, tends to happen naturally during the eruption of the permanent canines (Stage 7).

In the mandible, however, the incisors are most frequently in proximal contact from the time of their eruption. The interincisor diastema is rarely observed. Some crowding is considered normal, and when the spacing in this region is generous, the clinician should suspect an oral habit.

2.4.1 Dimensional changes in the dental arches at this stage

It should be noted that the dental arch length of the mandible is stable, with no significant changes after the eruption of the first permanent molars and permanent incisors. However, there is a significant increase in the intercanine distance, resulting from the distal displacement of the deciduous canines into the primate diastema [13, 24].

The maxillary arch length increases by approximately 1.5 mm due to increased labial tipping of the incisors and the greater labiolingual thickness of the crowns of these teeth. The intercanine distance is expected to increase by approximately 2 mm during the transition of deciduous to early mixed dentition [7], most likely due to appositional growth in this region. The greatest increase in the transverse dimension of the maxilla happens during the eruption of the central incisors [14].

2.4.2 Management of occlusal development at this stage

- **Oral habits:** To take advantage of dentoalveolar growth activity during the eruption of the incisors, it is imperative that interceptive approaches be performed to avoid the creation or the perpetuation of an anterior open bite.
- **Space maintenance:** The early loss of permanent incisors must be managed to maintain the original space.
- **Space regaining:** Space deficiency in the anterior region, with consequent misalignment and/or incisor crowding might be associated with oral habits causing constriction of the transverse dental arch (Figure 2.11) or with an intra-arch sagittal collapse (Figure 2.12). Interceptive orthodontic measures implemented to restore the transverse dimensions to their original dimensions as well as to reverse the lingual inclination of the incisors are indicated at this time, taking advantage of the dimensional changes that naturally occur in the anterior region during this stage (Figure 2.11).
- **Space creation:** Although techniques for creating space have been widely used in recent decades, the stability of arch development therapy is low and its use should be avoided.
- **Anterior crossbite:** The interceptive approach is highly recommended and should be addressed.
- **Posterior crossbite:** Same indications as in Stage 3.
- **Class II malocclusion:** When the overjet is greater than 5 mm, and the lips cannot protect the incisors, preventive measures are indicated to protect the newly erupted incisors from injury. If traumatic injury is not likely, and no aesthetic or psychological concern is reported, no treatment may be indicated at this stage as the effectiveness will not be greater than if it is done at a later time and the efficiency is less. Figure 2.13 shows an 8-year-old child with an increased overjet associated with Class II malocclusion. Despite the prepubertal stage of skeletal maturation (CS1), because of the increased risk of traumatic injury, orthodontic treatment was advocated.
- **Class III malocclusion:** Same indications as in Stage 3. However, the prognosis increasingly worsens with time—see Chapter 7.

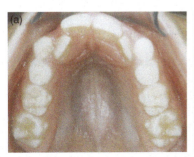 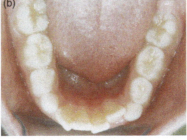

Figure 2.11 Incisors crowding associated with arch width reduction.

2 Development of the occlusion: what to do and when to do it

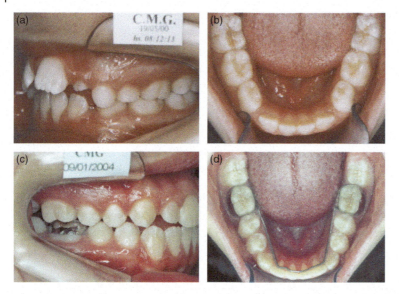

Figure 2.12 (a, b) An 8-year-old child presenting early loss of mandibular deciduous cuspid associated with negative space discrepancy. Arch perimeter loss with the incisors retroclination. (c, d) Early treatment consisted of rapid maxillary expansion, lip bumper, and E-space maintenance with a lower lingual holding arch. Differential diagnosis if the crossbite is associated with a simple dental malpositioning or a functional shift with a sagittal and/or lateral Class III pattern must be considered.

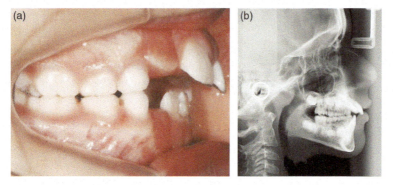

Figure 2.13 An 8-year-old child presenting increased overjet and a Class II dental relationship and proclaimed maxillary incisors. Prepubertal (CS1) stage of skeletal maturation.

2.5 Stage 5 — eruption of mandibular canines and first premolars

This stage marks the beginning of the second transitional period. From the point of view of occlusal development, eruption of the mandibular permanent canines prior to the adjacent first premolars is highly desirable, favoring space management and anterior tooth alignment. In panoramic radiographic examinations, it is common to see the germs of the mandibular canines below the germs of the first premolars in relation to the occlusal plane. Fortunately, however, in most cases, there is acceleration in the eruption of the mandibular canines, allowing a positive eruption sequence. The eruption of the mandibular first premolar before the canine is not rare and should be monitored. It is considered desirable in serial extraction procedures when the removal of the premolars should be performed before canine eruption (see Chapter 5).

Uncommonly, the first premolars present eruption difficulties. However, the maxillary first premolars frequently erupt buccally, due to the difficulty of exfoliation of their deciduous predecessors. Generally, the extraction of the first deciduous molar is sufficient to permit the redirection of an ectopic maxillary first premolar.

In the maxillary arch, we note that the intrabone large crowns of the first premolars often influence the eruption pattern of the adjacent permanent canines. Therefore, the early eruption of the maxillary first premolar plays an important role in preventing the permanent cuspid from being blocked out.

2.5.1 Management of occlusal development at this stage

- **Oral habits:** Ideally, at this stage of occlusal development, deleterious oral habits have already been eliminated.
- **Space maintenance:** Ensuring the eruption of the mandibular permanent canines before the first premolars is the space maintenance measure to be taken at this stage. Lower holding lingual arches (LHLA) may also be used to prevent mesial movement of the posterior teeth as well as natural retroinclination of the mandibular incisors.
- **Space regain:** Same indications as in Stage 4.
- **Space creation:** Same indications as in Stage 4.
- **Anterior crossbite:** If still present, should be intercepted promptly.
- **Posterior crossbite:** Same indications as in Stage 4. If root resorption is advanced, these deciduous teeth should not be used as anchors during arch expansion.
- **Class II malocclusion:** In some children, especially girls who have advanced skeletal maturation, it is possible that the peak of pubertal growth happens during Stage 5 of occlusal development. Skeletal assessment of each patient is warranted to take advantage of pubertal growth peak in the Class II orthopedic therapy.
- **Class III malocclusion:** Facemask therapy to intercept skeletal Class III malocclusions during this stage may be limited, although it can still be implemented. Recently, a technique to intercept this type of malocclusion through the use of intermaxillary elastics supported on skeletally anchored hooks (bolted to bone miniplates) has been introduced [25] and has been considered an alternative treatment for Class III malocclusions in more mature facial development.

2.6 Stage 6 – eruption of second premolars

By the age of 11, the exchange of deciduous second molars for the second premolars represents an important time for preventive/interceptive action by the preservation of the E-space. The well-documented difference in mesiodistal diameters of the crowns of the deciduous second molars and second premolars creates a free space known as the E-space or leeway space [26].

The concept of the leeway space was initially proposed by Nance [27] and included the dimensional differences between the deciduous canines and molars and their permanent successors. However, the deciduous canines are smaller than their successors, while the deciduous first molars are rarely larger than their successors. These facts induced Gianelly [28] to study this relationship and introduce the concept that the leeway space in the second transitional period is due mainly to the size difference of the crown of the deciduous second molars ("E's") and the second premolars.

There is evidence that the dental arch perimeter, especially of the mandibular arch,

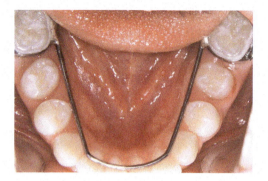

is reduced during the transition between the late mixed and permanent dentition, due to the mesial migration of the permanent first molars and the consequent occupation of the E-space. The clinician should evaluate the opportunity to maintain this precious space (Figure 2.14). The E-space can be used not only to improve intra-arch tooth alignment but also to facilitate the comprehensive orthodontic treatment of mild Class II and Class III dental relationships (Figures 2.15 and 2.16).

Figure 2.14 E-space maintenance with a lower lingual holding arch.

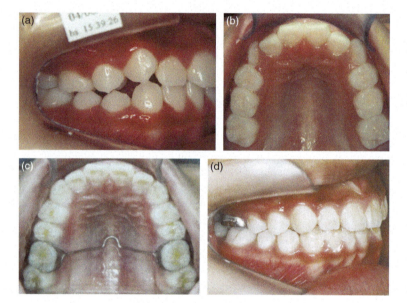

Figure 2.15 E-space preservation in the maxillary arch of Class II malocclusion patients may favor the improvement of the dental sagittal relationship.

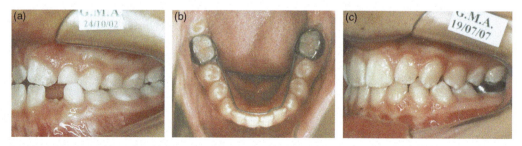

Figure 2.16 E-space preservation in the mandibular arch of Class III malocclusion patients is recommended to allow incisors retraction and the creation of adequate overjet.

2.6.1 Management of occlusal development at this stage

- **Oral habits:** Same indications as in Stage 5.
- **Space maintenance:** It is highly recommended that all children be examined, and the preservation of the E-space be considered before the exfoliation of the deciduous second molars. Maintenance of the dental arch perimeter by preserving the E-space provides adequate space for managing negative discrepancies in approximately 70% of cases [28].
- **Space regaining:** Any reduction in arch perimeter due to environmental factors may be intercepted during this stage. If a second deciduous molar is lost prematurely, regaining the perimeter may be indicated at this stage. The lingual inclination of the incisors may also be corrected at this stage, in preparation for the next stages.
- **Space creation:** Not recommended.
- **Anterior crossbite:** If still present, it should be corrected.
- **Posterior crossbite:** At this stage, it is expected that there will be no more posterior crossbites, especially those associated with a mandibular shift (functional).
- **Class II malocclusion:** Before the exfoliation of the maxillary second deciduous molars, children with a dental Class II malocclusion should have a comprehensive evaluation to determine the opportunity for using a palatal bar/Nance button or a headgear [19]. Moreover, at this stage, several children are near pubertal growth, the ideal time to treat this malocclusion.
- **Class III malocclusion:** Same indications as in Stage 5. The prognosis for a successful interceptive treatment worsens with time. If a skeletal Class III malocclusion is not intercepted before this stage, it may likely require camouflaging extraction treatment or even an orthognatic surgery plan. It may be too late to perform interceptive treatment techniques but the use of miniplates and bone anchorage may be tried to minimize the severity of the problem. Refer to Chapter 7.

2.7 Stage 7 – eruption of maxillary canines and second molars

The end of the second transitional period occurs with the eruption of the maxillary permanent canines and of the second molars. In the great majority of children, this happens around the age of 12. However, great variability in eruption chronology is observed and normally has no clinical meaning.

The complexity of the eruptive movements of the maxillary permanent canines creates a high risk of ectopic eruption and impaction. Therefore, as a preventive approach, it is important to perform annual panoramic radiographic monitoring.

Generally, the mandibular second molars erupt earlier than the maxillary second molars. In recent years, an increased incidence of impaction of the second permanent molars has been documented [29]. This fact has been associated with a reduced prevalence of extensive caries as well as the increasing use of interceptive orthodontic techniques for managing crowding in the anterior region. It is important that clinicians monitor the eruption of the permanent second molars until their complete intercuspation. In the maxillary arch, second molars can have their eruption blocked by ectopic third molars (see Chapter 8, Figure 8.28). In the mandibular arch, it is very common to observe obstruction of full eruption of the second molars by a locking in the distal surface of the first molars.

2.7.1 Management of occlusal development at this stage

- **Oral habits:** Same indications as in Stage 6.
- **Space maintenance:** At this stage, the continuity of the space maintenance process

must be maintained, in case the E-spaces have been preserved, to warrant better tooth alignment during the fixed appliance phase.
- **Space regaining:** To promote adequate eruption of the maxillary canines, space-opening intervention might be necessary. Generally, such procedures should be included in the corrective orthodontic phase.
- **Space creation:** Same indications as in space regaining.
- **Anterior crossbite:** Same indications as Stage 6.
- **Posterior crossbite:** Same indications as Stage 6.
- **Class II malocclusion:** This stage is an ideal time for correcting skeletal Class II malocclusions in many patients. Evaluation of the skeletal age is mandatory to establish the best time to approach Class II skeletal problems.
- **Class III malocclusion:** Same indications as in Stage 6.

2.8 Conclusions

Orthodontists, pediatric dentists, and general clinicians should see the importance of active supervision of the developing occlusion. Management of intraarch and interarch problems during the transition from deciduous to permanent dentition, as well as controlling environmental factors that contribute to malocclusion, are routine components of clinical dental care for children.

Clinicians must be aware that the assumptions of an ideal Class I occlusion on a Class I skeleton with good facial balance is a theoretical target that often does not occur in nature without orthodontic interceptive treatment. Recognition of our inability to verify whether the patient conforms to an ideal Class I pattern can only be retrospective, meaning that both diagnosis and treatment planning are empiric, even in our evidence-based era. This is not to say, "If in doubt, treat." Such an approach can most likely go both ways, doing as much harm as good. Some early treatment procedures have demonstrated good effects on skeletal and periodontal structures. However, it might be a disservice to persist in treating a child for minor crowding, a deep bite, a maxillary diastema or a skeletal Class II malocclusion.

A goal of orthodontists and of all dentists who take care of young patients should be to obtain diagnostically useful data to allow the evaluation of dental relationships at all stages of occlusal development. The use of a PIOM allows clinicians to successfully predict the changes that nature will produce in the future and to make the necessary adjustments through interceptive approaches wisely employing the effectiveness and efficiency concepts.

References

1 Moorrees CFA, Fanning EA, Hunt E. Age variation of formation stages for ten permanent teeth. *J Dent Res* 1963;**42**:1490–502.
2 Nanda RT. Eruption of human teeth. *Am J Orthod* 1960;**46**:363–78.
3 Gron AM. Prediction of tooth emergence. *J Dent Res* 1962;**41**:573–85.
4 Nickel JC, McLachlan KR, Smith DM. Eminence development of the postnatal human temporo-mandibular joint. *J Dent Res* 1988;**67**(6):896–902.
5 Nickel JC, McLachlan KR, Smith DM. A theoretical model of loading and eminence development of the postnatal human temporo-mandibular joint. *J Dent Res* 1988;**67**(6):903–10.
6 Hegde S, Panwar S, Bolar DR, Sanghavi MB. Characteristics of occlusion in primary dentition of preschool children of Udaipur, India. *Eur J Dent* 2012;**6**(1):51–5.
7 Bishara S, Ortho D, Jakobsen JR, et al. Arch width changes from 6 weeks to 45 years of age Maxillary Arch. *Am J Orthod* 1997;**111**(4):401–9.

8 Recommendations for the use of pacifiers. *Paediatr Child Health* 2003;**8**(8):515–28.

9 Warren JJ, Bishara SE. Duration of nutritive and non-nutritive sucking behaviors and their effects on the dental arches in the primary dentition. *Am J Orthod Dentofacial Orthop* 2002;**121**(4):347–56.

10 Cozza P, Baccetti T, Franchi L, et al. Sucking habits and facial hyperdivergency as risk factors for anterior open bite in the mixed dentition. *Am J Orthod Dentofacial Orthop* 2005;**128**(4):517–9.

11 Kumar KPS, Tamizharasi S. Significance of curve of Spee: an orthodontic review. *J Pharm Bioallied Sci* 2012;**4**(Suppl 2):S323–8.

12 Leighton BC. The early signs of malocclusion. *Eur J Orthod* 2007;**29**(Supplement 1):i89–95.

13 Moyers R. *Handbook of orthodontics*. 4th edn. Chicago, IL: YearBook Medical Publishers, Inc., 1988.

14 Baume L, Baume LJ. Physiological tooth migration and its significance for the development of occlusion. Part III The biogenesis of the successional dentition. *J Dent Res* 1950;**29**:331–7.

15 Warren JJ, Yonezu T, Bishara SE. Tooth wear patterns in the deciduous dentition. *Am J Orthod Dentofacial Orthop* 2002;**122**(6):614–8.

16 Infante PF. An epidemiologic study of deciduous molar relations in preschool children. *J Dent Res* 1975;**54**(4):723–7.

17 Urzal V, Braga AC, Ferreira AP. The prevalence of anterior open bite in Portuguese children during deciduous and mixed dentition–correlations for a prevention strategy. *Int Orthod* 2013;**11**(1):93–103.

18 Moorrees CF, Gron a M, Lebret LM, et al. Growth studies of the dentition: a review. *Am J Orthod* 1969;**55**(6):600–16.

19 Baume LJ. Physiological tooth migration and its significance for the development of occlusion. Part I The biogenetic course of the deciduous dentition. *J Dent Res* 1950;**29**:123–32.

20 De Vasconcelos FMN, Massoni ACDLT, Heimer MV, et al. Non-nutritive sucking habits, anterior open bite and associated factors in Brazilian children aged 30–59 months. *Braz Dent J* 2011;**22**(2):140–5.

21 Ghafari J. Early treatment of dental arch problems. I. Space maintenance, space gaining. *Quintessence Int* 1986;**17**(7):423–32.

22 American Academy on Pediatric Dentistry Clinical Affairs Committee-Developing Dentition Subcommittee [Corporate Author]. Guideline on management of the developing dentition and occlusion in pediatric dentistry. *Pediatr Dent* 2009;**30**(7 Suppl):184–95.

23 Tanner JM. Human growth and constitution. In: Harrison GA, Tanner GM, Pilbeam DR, Baker PT. *Human biology: an introduction to human evolution, variation, growth, and adaptability*. 3. Oxford; Oxford University Press, 1988. p. 337–435.

24 Moorrees CFA, Chadha J. Available space for the incisors during dental development – A growth study based on physiologic age. *Angle Orthod* 1965;**35**(1):12–22.

25 Heymann GC, Cevidanes L, Cornelis M, et al. Three-dimensional analysis of maxillary protraction with intermaxillary elastics to miniplates. *Am J Orthod Dentofacial Orthop* 2010;**137**(2):274–84.

26 Gianelly A. Leeway space and the resolution of crowding in the mixed dentition. *Semin Orthod* 1995;**1**(3):188–94.

27 Nance H. The limitations of orthodontic treatment. Part I. Mixed dentition diagnosis and treatment. *Am J Orthod Oral Surg* 1947;**33**:177.

28 Brennan MM, Gianelly AA. The use of the lingual arch in the mixed dentition to resolve incisor crowding. *Am J Orthod Dentofacial Orthop* 2000;**117**(1):81–5.

29 Rubin RL, Baccetti T, McNamara JA. Mandibular second molar eruption difficulties related to the maintenance of arch perimeter in the mixed dentition. *Am J Orthod Dentofacial Orthop* 2012;**141**(2):146–52.

3

Mixed dentition diagnosis: assessing the degree of severity of a developing malocclusion

Eustáquio A. Araújo, DDS, MDS

Department of Orthodontics, Center for Advanced Dental Education, Saint Louis University, St. Louis, MO, USA

Questions on the efficacy and efficiency of early treatment have not been satisfactorily answered. *Efficacy* can be defined as the ability to produce a desired or intended result, and *efficiency* is a measurement of the time, effort, or cost used to achieve such a result. With regard to phase I treatment, efficacy is difficult to assess because most of the available literature is qualitative, based on the subjective information. As for efficiency, even though there is no consensus, it is possible to find valuable data. Many clinicians and researchers are still skeptical about the benefits of an early phase of treatment.

Phase I treatment has been widely referred to as *early treatment*. Its purpose is to prevent, intercept, or correct a specific orthodontic problem or problems.

Prevention refers to the maintenance of a favorable overall dental health condition. On the other hand, interceptive early treatment techniques are intended to interrupt the progress of a developing problem by the use of early corrective intervention. Interceptive treatment may completely correct a problem or simply attempt to minimize it in an effort to restore better conditions for normal growth and development.

The clinician involved in treating a younger patient should have clear objectives for the phase I treatment that should include establishing a better occlusion, preventing problems that could potentially damage the dentition and supporting structures, reducing trauma risk to anterior teeth, managing dental arch development, correcting any transverse deviation, and implementing evidence-based theories of growth and development [1–13].

In addition, it is important to be attentive to psychological factors affecting patients and families, a strong reason for seeking orthodontic help. Enhancing the self-confidence of a young child is a key factor in their psychosocial growth and for the development of a balanced personality [14]. The well-being of the patient is a priority in the decision-making process for any treatment. This is a new paradigm in all healthcare including orthodontics [15].

3.1 Assessing treatment need, complexity, and outcome

Can the severity of a developing malocclusion be decreased? What percentage of reduction of the severity of a malocclusion can be obtained with

---

Recognizing and Correcting Developing Malocclusions: A Problem-Oriented Approach to Orthodontics, Second Edition. Edited by Eustáquio A. Araújo and Peter H. Buschang.
© 2025 John Wiley & Sons, Inc. Published 2025 by John Wiley & Sons, Inc.

an interceptive orthodontic treatment? How can the benefits (if any) of a phase I treatment be quantitatively assessed?

The evaluation of treatment need and outcome can be both time-consuming and difficult.

Much attention has been given to the assessment of the severity of a malocclusion before orthodontic treatment is rendered. However, the assessment of an early intervention in orthodontics has been mostly subjective.

Over the years, many indices have been created to assess treatment need, complexity, and outcome. A good index must be reliable, reproducible, and accurate. Numerous orthodontic indices have attempted to determine the need for treatment including: the Summers' Occlusal Index, the Dental Aesthetic Index (DAI), the Peer Assessment Rating, Index of Orthodontic Treatment Need (IOTN), and the Index of Complexity, Outcome, and Need (ICON).

3.1.1 Summers' Occlusal Index

In 1966, Chester Summers developed the Occlusal Index to evaluate the severity of a malocclusion. The Occlusal Index begins by determining the dental age of the patient. Then occlusal categories such as molar relation, overbite, overjet, posterior crossbite, posterior open bite, tooth displacement (actual and potential), midline relationship, and missing permanent teeth are assessed for each case. Each category is scored and applied to the correct weighted equation based on the predetermined dental age [16].

3.1.2 Dental Aesthetic Index (DAI)

Unlike Summers' Occlusal Index, the DAI combines both the esthetic and physical aspects of the occlusion to develop a treatment-need score. The DAI was developed in 1986 by Jenny and Cons [17]. The DAI was created using the public's perception of esthetics from photographs of 200 different occlusions. The photographs included both a full face photo and intraoral views. The result was a mathematical regression equation combining both aesthetics and dental malocclusion.

3.1.3 Peer Assessment Rating (PAR)

In 1987, as no index had been created to measure both initial malocclusion severity and treatment outcome, a group of 10 orthodontists called the British Orthodontic Standards Working Party set out to create the Peer Assessment Rating (PAR).

The investigators evaluated over 200 pre- and posttreatment dental casts and identified features to be assessed. The 11 components of the PAR index are upper right segment, upper anterior segment, upper left segment, lower right segment, lower anterior segment, lower left segment, right buccal occlusion, overjet, overbite, centerline, and left buccal occlusion.

The PAR index estimates the deviation from normal. It has good reliability and validity but it excludes several aspects of a malocclusion. A PAR score of zero represents normal occlusion and alignment, while a higher score indicates a higher severity of malocclusion. The pre- and posttreatment PAR scores can be compared and used to assess treatment success [18, 19].

3.1.4 Index of Orthodontic Treatment Need (IOTN)

In 1989, Brook and Shaw developed the IOTN. Similar to the PAR Index, the IOTN has both an aesthetic component and a dental health component. The IOTN is used mostly in the United Kingdom [17, 20]. The esthetic component of the IOTN is scored by looking at photographs. The dental components are evaluated on a scale of five grades. Grade one includes minor dental problems, while grade five consists of complex dental problems indicating a high need for orthodontic treatment. The doctor is expected to score the malocclusion into the appropriate grade. Applying the IOTN to determine treatment need is done initially by using the dental component and then, if necessary, applying the aesthetic score.

3.1.5 Index of Complexity, Outcome, and Need (ICON)

The ICON was developed from components of the IOTN and PAR. The ICON was developed by Richmond and Daniels in 1998 and, similar to the PAR, it can be used to evaluate pretreatment difficulty and posttreatment success [21]. The ICON uses five occlusal characteristics each placed into a weighted mathematical formula to develop a summed score. The categories used are Brook and Shaw's esthetic component of the IOTN, crossbite, upper arch crowding/spacing, buccal segment anteroposterior relationships, and anterior vertical relationship. Pretreatment scores can be compared to posttreatment scores to determine clinical success [21].

As demonstrated, attempts have been made to create objective tools to establish the need for orthodontic treatment as well as to compare pre- and posttreatment scores to determine treatment outcome.

3.1.6 The American Board of Orthodontics complexity index and outcome assessment

The American Board of Orthodontics (ABO) concluded that the existing indices determined case difficulty rather than case complexity. As case difficulty could be subjective, the Board felt that the assessment of case complexity would be more quantifiable. Case complexity is defined as "a combination of factors, symptoms, or signs of a disease or disorder which forms a syndrome" [21, 22]. Although many accept the PAR index as quantifiable, the ABO felt that it was not able to detect minor variations. The ABO decided to develop two indices that were called the discrepancy index (DI) and the objective grading system (OGS) to quantitatively assess the initial severity and to quantify the outcome of orthodontic treatments. In 1998, a group of 14 ABO directors convened for the development of those indices [23, 24].

To determine the DI (Discrepancy Index), orthodontic records in the form of models, cephalometric and panoramic radiographs are required. Variables included in the DI are overjet, overbite, anterior open bite, lateral open bite, crowding, occlusion, lingual posterior crossbite, buccal posterior crossbite, ANB angle, IMPA, and SN-GoGn angle. In addition, in the category *Others*, factors such as missing or supernumerary teeth, midline discrepancy, impaction, transposition, and anomalies of tooth size and shape are also scored. The DI underwent significant field testing from 2000 to 2002. The following year, the DI was fully implemented and is currently used for determining case complexity in the ABO phase III examination as a part of its certification process.

Since the DI has been extensively tested and validated, it can be assumed that determining the discrepancy index prior to a phase I treatment and then repeating the procedure after phase I would be a valuable way to quantitatively assess the changes in the complexity of a malocclusion caused by an interceptive intervention. In many instances, it could be even regarded as an *improvement index* from before phase I to before phase II.

This thought spawned an extensive research effort with significant findings. Vasilakou [25] examined 300 pre- and postphase I treatment records.

This investigation was able to quantify the changes generated by the phase I intervention and determine how much improvement, if any, had occurred before the initiation of the second phase. All variables constituting the DI score were measured separately to investigate which components of the DI underwent the most change. Finally, the three angle classification groups were compared to evaluate if any of these groups benefitted more from an early treatment phase.

The results were interesting, and show that, though much has been achieved, a lot has yet to be investigated. The DI score was calculated on a sample size of 300 individuals,

164 females and 136 males, who started phase I treatment at a mean age of 9y 3m years and had a mean treatment duration of 14.5 months. Measurements were taken before phase I, and the exact same evaluation was performed before phase II.

Since all prephase I (T1) and many of the prephase II (T2) models were in mixed dentition, the Tanaka–Johnston prediction was used to calculate the amount of dental crowding [26]. Another area of special consideration was the evaluation of anterior and lateral open bite. As several teeth were in the process of eruption, no point deviations were scored for teeth that were not fully erupted.

The mean scores were computed for the total group for T1 and T2, and the mean differences between the initial and final scores were calculated. If the total DI score was reduced at T2, it would indicate *a reduction in the complexity* of the cases. If the total DI score increased at T2, it would indicate *a greater complexity* of the sample analyzed. Table 3.1 displays the initial and final mean values for the total score and the scores of each individual component of the DI as well as the mean differences of those scores. In addition, paired *t*-tests compared T1 and T2 means and a *p*-value indicates if the difference in points was statistically significant. All significant values are marked with an asterisk.

The mean total score at T1 was 17.26 points and the mean total score at T2 was 9.98 points. There was a mean reduction of 7.28 points in the DI score, which according to the *t*-test was a statistically significant change. These numbers indicate a reduction of 42.2% in the DI, meaning a reduction in the complexity of the total sample.

Each of the variables of the DI was assessed individually in the same way, and the statistically significant were overjet, anterior open bite, crowding, occlusal relationship, posterior lingual crossbite, ANB angle, and the category "Other." The variables that underwent nonsignificant changes were overbite, lateral open

Table 3.1 Overall DI score differences.

	Mean T1	Mean T2	Mean difference	SD	*p* value
Overjet	3.06	0.87	2.19	2.64	<0.001*
Overbite	0.94	0.77	0.17	1.13	0.008
Anterior openbite	1.32	0.41	0.9	3.00	<0.001*
Lateral openbite	0.21	0.21	0	1.59	0.971
Crowding	1.92	1.25	0.67	1.76	<0.001*
Occlusal relation	3.49	1.96	1.54	2.73	<0.001*
Posterior lingual crossbite	0.91	0.083	0.83	1.37	<0.001*
Posterior buccal crossbite	0.02	0.11	−0.09	0.62	0.16
ANB	1.32	0.75	0.57	2.04	<0.001*
SN-MP	2.15	2.27	−0.12	2.59	0.410
IMPA	0.66	0.85	−0.19	2.26	0.146
Other	1.26	0.46	0.80	1.29	<0.001*
Total	17.26	9.98	7.28	7.06	<0.001*

* Statistically significant difference at *p* < 0.004.

Table 3.2 Percentages of change (%).

	Class I	Class II	Class III	Overall
Total	49.3*	34.5*	58.5*	42.2*

* Statistically significant differences as shown by the *t*-tests at $p < 0.004$.

bite, posterior buccal crossbite, and SN-MP and IMPA angles.

Next, the sample was categorized in three different groups according to the angle classification (Class I, II, and III), and the percentage of the reduction of the complexity measured by the DI is given in Table 3.2.

3.2 Assessing interceptive treatment outcome

How did each type of malocclusion respond to the interceptive treatment? Which variables demonstrated greater response to treatment?

3.2.1 Class I

The Class I group included 81 subjects. The mean total DI score at T1 was 11.74 points and at T2 it was 5.94 points, with a mean reduction of 5.79 points, which also proved to be statistically significant. These numbers indicate a reduction of 49.3% in the DI, meaning a reduction in the complexity of that sample. All variables in the index were analyzed with the same methodology, and the ones statistically significant were overjet, anterior open bite, crowding, occlusal relationship, posterior lingual crossbite, and the category "Other." All the significant changes meant a reduction of the DI score at T2. The nonsignificant changes were overbite, lateral open bite, posterior buccal crossbite, and all cephalometric measurements (ANB, SN-MP, IMPA) (see Table 3.3).

3.2.2 Class II

The Class II group included 165 subjects. The mean total DI score at T1 was 19.13 points and at T2 it was 12.53 points, showing a mean

Table 3.3 Discrepancy Index Score differences for the Class I group.

	Mean T1	Mean T2	Mean difference	SD	*p* value
Overjet	2.27	0.57	1.7	1.6	<0.001*
Overbite	0.53	0.39	0.14	0.89	0.174
Anterior openbite	2.04	0.42	1.62	3.49	<0.001*
Lateral openbite	0.32	0.07	0.25	1.53	0.150
Crowding	1.49	0.87	0.62	1.76	0.001*
Occlusal relation	0	0.35	−0.35	1.58	0.002*
Posterior lingual crossbite	0.89	0.10	0.79	1.31	<0.001*
Posterior buccal crossbite	0	0.02	−0.02	0.22	0.320
ANB	0.57	0.58	−0.01	1.57	0.944
SN-MP	1.96	2.08	−0.12	2.44	0.650
IMPA	0.55	0.33	0.22	1.73	0.252
Other	1.11	0.15	0.96	1.52	<0.001*
Total	11.74	5.95	5.79	5.30	<0.001*

* Statistically significant difference at $p < 0.004$.

reduction of 6.60 points, which also proved to be statistically significant. These numbers indicate a reduction of 34.5% in the DI, meaning a decrease in the evaluated complexity. All features of the DI were analyzed, and the ones that showed a significant reduction in DI score were overjet, anterior open bite, crowding, occlusal relationship, posterior lingual crossbite, ANB, and the category "Other." In this group, the IMPA angle demonstrated a statistically significant *increase* in score, which indicates that after treatment the position of the lower incisors was *less* favorable. The nonsignificant changes were overbite, lateral open bite, posterior buccal crossbite, and SN-MP angle (see Table 3.4).

3.2.3 Class III

The Class III group was composed of 54 subjects. The mean total score at T1 was 19.85 points, which was reduced to 8.24 points at T2. The mean difference was 11.6 points, a statistically significant change. These numbers indicate a reduction of 58.5% in the DI, which represents a considerable decrease in the complexity of the sample. The statistically significant changes were overjet, crowding, occlusal relationship, posterior lingual crossbite, and the category "Other." The nonsignificant changes were overbite, anterior open bite, lateral open bite, and all cephalometric measurements (ANB, SN-MP, and IMPA). The *t*-test for the posterior buccal crossbite was not viable as no patients presented with the deviation at T1 or T2 (see Table 3.5).

These observations may minimize the controversy on the effectiveness of interceptive treatment, but although they do bring some answers, they also generate other questions. The numbers for the Class I deviations were surely expected as a result of improvements in the transverse and vertical dental dimensions as well as crowding and overjet. Chapter 5 thoroughly describes Class I.

Early intervention in Class II malocclusions is undoubtedly one of the most controversial procedures in orthodontics. Class II corrections are highly affected by growth. Interesting to observe that based on these results, Class II

Table 3.4 Discrepancy Index Score differences for the Class II group.

	Mean T1	Mean T2	Mean difference	SD	*p* value
Overjet	2.62	1.08	1.54	1.76	<0.001*
Overbite	1.41	1.15	0.26	1.32	0.01
Anterior openbite	0.91	0.24	0.67	2.43	<0.001*
Lateral openbite	0.17	0.27	−0.10	1.63	0.418
Crowding	2.33	1.68	0.65	1.88	<0.001*
Occlusal relation	5.13	2.80	2.33	2.87	<0.001*
Posterior lingual crossbite	0.62	0.07	0.55	1.12	<0.001*
Posterior buccal crossbite	0.04	0.18	−0.14	0.81	0.023
ANB	1.57	0.82	0.75	2.03	<0.001*
SN-MP	2.31	2.42	−0.11	2.31	0.523
IMPA	0.78	1.37	−0.59	2.58	0.004*
Other	1.25	0.44	0.81	1.25	<0.001*
Total	19.13	12.53	6.60	6.60	<0.001*

* Statistically significant difference at $p<0.004$.

Table 3.5 Discrepancy Index Score differences for the Class III group.

	Mean T1	Mean T2	Mean difference	SD	p value
Overjet	5.61	0.68	4.93	4.05	<0.001*
Overbite	0.13	0.18	−0.05	0.73	0.582
Anterior openbite	1.48	0.92	0.56	3.64	0.267
Lateral openbite	0.148	0.18	−0.03	1.58	0.864
Crowding	1.33	0.48	0.85	1.64	<0.001*
Occlusal relation	3.74	1.78	1.96	2.73	<0.001*
Posterior lingual crossbite	1.83	0.11	1.72	1.76	<0.001*
Posterior buccal crossbite	0	0	0	0	—
ANB	1.67	0.74	0.92	2.5	0.009
SN-MP	1.94	2.09	−0.15	3.50	0.757
IMPA	0.46	0.05	0.41	1.61	0.068
Other	1.5	1	0.50	0.95	<0.001*
Total	19.85	8.24	11.6	8.96	<0.001*

* Statistically significant difference at $p < 0.004$.

malocclusions are the ones that benefit the least from early intervention. It is also clear that much of the correction observed was due to the proclination of the mandibular incisors. That certainly reinforces the need for a deep reflection on the benefits of an early intervention. Trauma to the maxillary incisors, psychological issues, and patients' well-being and developing hyperdivergence are among the recommended reasons to intervene early in Class IIs as discussed in Chapter 6.

The results also confirm the fact that the malocclusion that benefits most from an early intervention is the Class III. However, it may be the most unstable. It is the one most likely to lose more in the long run due to the adversities of unfavorable growth. Class III theories and interventions are described in Chapter 7.

References

1 Pancherz H. Treatment timing and outcome. *Am J Orthod Dentofac Orthop* 2002 Jun;**121**(6):559.
2 Ngan P. Biomechanics of maxillary expansion and protraction in Class III patients. *Am J Orthod Dentofacial Orthop* 2002 Jun;**121**(6):582–3.
3 Mitani H. Early application of chincap therapy to skeletal Class III malocclusion. *Am J Orthod Dentofacial Orthop* 2002 Jun;**121**(6):584–5.
4 McNamara JA Jr. Early intervention in the transverse dimension: is it worth the effort? *Am J Orthod Dentofacial Orthop* 2002 Jun;**121**(6):572–4.
5 Little RM. Stability and relapse: early treatment of arch length deficiency. *Am J Orthod Dentofacial Orthop* 2002 Jun;**121**(6):578–81.
6 Lindsten R. Early orthodontic treatment and interceptive treatment strategies. *Eur J Orthod* 2013 Apr;**35**(2):190.
7 Kurol J. Early treatment of tooth-eruption disturbances. *Am J Orthod Dentofac Orthop* 2002 Jun;**121**(6):588–91.
8 Kokich VO Jr. Congenitally missing teeth: orthodontic management in the adolescent

patient. *Am J Orthod Dentofacial Orthop* 2002 Jun;**121**(6):594–5.

9 Keski-Nisula K, Hernesniemi R, Heiskanen M, et al. Orthodontic intervention in the early mixed dentition: a prospective, controlled study on the effects of the eruption guidance appliance. *Am J Orthod Dentofacial Orthop* 2008 Feb;**133**(2):254–60; quiz 328.e2.

10 Gianelly AA. Treatment of crowding in the mixed dentition. *Am J Orthod Dentofacial Orthop* 2002 Jun;**121**(6):569–71.

11 English JD. Early treatment of skeletal open bite malocclusions. *Am J Orthod Dentofacial Orthop* 2002 Jun;**121**(6):563–5.

12 Boley JC. Serial extraction revisited: 30 years in retrospect. *Am J Orthod Dentofacial Orthop* 2002 Jun;**121**(6):575–7.

13 Chongthanavanit N. (2013). Effect of early headgear and lower arch treatment on the development of occlusion. Master's Thesis, St. Louis, MO, Saint Louis University.

14 Proffit WR, Tulloch JFC. Preadolescent Class II problems: treat now or wait? *Am J Orthod Dentofacial Orthop* 2002 Jun;**121**(6):560–2.

15 Sarver D, Yanosky M. *Special considerations in diagnosis and treatment planning. Orthodontics current principles and techniques.* 5th edn. St. Louis, MO: Mosby, Inc., 2012. p. 59–98.

16 Summers CJ. The occlusal index: a system for identifying and scoring occlusal disorders. *Am J Orthod* 1971 Jun;**59**(6):552–67.

17 Jenny J, Cons NC. Comparing and contrasting two orthodontic indices, the Index of Orthodontic Treatment need and the Dental Aesthetic Index. *Am J Orthod Dentofacial Orthop* 1996 Oct;**110**(4):410–6.

18 Richmond S, Shaw WC, O'Brien KD, et al. The development of the PAR Index (Peer Assessment Rating): reliability and validity. *Eur J Orthod* 1992 Apr;**14**(2):125–39.

19 Richmond S, Shaw WC, Roberts CT, Andrews M. The PAR Index (Peer Assessment Rating): methods to determine outcome of orthodontic treatment in terms of improvement and standards. *Eur J Orthod* 1992 Jun;**14**(3):180–7.

20 McGuinness NJ, Stephens CD. An introduction to indices of malocclusion. *Dent Update* 1994 May;**21**(4):140–4.

21 Daniels C, Richmond S. The development of the index of complexity, outcome and need (ICON). *J Orthod* 2000 Jun;**27**(2):149–62.

22 Cangialosi TJ, Riolo ML, Owens SE Jr, et al. The American Board of Orthodontics and specialty certification: the first 50 years. *Am J Orthod Dentofacial Orthop* 2004 Jul;**126**(1):3–6.

23 Cangialosi TJ, Riolo ML, Owens SE Jr, et al. The ABO discrepancy index: a measure of case complexity. *Am J Orthod Dentofacial Orthop* 2004 Mar;**125**(3):270–8.

24 Casko JS, Vaden JL, Kokich VG, et al. Objective grading system for dental casts and panoramic radiographs. American Board of Orthodontics. *Am J Orthod Dentofacial Orthop* 1998 Nov;**114**(5):589–99.

25 Vasilakou N. Quantitative assessment of the effectiveness of phase 1 orthodontic treatment utilizing the ABO discrepancy index. Master's Thesis, St. Louis, MO, Saint Louis University, 2013.

26 Tanaka MM, Johnston LE. The prediction of the size of unerupted canines and premolars in a contemporary orthodontic population. *J Am Dent Assoc* 1974 Apr;**88**(4):798–801.

4

The genetics of the dental occlusion and malocclusion

Robyn Silberstein[1], DDS, PhD and Mary MacDougall[2], PhD

[1] Department of Orthodontics, College of Dentistry (retired), University of Illinois at Chicago, Chicago, IL, USA
[2] Faculty of Dentistry, University of British Columbia, Canada

4.1 Introduction

Birth defects are due to a combination of environmental and genetic factors. Associations can be with a known cause, such as chromosomal abnormalities, single gene defects, or a teratogenic exposure, but equally they are of unknown etiology [1]. This chapter will give examples of some common craniofacial, orofacial, and dental anomalies and special treatment considerations required by orthodontists. Excellent sources for comprehensive reviews of genetic anomalies and associated craniofacial features can be found in the online database relating to human genes, traits, and genetic disorders, such as Online Mendelian Inheritance in Man (OMIM, https://www.omim.org) and Medlineplus.gov (https://www.medlineplus.gov; search genetics) or review articles [2–4] found in PubMed (https://pubmed.ncbi.nlm.nih.gov). The focus of this chapter will be on some of the most common genetic defects you may encounter as an orthodontist.

4.1.1 Personalized medicine

Identifying contributions of genome and environment to the variation observed in phenotypic traits is advancing at a tremendous rate due to high-tech analytic tools, linkage analysis with large family studies, and genome-wide association studies. Human DNA sequencing is fast, affordable, and sophisticated. Genetic testing for dental diseases lists worldwide labs in the genetic testing registry of the National Center for Biotechnology Information (NCBI, https://www.ncbi.nlm.gov). In addition, the emphasis on patient-centered clinical research combines genetic background and appropriate research design so there is the potential to support recommendations grounded in science and better patient outcomes [5–7].

4.1.2 Clinical examination

A patient may present with a confirmed genetic diagnosis, but observant clinical examination is often the initial clue to an important genetic contribution. There is a tremendous amount of information that can be gleaned from careful observation of a patient before they open their mouth. Minor anomalies, which are of limited aesthetic or functional significance, occur approximately 65% of the time in the head and neck region and nearly 85% if skin and hands are included. This is important, since a newborn who has three or more minor anomalies is at increased risk of having a major malformation. Detecting minor anomalies might aid

---

Recognizing and Correcting Developing Malocclusions: A Problem-Oriented Approach to Orthodontics,
Second Edition. Edited by Eustáquio A. Araújo and Peter H. Buschang.
© 2025 John Wiley & Sons, Inc. Published 2025 by John Wiley & Sons, Inc.

in recognition of syndromes or major malformations (Figure 4.1) [8, 9]. Head shape, frontal bossing, orbital distortion, mandibular shape and size, ear anomalies, nerve involvement, soft tissue involvement, hand anomalies, nail dysplasia, and asymmetries are examples of features that can be assessed in the initial patient meeting. Additional photographs may be helpful in diagnosis and treatment planning, since many corrective surgeries occur at a young age and even the scar is a record (Figure 4.2).

4.1.3 Principles of dysmorphology: variable expressivity and etiologic heterogeneity

Consequences of the presence of any single etiologic factor differ from one embryologic environment to another. "That is, the developing fetus is the product of both its unique genetic background and the environment in which this background is forced to operate" as summarized by Melnick [10]. Even in cases where etiology is strongly associated with a

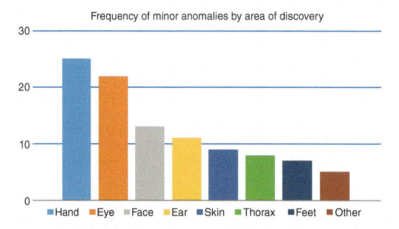

Figure 4.1 Minor anomalies detected by the area of discovery.

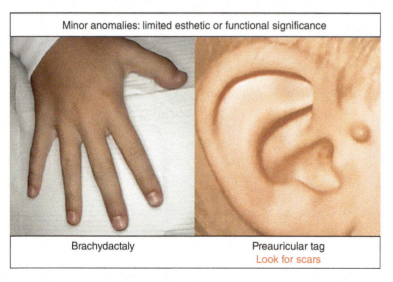

Figure 4.2 Approximately 15–20% of newborn infants in the United States are found to have at least one minor anomaly. The presence of three or more minor anomalies is associated with an increased incidence of a major malformation.

gene, such as achondroplasia or cleidocranial dysplasia (CCD), there is variation in phenotype. There is evidence for genomic variation attributable to single nucleotide polymorphisms (SNPs) and mutations in noncoding gene regions [11]. Furthermore, epigenetic modifications such as DNA methylation determine when and where genes are expressed during development and even throughout a lifetime. Examples of this contribute to phenotypic variation as well as the potential to influence personal response to treatment [12, 13].

Etiologic heterogeneity is a basic theme when evaluating many craniofacial and dental anomalies. The developing embryo has only a limited number of reactions, and there are a multitude of agents that can initiate these reactions (Figure 4.3) [8]. A dental example is seen with enamel opacities. Amelogenesis imperfecta (AI) with a strong genetic association has phenotypes similar to fluorosis, which has a strong environmental association (Figure 4.4).

4.2 Chromosomal abnormalities

Trisomy 21, Down syndrome (OMIM #190685), is the most common of all autosomal (nonsex chromosomes) chromosomal abnormalities. The syndrome can be displayed in varying degrees depending upon the amount of extra genetic material associated with chromosome 21. This syndrome is common across all ethnic origins and occurs approximately 1 in 750 births [3, 4]. There are a myriad of mental, physical, and developmental traits associated with the syndrome. Facial features include midface deficiency, muscle hypotonia and flaccid lip tonicity, protruding tongue, almond-shaped eyes with prominent epicanthal folds, ocular hypotelorism, and platybasia (an obtuse nasion-sella-basion angle). Orthodontic considerations need to account for significantly delayed dental development, delayed physical maturation, mouth breathing, chronic periodontitis, xerostomia, microdontia, dental agenesis, and general health considerations for each individual [14, 15].

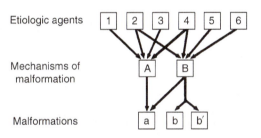

Figure 4.3 The continuum of dysmorphogenesis. Refer to text on principles of dysmorphology: variable expressivity and etiologic heterogeneity.

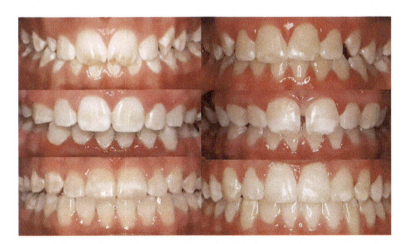

Figure 4.4 Phenotypic heterogeneity of enamel defects.

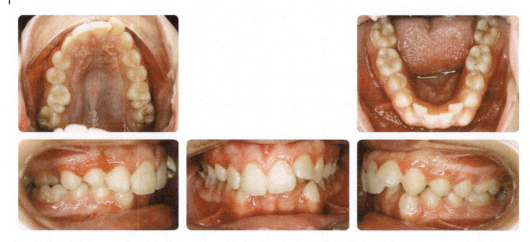

Figure 4.5 The orofacial manifestations of Marfan syndrome includes dolichocephaly, retrognathia, high arched palate, narrow maxilla, and Class II malocclusion.

4.3 Single gene defects

The number of single gene mutations associated with craniofacial anomalies is extensive. "Single gene mutations are not mechanisms in themselves but agents which may initiate mechanisms of malformation or disease at the subcellular, cellular, or tissue levels" [16].

Marfan syndrome (MFS, OMIM #154700) is an autosomal dominant connective tissue defect. The mutation in the fibrillin-1 gene (*FBN1*) affects skeletal, ocular, and cardiovascular systems. Many mutations in the *FBN1* gene have been reported with highly variable phenotypes and may be identified as MFS or fibrillinopathies [17]. Prevalence of MFS is approximately 4–6 in 100,000 births. The orofacial manifestations include dolichocephaly, retrognathia, a high arched palate, narrow maxilla, and Class II malocclusion (Figure 4.5). The critical issue prior to orthodontic treatment is cardiovascular, and clearance from the treating cardiologist is indicated. Gingival health is extremely important since there is a concern about bacteremia [18].

CCD (OMIM CLCD1 #119600) is an autosomal dominant skeletal dysplasia mapped to a mutation in the *RUNX2* gene, previously known as *CBFA1*, a member of the runt family of transcription factors. The clinical features of CCD reflect a defect in osteoblastic differentiation that include short stature, abnormal clavicles, patent or late closure of sutures, frontal bossing, hypertelorism, supernumerary teeth, and delayed tooth eruption (Figure 4.6) [19]. RUNX2 is essential for both endochondral and membranous bone formation. For orthodontic treatment planning, it is critical to understand that the underlying skeletal dysplasia results in markedly delayed tooth eruption; it is not simply supernumerary teeth (the mechanical interference) but actual slow and delayed tooth eruption. Removal of supernumerary teeth does not provide immediate eruption of the permanent dentition as would be expected. Dental eruption may be delayed significantly, even by many years (Figure 4.7). Heterogeneous coding mutations of *RUNX2* or *RUNX2* gene deletions have been identified with various phenotypes from severe to mild and undiagnosed, hence an orthodontist may encounter a mild case [20–23].

4.4 Multifactorial inheritance

Many craniofacial features and traits are a combination of multiple genetic and environmental factors. Complex inheritance patterns

4.4 Multifactorial inheritance | 39

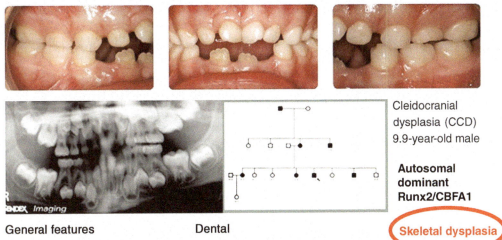

Cleidocranial dysplasia (CCD) 9.9-year-old male

Autosomal dominant Runx2/CBFA1

General features

- Short stature
- Aplasia of clavicles
- Late closure of sutures
- Low nasal bridge

Dental

- Supernumerary teeth
- Delayed eruption***

Skeletal dysplasia

Figure 4.6 Cleidocranial dysplasia (CCD) patients demonstrate enlarged calvarium, hypertelorism, low nasal bridge, supernumerary teeth, markedly delayed dental eruption, and an autosomal dominant inheritance pattern. *In this case the lower incisor eruption was delayed by 3–4 years at which time the upper mesiodens was removed and it was another 5 years until the upper anterior incisors were ultimately exposed and extruded into the arch.

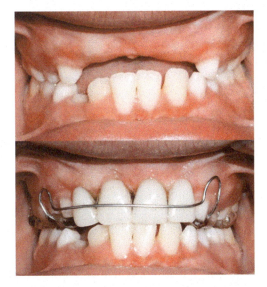

Figure 4.7 Delayed craniofacial development in cleidocranial dysplasia complicates orthodontic treatment planning. Retainers with teeth are an option for aesthetic facial appearance during adolescence, while waiting for dental eruption, or timing surgical exposure and extrusion.

follow a multifactorial model of genetic and environmental risk factors. The following examples are included owing to their prevalence in craniofacial anomalies, the etiologic heterogeneity and complexity [24].

Orofacial clefts (OMIM #119530): Cleft lip, with or without cleft palate (CL ± P) and isolated cleft palate (CP) are the most common orofacial defects in newborn infants, occurring approximately 1 in every 575 live births in the United States and 1 in every 500–1000 births worldwide. Clefting is a primary feature identified in hundreds of syndromes, but the majority of cases are classified as nonsyndromic. There are prevalence differences between geographic regions, with the highest incidence occurring in Native Americans and Asians, followed by Caucasians and the lowest occurrence rate in African Americans. There is also evidence for environmental risk factors such as phenytoin and vitamin A, socioeconomic, and lifestyle risk factors. Maternal smoking in the first trimester of pregnancy has been shown to increase the risk of clefting ninefold in certain genotypes. Clefting can also occur occasionally as part of fetal alcohol syndrome [25–27].

Orthodontic treatment challenges include transverse maxillary constriction and posterior crossbites, hypodontia, and midface deficiency. Expansion appliances are capable of correcting the problem in spite of an absent midpalatal suture and stretching of palatal scar tissue rather than a suture separation. The same strategies are applied to expansion and Class III malocclusions in patients with and without clefts but should include consideration for additional resistance and instability associated with palatal scarring and poorer prognosis for normal post treatment growth. Aligning incisors adjacent to the alveolar cleft site requires control of root angulation to avoid perforating into the cleft site, especially if done before alveolar bone grafting. Hypodontia and Class III dental and skeletal malocclusion is much more prevalent in clefts than in the general population. The orthodontist is one of many specialists from birth to young adult and it is important to keep long-term growth and burden of treatment in mind. Communication with the craniofacial team and other specialists is critical to these unique treatment considerations [28, 29].

Craniosynostosis (OMIM #12310), the premature closure of one or more cranial sutures, occurs approximately 1 in 2000 births and shows genetic heterogeneity being associated with over 130 syndromes. It can also be found without a syndromic association and varying patterns of inheritance. As the treating orthodontist, communication with the craniofacial team caring for that patient is critical. There might have been early cranial corrective surgery (surgeries) and future growth may significantly impact prognosis. Since growth is not predictable, staged observations and interventions help minimize extended treatment time (Figure 4.8) [30].

Craniofacial microsomia (CFM, OMIM #164210) is a congenital craniofacial anomaly occurring 1 in 4000–5600 births. Hemifacial microsomia (HFM) or CFM is sporadic, although there is some documented familial transmission and etiology, and pathogenesis is unknown. Structures of the first and second branchial arches are involved in HFM. Classic involvement includes orbit, mandible, ear, nerve, soft tissue (OMENS) and may be referred to as oculo-auriculo-vertebral syndrome. Hypodontia is more prevalent in HFM. Often craniofacial teams manage these patients, but it is possible that milder phenotypes are undiagnosed in the general orthodontic population. Differential diagnosis for mandibular microsomia includes many chromosomal aberrations, single gene defects such as Treacher Collins syndrome, environmental exposures such as methotrexate, Pierre Robin anomaly or familial microsomia. Explaining the limitations of orthodontics alone with skeletal asymmetry in HFM aids patient expectations and realistic treatment goals [31]. Considerations of orthognathic surgery, genioplasty, and soft tissue augmentations may be indicated (Figure 4.9).

4.5 Genetics of nonsyndromic malocclusion

The complexity of determining contributions of multiple genetic, environmental, and growth interactions to the complex inheritance traits of a Class II or III malocclusion is a challenge. There is data suggesting a genetic association with Class II division 2 (Class II/2) and Class III malocclusion. Class II/2 individuals show an increased risk of first-degree relatives with a Class II/2 malocclusion greater than found in the general population (approximately 16% versus 3%). Class III malocclusions show significant skeletal heterogeneity: mandibular prognathism, maxillary retrognathism, or a combination of the two. Data for possible gene contributions to Class III malocclusions comes from worldwide prevalence data, anatomical, and ethnic reports in the literature

4.5 Genetics of nonsyndromic malocclusion

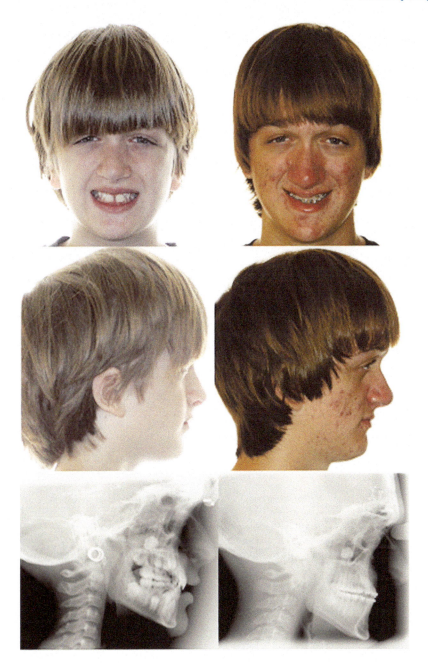

Figure 4.8 Orthodontic patient with a diagnosis of craniosynostosis and significantly disproportionate facial growth.

with population based association studies and family based linkage studies. The highest prevalence rates of Class III malocclusions are recorded in Asian, Inuit, and African populations and the lowest among Indian, US American Indian and European populations. There are several genetic loci, patterns of inheritance, and environmental factors that are thought to play a role in nonsyndromic Class III malocclusion [32–36].

4 The genetics of the dental occlusion and malocclusion

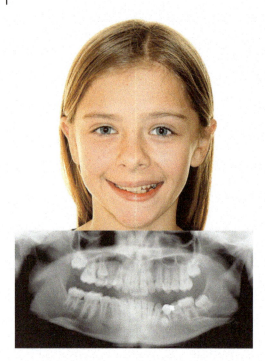

Figure 4.9 Hemifacial microsomia (HFM) or craniofacial microsomia (CFM) is of unknown etiology and presents in a range of severe to mild forms. Involvement includes orbit, mandible, ear, nerve, and soft tissue. Hypodontia and an anomalous left condyle are noted in addition to left microsomia, orbital, soft tissue, and muscle variations. This patient was ultimately diagnosed with mild hemifacial microsomia.

4.6 Altered tooth number

Alterations of tooth number, size, and shape are common craniofacial anomalies, while structure and eruption problems are less frequent. As with other anomalies, alterations resulting in agenesis, aplasia, or dysplasia of the tooth germ are sometimes Mendelian but often not clearly Mendelian and there are environmental associations as well. There is a close association between tooth agenesis, microdontia, and anomalous tooth shape evidenced in both human syndromic conditions such as ectodermal dysplasia (ED) as well as found in mutant and transgenic mice [37].

Supernumerary teeth, or hyperdontia, occur in the permanent dentition in white Caucasian populations 1–3% (slightly higher in Japanese populations). Syndromes associated with supernumerary teeth are CCD as previously outlined and Gardner syndrome, but there are more complete lists as reference [4].

Tooth agenesis is the most prevalent craniofacial malformation and occurs in isolation as part of a nonsyndromic trait but also occurs in association with many syndromes (comprehensive reports found at OMIM, www.ncbi.nlm.nih.gov/omim). Many genes have been identified with missing teeth including transcription factors MSX1 and PAX9, Wnt signaling factor AXIN2 as well as various genes in the EDA signaling pathway including EDA, EDAR, EDARADD [38].

Complete absence of teeth (anodontia) in the primary or permanent dentition is extremely rare and is often associated with hypohidrotic ectodermal dysplasia (HED) [39]. ED is defined as any syndrome exhibiting at least two defects of ectodermal origin, that is, abnormal hair, teeth, nails, or sweat glands. There is huge variability in phenotypes and more than 100 different ED syndromes (Figure 4.10) [39].

Selective tooth agenesis (STHAG) hypodontia (<6 teeth absent, excluding third molars) occurs most frequently in second premolars and maxillary laterals (approximately 3–5%). Oligodontia (≥6 teeth absent, excluding third molars) seen in less than 1% of the population [40, 41]. Absence of third molars occurs in approximately 20% of the population.

An AXIN2 mutation with familial tooth agenesis is associated with colorectal cancer [42]. While there are several known genes associated with oligodontia (AXIN2, MSX1, PAX9, EDA, EDAR, EDARADD), it is prudent to refer and test for the AXIN2 mutation, especially if there is family history of colorectal cancer, since expression of agenesis with AXIN2 mutation is highly penetrant and shows a predisposition to colorectal cancer [42, 43].

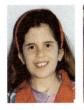
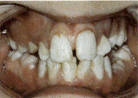
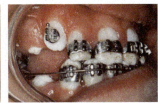
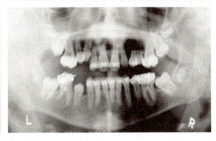

- Hypotelorism, macrocephaly
- Enamel chips, pits
- Discolored enamel
- Hypoplasia, hypomineralization
- Root resorption
- Eruption problems

Figure 4.10 Orthodontic patient exhibits amelogenesis imperfecta, cranial and eye anomalies but no identified syndrome. Weak bond strengths required banding. Root malformations, eruption issues, and root resorption were observed during treatment.

4.7 Altered tooth structure

Anomalies of tooth structure involve three specialized calcified hard tissues: enamel, dentin, and cementum. These anomalies can be genetic or caused by local or systemic environmental factors.

AI can be inherited as an autosomal dominant, autosomal recessive, sex-linked, or sporadic trait with both syndromic and non-syndromic forms. Prevalence ranges from 1:1000 to 1:14,000 in different populations. There are currently 43 genes identified in association with various AI forms [44, 45]. Orthodontic concerns include lower bond strengths leading to multiple bond failures. This may require banding or in severe cases stainless steel crowns with welded brackets or tubes. Patient management may include informing patients of increased treatment times and weak enamel due to the forces of treatment and removing appliances causing fractures. Root malformations may be present, and rigorous monitoring of root resorption is necessary (Figure 4.10). The literature has revealed a possible association of AI with open bite [46, 47]. Classification of AI is very challenging due to phenotypic variability even within pedigrees and poor phenotypic–genotypic correlations (Figure 4.11) [48].

Dentinogenesis imperfecta (DGI) is historically classified using Shields types, I–III. Broadly, type I is osteogenesis imperfecta with DGI, type II "opalescent" dentin, and type III Brandywine isolate, or "shell teeth" found in a tri-racial population originating in southern Maryland. Teeth are marked by a bluish opalescent discoloration, attrition, fractures and chipping, and pulpal obliteration. Advances in molecular genetics demonstrate heterozygous mutations in the dentin sialophosphoprotein (*DSPP*) gene linking DGI types II, III, and type II dentin dysplasia [49, 50]. Orthodontic concerns of DGI and dentin dysplasia include risk of crown fractures, which requires cautiousness and in severe cases restraint. There are also aesthetic challenges due to the discoloration (Figure 4.12).

4.8 Altered eruption

Primary failure of eruption (PFE) is an isolated condition with a localized failure of eruption in the absence of impactions or other mechanical interference. PFE commonly

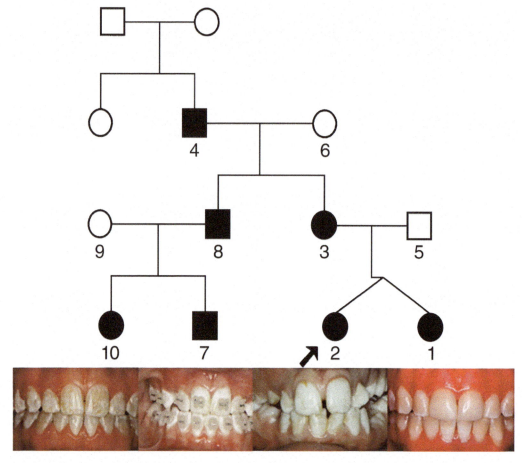

Figure 4.11 This pedigree shows proband from Figure 4.10 and her twin sister who has bonding on the centrals to cover the enamel defects and cousins with enamel opacities. Phenotypic variability exists within pedigrees with poor phenotypic–genotypic correlations.

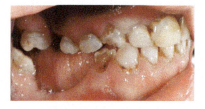

Figure 4.12 Orthodontic concerns of dentinogenesis imperfecta (DGI) include risk of crown fractures and esthetic challenges due to discoloration.

affects the posterior teeth and almost always affects a molar tooth. Previously a diagnosis of PFE was made when the lack of eruption was noted with no mechanical, pathological, or environmental responsible factors. Often the diagnosis is not made until the affected teeth are ankylosed and the adjacent teeth respond negatively. Recently, the parathyroid receptor 1 (PTHR1) has been associated with familial nonsyndromic PFE in many but not all of the diagnosed cases. Testing for a mutation in this gene can now be done prior to initiating lengthy, futile, and even damaging orthodontic treatment [51–54]. If PFE is suspected, treatment benefits from sectionals to align teeth for prosthetic or surgical management and minimize collateral damage, or in some cases extraction of the affected tooth/teeth (Figure 4.13).

Premature exfoliation of primary teeth can be an indication of a systemic issue either

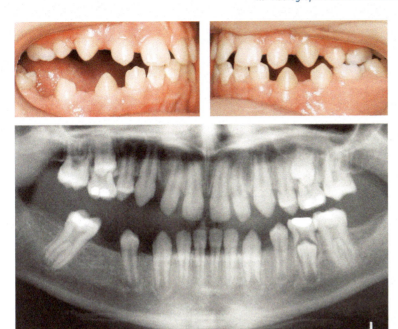

Figure 4.13 Primary failure of eruption (PFE) is most often an isolated condition with a localized failure of eruption in the absence of impactions or other mechanical interferences.

hereditary or environmentally generated. Primary tooth loss in children younger than 5 years of age in the absence of trauma suggests a genetic or systemic disease. If it does not appear as juvenile periodontitis or a dental cause such as radicular dentin dysplasia, referral to the pediatrician is indicated, since there may be hypophosphatasia, immune deficiencies, or collagen disorders (Figure 4.14) [55].

4.9 Radiographic deviations associated with genetic conditions

Inspecting radiographs as part of the dental and orthodontic records may offer clues to the overall diagnosis and prognosis that are not obvious from routine measurements. There are unique markers recognized as different from patterns generally encountered.

Fibrous dysplasia (FD) exhibits genetic heterogeneity. In one nonmalignant condition, a mutation of the *GNAS* gene results in the replacement of normal bone and marrow by fibrous tissue and woven bone. The phenotype is variable and may be limited to one site or many sites. Many patients are asymptomatic and the diagnosis is made from a finding of craniofacial asymmetry or an abnormality on dental X-rays. Lesions may have a typical "ground glass" appearance, but there are examples where there is a subtle variation observed in the maxilla or mandible (Figure 4.15). There are cases with aggressive growth of lesions, but it is more common to find a conservative growth pattern that tapers off at skeletal maturity [56]. Orthodontic considerations require caution for traumatic treatment plans such as injections and extractions, which might exacerbate lesions. In many cases, however, orthodontic treatment is not contraindicated [57].

Taurodontism (OMIM 27200) is characterized by molar tooth morphology in which the crown root ratio of the tooth is larger than normal. It occurs in approximately 2.5% of Caucasian adults as an isolated (nonsyndromic) trait [58]. Individuals with nonsyndromic hypodontia are more likely to show

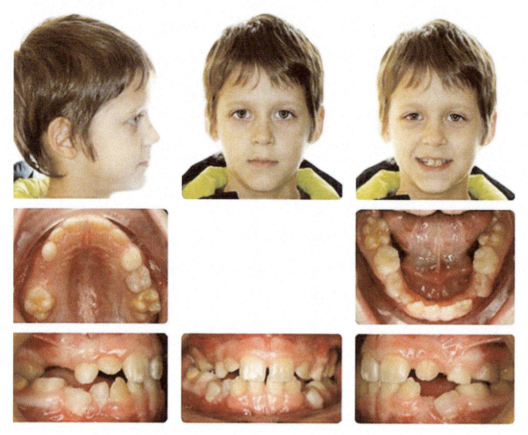

Figure 4.14 This 7-year-old patient presented with molar and incisor enamel defects. His mother reported early loss of his primary teeth beginning at age 2 in the absence of trauma. Premature primary tooth exfoliation suggests a genetic or systemic disease, which might warrant referral to the pediatrician for consideration of hypophosphatasia, collagen, and immune disorders.

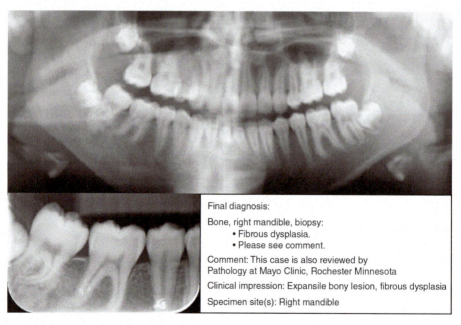

Figure 4.15 Diagnosis of fibrous dysplasia was made after referral for evaluation of a radiographic lesion at the apex of the mandibular right second molar. Often the orthodontist is the first practitioner to recognize facial asymmetry and/or radiographic evidence suggestive of fibrous dysplasia.

taurodontism of the permanent first molars [59]. Taurodontism can also be found in several syndromes, including tricho-dento-osseous (TDO) syndrome, otodental dysplasia, and chromosomal anomalies such as Klinefelter syndrome and Down syndrome [60]. TDO is caused by mutations in the *DLX3* gene [61, 62]. Amelogenesis imperfecta with taurodontism (AIHT) is caused by a different DLX3 mutation. The structural finding of taurodontism does not usually require action but hints at an occasional syndromic association.

Short root anomaly (SRA) is characterized mainly in maxillary incisor tooth morphology in which the roots are short and blunt. The crown root ratio in SRA is significantly reduced [63]. There is evidence of a genetic/familial component to SRA [64–67]. Given the presence of anatomically short roots, understanding current available genetic markers can only help in making nuanced treatment choices when dealing with such mysterious and devastating sequelae of orthodontic treatment as root resorption. There is evidence that variation in the interleukin 1 beta gene in orthodontically treated individuals accounts for at least some of the differences seen in the amount of external apical root resorption (EARR) [68].

4.10 Conclusion

Orthodontists are in a fortunate position to identify unusual patterns in skeletal, dental, and radiographic conditions and make appropriate referrals for gene testing and work with other specialists. Careful observation, a thorough medical history and knowledge of genetic conditions directly affect prognosis and orthodontic treatment planning. Examples include clearance from the cardiologist with MFS, treatment timing decisions with CCD, evaluation of orthodontic treatment goals with HFM and craniosynostosis, and caution and genetic testing with PFE and oligodontia. Growing knowledge and testing of variations in target genes and collaborations with indicated specialists contribute to personalized orthodontic treatment planning.

References

1. Christianson A, Howson CP, Modell B. *March of dimes: global report on birth defects, the hidden toll of dying and disabled children*. 2005.
2. Hartsfield JK Jr. The benefits of obtaining the opinion of a clinical geneticist regarding orthodontic patients. *Integrated Clinical Orthodontics* 2011:109–31.
3. Goodman RM, Gorlin RJ, Meyer D. *The malformed infant and child: an illustrated guide*. New York: Oxford University Press, 1983.
4. Khandekar S, Dive A, Munde P. Chromosomal abnormalities-a review. *Central India J Dent Sci* 2013;**4**(1):35–40.
5. Cobourne MT, Sharpe PT. Diseases of the tooth: the genetic and molecular basis of inherited anomalies affecting the dentition. *Wiley Interdiscip Rev Dev Biol* 2013;**2**(2):183–212.
6. Slavkin HC, Santa Fe Group. Revising the scope of practice for oral health professionals: enter genomics. *J Am Dent Assoc* 2014 Mar;**145**(3):228–30.
7. Collins FS, Hudson KL, Briggs JP, Lauer MS. PCORnet: turning a dream into reality. *J Am Med Inform Assoc* 2014 July;**21**(4):576–7.
8. Shields ED, Burzynski NJ. *Clinical dysmorphology of oral-facial structures*. J. Wright, PSG Inc, 1982.
9. Stevenson AC, Johnston HA, Stewart MI, et al. A report of a study of a series of consecutive births in 24 centers. *Bull World Health Organ* 1966;**34**(Suppl):9–127.
10. Melnick M. The doctrine of multifactorial association: gene-environment interaction.

In: Shields ED, Burzynski NJ (eds), *Clinical Dysmorphology of Oral-Facial Structures*. Massachusetts, USA: John Wright, PSG Inc., 1982. p. 28.

11 Altshuler D, Pollara VJ, Cowles CR, et al. An SNP map of the human genome generated by reduced representation shot-gun sequencing. *Nature* 2000;**407**(6803):513–6.

12 Hughes T, Bockmann M, Mihailidis S, et al. Genetic, epigenetic, and environmental influences on dentofacial structures and oral health: ongoing studies of Australian twins and their families. *Twin Research and Human Genetics* 2013;**16**(01):43–51.

13 Williams S, Hughes T, Adler C, et al. Epigenetics: a new frontier in dentistry. *Aust Dent J* 2014;**59**(s1):23–33.

14 Korayem MA, Alkofide EA. Characteristics of Down syndrome subjects in a Saudi sample. *Angle Orthod* 2013;**84**(1):30–7.

15 Desai SS, Flanagan TJ. Orthodontic considerations in individuals with Down syndrome: A case report. *Angle Orthod* 1999;**69**(1):85–8.

16 Poswillo D. Mechanisms and pathogenesis of malformation. *Br Med Bull* 1976;**32**(1):59–64.

17 Robinson PN, Booms P, Katzke S, et al. Mutations of FBN1 and genotype–phenotype correlations in Marfan syndrome and related fibrillinopathies. *Hum Mutat* 2002;**20**(3):153–61.

18 Utreja A, Evans CA. Marfan syndrome-an orthodontic perspective. *Angle Orthod* 2009;**79**(2):394–400.

19 Mundlos S. Cleidocranial dysplasia: clinical and molecular genetics. *J Med Genet* 1999 Mar;**36**(3):177–82.

20 Otto F, Kanegane H, Mundlos S. Mutations in the RUNX2 gene in patients with cleidocranial dysplasia. *Hum Mutat* 2002;**19**(3):209–16.

21 Silberstein R, Dong J, Chary-Reddy S, et al. *CBFA1 (RUNX2) Exon 1 Mutation Associated with CCD*. 2006.

22 Zhou G, Chen Y, Zhou L, et al. CBFA1 mutation analysis and functional correlation with phenotypic variability in cleidocranial dysplasia. *Hum Mol Genet* 1999 Nov;**8**(12):2311–6.

23 Lee KE, Seymen F, Ko J, et al. RUNX2 mutations in cleidocranial dysplasia. *Genet Mol Res* 2013 Oct 15;**12**(4):4567–74.

24 Dixon MJ, Marazita ML, Beaty TH, Murray JC. Cleft lip and palate: understanding genetic and environmental influences. *Nat Rev Genet* 2011;**12**(3):167–78.

25 Genetics of cleft lip and cleft palate. *American Journal of Medical Genetics Part C: Seminars in Medical Genetics: Wiley Online Library*, 2013.

26 Marazita ML. The evolution of human genetic studies of cleft lip and cleft palate. *Annu Rev Genomics Hum Genet* 2012;**13**:263–83.

27 Murray J. Gene/environment causes of cleft lip and/or palate. *Clin Genet* 2002;**61**(4):248–56.

28 Kernahan DA, Rosenstein SW. *Cleft lip and palate: a system of management*. Williams & Wilkins, 1990.

29 Long RE, Semb G, Shaw WC. Orthodontic treatment of the patient with complete clefts of lip, alveolus, and palate: lessons of the past 60 years. *Cleft Palate Craniofac J* 2000;**37**(6):533.

30 Vargervik K, Rubin MS, Grayson BH, et al. Parameters of care for craniosynostosis: Dental and orthodontic perspectives. *Am J Orthod and Dent Orthop* 2012;**141**(4):S68–73.

31 Ohtani J, Hoffman WY, Vargervik K, Oberoi S. Team management and treatment outcomes for patients with hemifacial microsomia. *Am J Orthod and Dent Orthop* 2012;**141**(4):S74–81.

32 LaBuda MC, Gottesman I, Pauls DL. Usefulness of twin studies for exploring the etiology of childhood and adolescent psychiatric disorders. *Am J Med Genet* 1993;**48**(1):47–59.

33 *Personalized orthodontics, the future of genetics in practice. Seminars in Orthodontics*. Elsevier, 2008.

34 Hartsfield JK, Morford LA, Otero LM, Fardo DW. Genetics and non-syndromic facial growth. *J Pediatr Genet* 2013;**2**(1):9–20.

35 Zhou X, Zhang C, Yao S, et al. Genetic architecture of non-syndromic skeletal class III malocclusion. *Oral Dis* 2023 Sep;**29**(6):2423–37.

36 Harris JE, Kowalski CJ, Walker SJ. Intrafamilial dentofacial associations for Class II, Division 1 probands. *Am J Orthod* 1975;**67**(5):563–70.

37 Kangas AT, Evans AR, Thesleff I, Jernvall J. Nonindependence of mammalian dental characters. *Nature* 2004;**432**(7014):211–4.

38 Azza Husam Al-Ani, Joseph Safwat Antoun, William Murray Thomson, Tony Raymond Merriman, Mauro Farella, "Hypodontia: An Update on Its Etiology, Classification, and Clinical Management", *Biomed Res Int*, vol. 2017, Article ID 9378325, 9 pages, 2017.

39 Nakata M, Koshiba H, Eto K, Nance WE. A genetic study of anodontia in X-linked hypohidrotic ectodermal dysplasia. *Am J Hum Genet* 1980 Nov;**32**(6):908–19.

40 Pinheiro M, Freire-Maia N. Ectodermal dysplasias: a clinical classification and a causal review. *Am J Med Genet* 1994;**53**(2):153–62.

41 Larmour CJ, Mossey PA, Thind BS, et al. Hypodontia—a retrospective review of prevalence and etiology. Part I *Quintessence Int* 2005;**36**(4):263–70.

42 Lammi L, Arte S, Somer M, et al. Mutations in AXIN2 cause familial tooth agenesis and predispose to colorectal cancer. *Am J Hum Genet* 2004;**74**(5):1043–50.

43 Bergendal B, Klar J, Stecksén-Blicks C, et al. Isolated oligodontia associated with mutations in EDARADD, AXIN2, MSX1, and PAX9 genes. *Am Journal Med Genet Part A* 2011;**155**(7):1616–22.

44 Wright JT, Torain M, Long K, et al. Amelogenesis imperfecta: genotype-phenotype studies in 71 families. *Cells Tissues Organs* 2011;**194**(2–4):279–83.

45 Dong J, Ruan W, Duan X. Molecular-based phenotype variations in amelogenesis imperfecta. *Oral Dis* 2023;**29**:2334–65.

46 Alachioti XS, Dimopoulou E, Vlasakidou A, Athanasiou AE. Amelogenesis imperfecta and anterior open bite: Etiological, classification, clinical and management interrelationships. *J Orthod Sci* 2014 Jan;**3**(1):1–6.

47 Messaoudi Y, Kiliaridis S, Antonarakis GS. Craniofacial Cephalometric Characteristics and Open Bite Deformity in Individuals with Amelogenesis Imperfecta-A Systematic Review and Meta-Analysis. *J Clin Med* 2023 Jun 2;**12**(11):3826.

48 Arkutu N, Gadhia K, McDonald S, et al. Amelogenesis imperfecta: the orthodontic perspective. *Br Dent J* 2012;**212**(10):485–9.

49 de La Dure-Molla M, Fournier BP, Berdal A. Isolated dentinogenesis imperfecta and dentin dysplasia: revision of the classification. *Eur Jo. Hum Genet* 2014.

50 MacDougall M, Dong J, Acevedo AC. Molecular Basis of Human Dentin Diseases. *Am J Med Genet A* 2006;**140A**:2536–46.

51 Frazier-Bowers SA, Koehler KE, Ackerman JL, Proffit WR. Primary failure of eruption: further characterization of a rare eruption disorder. *Am J Orthod Dent Orthop* 2007;**131**(5):578. e1–578. e11.

52 Proffit WR, Vig KW. Primary failure of eruption: a possible cause of posterior open bite. *Am J Orthod* 1981;**80**(2):173–90.

53 Frazier-Bowers SA, Simmons D, Wright JT, et al. Primary failure of eruption and PTH1R: The importance of a genetic diagnosis for orthodontic treatment planning. *Am J Orthod Dento Orthop* 2010;**137**(2):160.

54 Frazier-Bowers SA, Hendricks HM, Wright JT, et al. Novel mutations in PTH1R associated with primary failure of eruption and osteoarthritis. *J Dent Res* 2014 Feb;**93**(2):134–9.

55 Hartsfield JK Jr. Premature Exfoliation of Teeth in Childhood and Adolescence. *Adv Pediatr Infect Dis* 1994;**41**:453.

56 Lee J, FitzGibbon E, Chen Y, et al. Clinical guidelines for the management of

craniofacial fibrous dysplasia. *Orphanet J Rare Dis* 2012;**7**(Suppl 1):S2.
57 Akintoye SO, Lee JS, Feimster T, et al. Dental characteristics of fibrous dysplasia and McCune-Albright syndrome. *Oral Surg Oral Med Oral Pathol Oral Radiol Endod* 2003;**96**(3):275–82.
58 Jaspers MT, Witkop CJ Jr. Taurodontism, an isolated trait associated with syndromes and X-chromosomal aneuploidy. *Am J Hum Genet* 1980 May;**32**(3):396–413.
59 Stenvik A, Zachrisson B, Svatun B. Taurodontism and concomitant hypodontia in siblings. *Oral Surg, Oral Med, Oral Pathol* 1972;**33**(5):841–5.
60 Schulman GS, Redford-Badwal D, Poole A, et al. Taurodontism and learning disabilities in patients with Klinefelter syndrome. *Pediatr Dent* 2005;**27**(5):389–94.
61 Price JA, Bowden DW, Wright JT, et al. Identification of a mutation in DLX3 associated with tricho-dento-osseous (TDO) syndrome. *Hum Mol Genet* 1998 Mar;**7**(3):563–9.
62 Bloch-Zupan A, Goodman JR. Otodental syndrome. *Orphanet J Rare Dis* 2006;**1**:5.
63 Apajalahti S, Hölttä P, Turtola L, Pirinen S. Prevalence of short-root anomaly in healthy young adults. *Acta Odontol Scand* 2002;**60**(1):56–9.
64 Puranik CP, Hill A, Henderson Jeffries K, et al. Characterization of short root anomaly in a Mexican cohort – hereditary idiopathic root malformation. *Orthod Craniofacial Res* 2015;**18**(Suppl.1):62–70.
65 Wang J, Rousso C, Christensen BI, et al. Ethnic differences in the root to crown ratios of the permanent dentition. *Orthod Craniofacial Res* 2019;**22**:99–104.
66 Yu M, Jiang Z, Wang Y, et al. Molecular mechanisms for short root anomaly. *Oral Dis* 2021;**27**:142–50.
67 Baghaei NN, Zhai G, Lamani E. Genetic and other factors contributing to external apical root resorption in orthodontic patients. *Orthod Craniofacial Res* 2023;**26**(Suppl. 1):64–72.
68 Hartsfield JK, Everett ET, Al-Qawasmi RA. Genetic Factors in External Apical Root Resorption and Orthodontic Treatment. *Crit Rev Oral Biol Med* 2004;**15**(2):115–22.

5

Class I: Recognizing and correcting intraarch deviations

5.1

Section I: The development and etiology of a Class I malocclusion

Peter H. Buschang, MA, PhD

Regents Professor Emeritus, Department of Orthodontics, Texas A&M University School of Dentistry, Dallas, TX, USA

5.1 Introduction

Class I molar relationships, also referred to as neutrocclusion, are based on having the mesiobuccal cusps of the maxillary first molars occluding in line with the buccal grooves of the mandibular first molars. Permanent Class I molar relationships develop from either flush terminal plane or mesial step deciduous molar relationships (Figure 5.1). Most children with flush terminal plane relationships develop cusp-to-cusp molar relationships in the early mixed dentition, while a few will develop normal molar relationships. Most mesial step relationships develop into normal relationships in the mixed dentition, and some will develop cusp-to-cusp relationships. Most cusp-to-cusp and normal mixed dentition relationships will become Class I permanent molar relationships. Some of those with cusp-to-cusp relationships will develop Class II malocclusion and a few of those with normal relationships in the mixed dentition will develop into Class III malocclusion.

Individuals with Class I malocclusion have normal molar relationships, but their teeth are not correctly positioned in the line of occlusion, due to malalignments, rotations, overbites, open bites, posterior crossbites, or anterior crossbites. Class I malocclusion is the most prevalent form of malocclusion, even more common than normal occlusion. Maxillary and mandibular malalignments are by far the most prevalent forms of Class I malocclusion.

Two basic measures have been developed to quantify the malalignment that characterizes Class I malocclusion: tooth size arch length discrepancies (TSALD) and the irregularity index. Importantly, these two indices do not measure the same attributes. Incisor irregularity only explains 25–36% of the variation in TSALD [1, 2]. Because the mandibular incisors have similar mesiodistal and buccolingual dimensions [3], incisor rotation can have a substantial impact on incisor irregularity without impacting TSALD. Displacements of teeth that maintain the space needed for correction will also affect irregularity, but not TSALD. Due to these differences, incisor irregularity and changes in irregularity over time are usually greater than TSALD and changes in TSALD. Regardless, TSALD provides a better measure of crowding than incisor irregularity.

The distinction between incisor irregularity and TSALD is particularly important during the mixed dentition when the size of the teeth in the mouth is typically larger than the space available. To determine whether or not there will be a space problem in the permanent dentition, it is necessary to obtain accurate size estimates

Recognizing and Correcting Developing Malocclusions: A Problem-Oriented Approach to Orthodontics,
Second Edition. Edited by Eustáquio A. Araújo and Peter H. Buschang.
© 2025 John Wiley & Sons, Inc. Published 2025 by John Wiley & Sons, Inc.

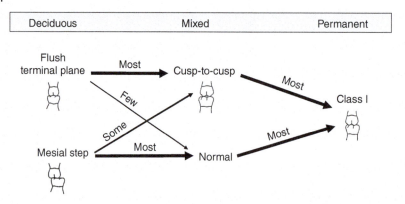

Figure 5.1 Development of Class I molar relationships between the deciduous (illustration of deciduous mesial steps larger than 0.5–1.0 mm), early mixed, and permanent dentitions.

of the teeth that have not yet emerged. Accurate estimates of the mesiodistal widths of the unerupted permanent teeth are an essential aspect of the mixed-dentition arch analysis.

Various methods exist for estimating the sizes of the unerupted teeth. Some are based solely on measurements taken of erupted teeth, some use only radiographic measurements, and others measure both the erupted and unerupted teeth. Methods based on both are considered more accurate [4, 5]. Gardner [6], who evaluated four of the most commonly used methods, showed that the Hixon and Oldfather [7] approach was the most accurate. This approach is based on the mesiodistal diameters of the erupted permanent incisors and unerupted premolars, evaluated with periapical X-rays. Because the original method underestimated the sizes of the unerupted canines and premolars, a revised, more accurate, Hixon and Oldfather method was developed [8].

5.2 Prevalence of Class I malocclusion and changes in arch form

The National Center of Health Statistics (NCHS) nationwide survey indicated that approximately 50% of Caucasians and 70% of African Americans 6–11 years of age have Class I buccal segment relationships [9]. The data from the Third National Health and Nutrition Examination Survey (NHANES III), conducted between 1988 and 1991, showed that 45.5% of children of 8–11 years possess irregular lower incisors [10]. In the maxilla, approximately 22% have clinically significant amounts (≥ 4 mm) of incisor irregularities and 8.7% have severe (≥ 7 mm) irregularities; the corresponding prevalences in the mandible are approximately 20.6% and 4.7%, respectively. The prevalence of both maxillary and mandibular incisor irregularity increases with age. Clinically significant amounts of maxillary irregularity increase to 31% among 12–17-years-olds, and then decrease slightly to 30.4% among adults 18–50 years of age. Clinically significant mandibular irregularities increase to 31% among adolescents, and then to 39% among adults.

While generalized spacing has often been reported to occur during the primary dentition [11], secular changes in mandibular spacing are happening. A sample of 184 North American white children evaluated in 1965 showed 2.2–2.6 mm of maxillary spacing and 1.8–2.1 mm of mandibular spacing in the deciduous dentition [12]. Based on 526 Iowan children 4–6 years of age evaluated in 2003, the primary maxillary teeth of boys and girls exhibited 2.7 and 1.9 mm of extra space, and the primary mandibular teeth exhibited 0.1 and 1.4 mm of space deficiency, respectively [13]. Approximately, 58% of the boys and 76% of the

5.2 Prevalence of Class I malocclusion and changes in arch form

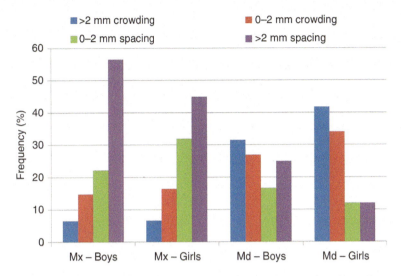

Figure 5.2 Percentages of boys and girls 4–6 years of age with spacing and crowding in the maxilla (mx) and mandible (md) (Warren et al. [13]/with permission of Elsevier).

girls had some degree of TSALD in the lower jaw (Figure 5.2); 32% of the boys and 42% of the girls had TSALD >2.0 mm. A historical cohort of children from the Iowa Growth Study whose records were collected 50 years earlier showed twice as much maxillary spacing than their more current counterparts, and 4–4.7 mm more spacing in the mandible. Thus, there appears to have been a secular trend toward increased space deficiencies in both jaws.

Crowding of the deciduous dentition is important because it often produces crowding in the mixed dentition [14]. However, it should not be assumed that all children without spaces in the primary dentition will develop incisor crowding. Baume [15] showed that most (57%) children without space in the primary dentition do not develop incisor crowding. Similarly, most of the children evaluated by Moorrees and Chadha [12] who had no spacing or slight crowding in the primary dentition exhibited normal alignment or only slight crowding in the mixed dentition.

Increases in anterior crowding should be expected during the transition from primary to early mixed dentition [16], which worldwide data shows starts to occur at approximately 6 years of age (Figure 5.3). During this transition, the spaces commonly seen in the primary dentition are lost with the emergence of the permanent incisors, and crowding typically develops, even among those children who will eventually have acceptable anterior alignment [12]. The crowding occurs because the deciduous incisors are considerably smaller than their permanent successors. The differences in tooth sizes, commonly referred to as incisor liability, are approximately 7–8 mm in the maxilla and 5–6 mm in the mandible.

Importantly, the amount of crowding that occurs is substantially less than might be expected based on incisor liability. On average, there is approximately 2–3 mm and 1–1.5 mm of anterior TSALD in the maxilla and mandible, respectively, after the full emergence of the permanent incisors [17]. It should be emphasized that the emergence of the permanent incisors is a relatively slow process, during which a substantial amount of growth takes place (Figure 5.4). The incisors require approximately 6–7 months and 19 months to attain 70% and 90%, respectively, of their maximum intraoral heights [18]. This provides time for dentoalveolar compensations (i.e. adjustments for the larger incisors that are erupting) to occur.

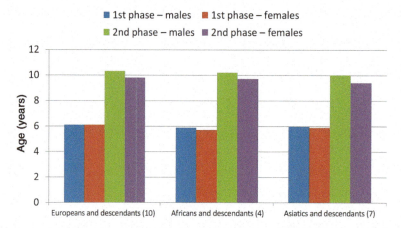

Figure 5.3 Average ages at which first and second phases of permanent tooth emergence start (values in brackets indicate the number of samples for each group) (Eveleth and Tanner [69]/Cambridge University Press).

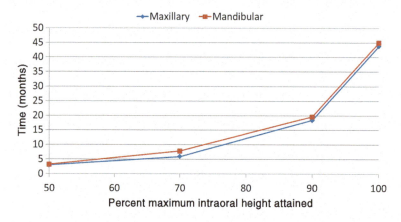

Figure 5.4 Time required for the permanent maxillary left central and mandibular left central incisors to erupt various amounts of their maximum intraoral heights (adapted from Giles et al. [18]).

Crowding is substantially less than incisor liability because the arch form changes during the transition. The anterior part of the arch widens substantially with the emergence of the permanent incisors (Figure 5.5). Intercanine width increases by approximately 3 mm in the maxilla and 2 mm in the mandible [19]. In addition, the limited amount of space available causes the permanent maxillary incisors to emerge more labially inclined. This increases maxillary arch depth. Together, these compensations increase anterior arch perimeter, especially in the maxilla. During the eruption of the incisors into functional occlusion, maxillary arch perimeter increases by 4–5 mm, and mandibular perimeter increases by approximately 2 mm (Figure 5.6). The difference between incisor liability and the increase in arch perimeters explains the less-than-expected amount of crowding seen after the transition to the mixed dentition.

The crowding that occurs during the early transition is temporary for most children. Crowding decreases during the late mixed dentition phase, when the larger deciduous molars are replaced by smaller permanent premolars [12, 16, 20, 21]. This phase typically starts

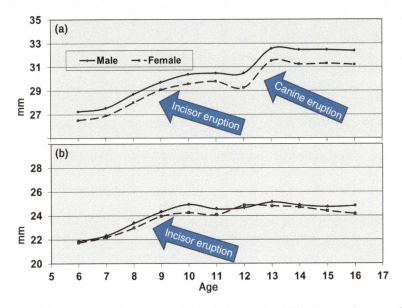

Figure 5.5 Maxillary (a) and mandibular (b) intercanine width changes between 6 and 16 years of age (adapted from Moyers et al. [19]).

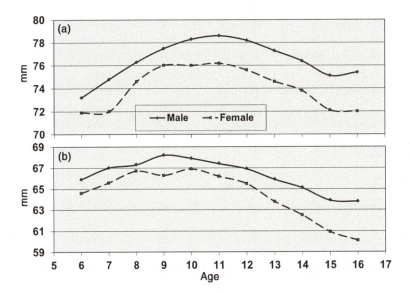

Figure 5.6 Maxillary (a) and mandibular (b) arch perimeter (first molar to first molar) changes between 6 and 16 years of age (adapted from Moyers et al. [19]).

slightly later in males (just after 10 years) than females (just before 10 years) (Figure 5.3). The decreases in crowding that occur have been reported to range from 0.2 mm [20] to 1–1.5 mm [12]. There are greater decreases in mandibular than maxillary crowding. The difference is related to Leeway spaces, which provide approximately 2.5 mm in the maxilla and 5 mm in the mandible [17, 19]. For many children, the Leeway spaces are sufficient to resolve anterior crowding in the majority of cases.

Crowding again increases during the early permanent dentition. Based on the available longitudinal data, the greatest increases in malalignment occur during the teenage years and then taper off during the early 20s (Figure 5.7). Bishara et al. [22, 23] provide some of the best long-term longitudinal data for untreated subjects, showing a 2.4 mm increase in anterior TSALD between 14 and 25 years of age, and another 0.7 mm increase between 25 and 46 years of age. Bondevik [24] reported increases of 2.0 mm in anterior TSALD in untreated subjects between 23 and 34 years of age, while Richardson [25] showed increases of 2.3 mm in anterior and posterior TSALD between 13 and 18 years of age.

Importantly, increases in TSALD and incisor irregularity in untreated subjects have been consistently associated with decreases in intercanine width, arch depth, and arch perimeter. The 0.7 mm increase in irregularity reported by Sinclair and Little [20] in the permanent dentition was associated with a 2 mm decrease in arch length and a 1.5 mm decrease in intercanine width. Bishara et al. [22, 23] showed that the greater the increases in malalignment, the greater the decreases in arch length (Figure 5.8). This association might be expected because the posterior teeth usually migrate mesially into a narrower part of the arch as anterior crowding increases, filling the spaces created [24, 25].

The malalignments that occur between adjacent pairs of teeth vary considerably. Based on 9044 adults who participated in the NHANES III, contact displacements (i.e. distances between contact points) between the maxillary canines and lateral incisors, showed only slightly greater discrepancies than the contact displacements between the maxillary lateral and central incisors (Figure 5.9), both of which were substantially greater than the contact displacements between the central incisors. Subjects with severe incisor irregularities showed the greatest contact irregularities between the lateral and central incisors. In the mandible, the contacts between the canines and lateral incisors showed the greatest discrepancies; the discrepancies for the contacts between the laterals and centrals were only slightly greater than those between the centrals. Regardless of whether crowding is severe or slight, the same patterns always occur in the mandible. Orthodontic patients show the same patterns of posttreatment changes [26]. This emphasizes the fact that longitudinal changes

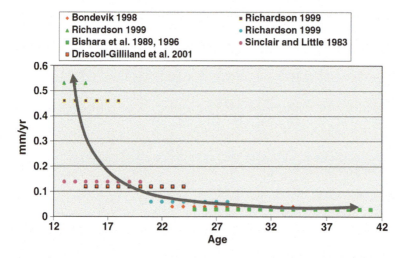

Figure 5.7 Annualized (total Δ/total duration) rates of malalignment of untreated samples 13–41 years of age, including data from Bondevik [49], Richardson [48], Bishara et al. [22, 23], Sinclair and Little [20], and Driscoll-Gilliland et al. [27].

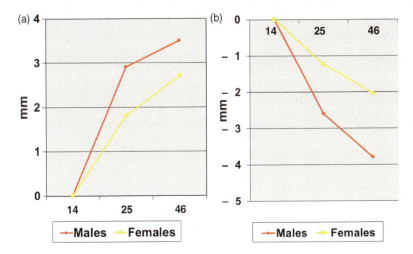

Figure 5.8 (a) Anterior TSALD and (b) arch length changes of untreated subjects between 14 and 46 years of age (data from Bishara et al. [22, 23]).

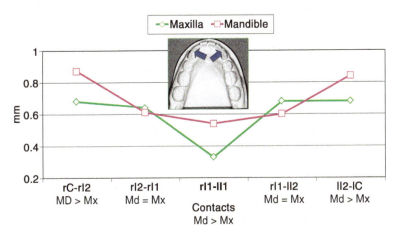

Figure 5.9 Anterior contact irregularity (distances between contacts) of untreated and treated US adults measured by the NHANES III. Note that the greatest contact irregularity occurs between the mandibular canines and lateral incisors.

in incisor alignment follow the same patterns for treated and untreated subjects.

The most recent epidemiology survey of the USA (NHANES III) also provided prevalence estimates of clinically significant overbite, open bites, maxillary diastemas, and posterior crossbites. Based on the survey conducted between 1988 and 1991, approximately 16.9% of individuals 8–50 years of age had overbites greater than 4 mm, 3.3% had open bites, 6.5% maxillary diastemas greater than 2 mm, and 9.4% had posterior crossbites [10, 27]. Between childhood (8–11 years) and adulthood (18–50 years), clinically meaningful overbites decreased from 20% to 15.2%, open bites decreased from 3.6% to 3.3%, maxillary diastema decreased from 19.3% to 4.8%, and posterior crossbites increased from 8.5% to 9.9%. A more recent evaluation of the NHANES data collected from 1988 to 1994 showed that overbite increased from 10.6% to 13% between early adulthood (17–26 years) and mid-adulthood (27–46 years) [28]. Over the same period, open bites decreased from 4.4% to 3.1%, and posterior crossbites decreased from 10.1% to 7%.

5.3 Class I malocclusion and the dental compensatory mechanism

Malalignments should be thought of as forms of dentoalveolar compensation. Most of the time, teeth are maintained in positions of equilibrium between the lingual, labial, and vestibular muscles [29]. Dentoalveolar compensations are the changes in tooth positions that occur between periods of equilibrium. Compensations often represent positive adaptive changes necessary to maintain normal interarch relations under varying skeletal relationships [30]. But compensations can also produce negative, maladaptive, changes that account for the high prevalence of Class I malocclusion in today's populations. The factors responsible for dentoalveolar adaptations include: 1) a normal eruptive system; 2) soft-tissue forces exerted on the teeth; and 3) the influence of the neighboring teeth [30]. When one or more of these factors breaks down, malocclusion results. For example, subjects with systematic problems that interfere with the eruptive system have a less efficient dentoalveolar compensatory mechanism.

Teeth continue to move after they emerge and erupt into functional occlusion. The clinical importance of continuous eruption and migration that occur is often unappreciated; tooth movements play an important role in the development of malalignment. Superimposing on small metallic implants, Björk and Skieller [31] reported that the maxillary first molars erupt and migrate 1.1–2.2 mm/yr in girls 10–14 years of age; somewhat lesser amounts of incisor eruption/migration occur over the same period. Using naturally stable reference structures superimpositions, it has been shown that the maxillary first molars undergo approximately 1.2–1.5 mm/yr of vertical eruption and 0.4–0.6 mm/yr mesial migration between 10 and 15 years of age; the mandibular first molars show less eruption over the same period, averaging 0.6–0.8 mm/yr, and slightly more mesial migration (0.6–0.7 mm/yr) [32]. Between 6 and 12 years of age, the maxillary teeth drift anteriorly more than the mandibular teeth, but the mandibular teeth undergo greater anterior growth displacement [33]. Vertically, the maxillary incisors and molars erupt approximately 1 mm/yr (Figure 5.10); they are displaced inferiorly approximately 0.8–1.0 mm/yr. The mandibular teeth are displaced inferiorly 2.0–2.3 mm/yr and erupt 0.5–0.6 mm/yr.

The amount of eruption that occurs after the teeth achieve occlusal contact depends primarily on the amount of space created by the vertical growth displacement of the jaws. The mandible is usually displaced down more than the maxilla. Inferior growth displacements of the posterior mandible explain approximately 54% of the variation in lower molar eruption [34]. The greater the inferior displacement of the mandible, the greater the superior eruption of the molars. Importantly, inferior mandibular displacement and vertical molar eruption exhibit adolescent spurts at slightly different times, with displacement and eruption peaking at 11y 8m and 12y 1m, respectively. This substantiates the fact that eruption compensates for, or adapts to, the growth displacements.

Teeth move to fill spaces, created by growth, occlusal wear, interproximal wear, or tooth loss. Supraeruption is a normal compensatory response to offset occlusal attrition and maintain efficient mastication [35, 36]. Rhesus monkeys, both growing and nongrowing, with bite splints cemented to their posterior teeth showed significantly greater incisor supraeruption than control monkeys [37]. Similarly, interproximal wear produces broader contacts and greater mesial migration of the dentition. Mesial migration also occurs when there are extensive carious lesions and when teeth are lost prematurely [38]. The movements are compensating for the spaces that are created.

5.3 Class I malocclusion and the dental compensatory mechanism

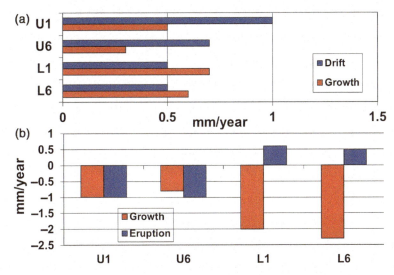

Figure 5.10 (a) Horizontal growth displacement and drift and (b) vertical growth displacement and eruption of the central incisors and first molars of males 6–12 years of age (Craig [33]/OAKTrust).

When space is created, teeth compensate by partially and spontaneously resolving crowding. When first premolars are extracted – and no other form of treatment is performed – in younger (10y 4m) and older (14y 2m) subjects, there were marked differences in the anterior compensations that occurred. The compensations depended on the amount of initial crowding [39]. In both groups, the canines drifted laterally and distally into the extraction sites. Irregularity in the younger group decreased from 5.5 to 3.3 mm; the older group showed greater compensations, with incisor irregularity decreasing from 8.3 to 4.2 mm. Similarly, the changes in arch dimensions that occur when patients are treated with lip bumpers also serve to partially resolve crowding. On average, approximately 3.5 mm spontaneous resolution of crowding occurs (Figure 5.11) with lip-bumper-only treatments.

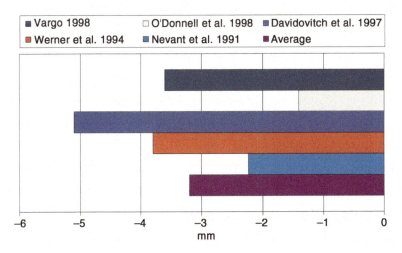

Figure 5.11 Improvements in anterior alignment when only lip bumper therapy is performed, as shown by Vargo et al. [70], O'Donnell et al. [71], Davidovitch et al. [72], Werner et al. [73], and Nevant et al. [74].

5.4 What is anterior mandibular malalignment is related to?

At the most basic levels, anterior mandibular malalignment is due to: 1) teeth erupting into abnormal positions due to the lack of space or space loss and 2) contact displacements due to relapse and unwanted tooth movements (Figure 5.12). The anterior teeth move out of alignment when contacts are broken. Teeth usually move mesially until a new equilibrium is established.

5.4.1 Predisposing factors

Several predisposing factors need to be considered to appreciate why and how malalignments occur (Figure 5.12). Among the most important for the malalignment of the anterior teeth are point-to-point interdental contacts. It simply stands to reason that broader surface contacts are more stable than point-to-point contacts. Simulated arches with teeth that have concave/convex contact surfaces have been shown to be considerably more stable than arches that have point-to-point contacts [40]. Importantly, the teeth located in the anterior, more curved, part of the simulated arches were the least stable. Contemporary populations exhibit thinner enamel on the mesial than distal surfaces of the molars and premolars [41], with the mesial surfaces tending to be more concave. This, along with their broader contacts and limited arch curvature, helps to explain why the alignment of the posterior teeth is more stable than the alignment of the anterior teeth. Broader contacts of the anterior teeth result in less crowding and irregularity. This explains why posttreatment irregularity changes were significantly less (≈ 1.4 mm) in patients who had anterior interproximal reductions at the end of retention than in patients who did not have enamel reductions [42].

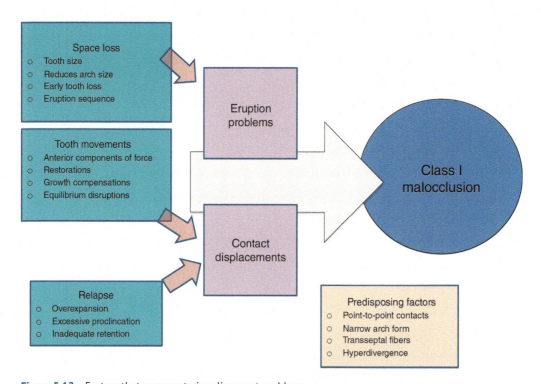

Figure 5.12 Factors that cause anterior alignment problems.

As previously suggested, the stability of point-to-point contacts depends, at least in part, on the shape of the arch. The risk of postretention crowding is greater in patients with narrower arch forms than in patients with broader arches [2]. Differences in mandibular arch shape explain why there is slightly, but significantly, more (0.8 mm) postretention irregularity in extraction patients than in nonextraction patients [2]. The difference was because extraction patients had narrower arch forms. Moreover, adjacent teeth that have smaller interdental angles are at greater risk of posttreatment crowding than teeth with larger interdental angles. The canine and lateral incisors have, as previously indicated, the greatest discrepancies between contact points posttreatment and the smallest interdental angles.

Due to their ability to move teeth, transseptal fibers play an important role in the development of crowding. The fibers extend from the cementum of one tooth, over the interdental bone, to the cementum of the adjacent tooth. Transseptal fibers, which link all of the teeth together, serve to maintain interdental contacts [43]. Their function is to keep the teeth together; transseptal fibers serve as a biological splint (i.e. nature's retainers). To maintain tooth contacts, the transseptal fibers must be able to move teeth and close spaces. Moss and Picton [44] showed that the transseptal fibers were responsible for moving the teeth after space is created. When the occlusal surfaces were ground out of occlusion, and the interproximal surfaces were ground to create interdental spaces, the teeth moved mesially to reestablish contact. The mesial drift of the teeth is due to the contractile mechanism of the transseptal ligament [45].

Finally, hyperdivergence also predisposes individuals to greater amounts of crowding. Goldberg et al. [46] showed that individuals with greater pretreatment mandibular plane angles, anterior-to-posterior facial height ratios, and anterior facial heights also had greater posttreatment increases in incisor irregularity and TSALD. Others have also established relationships between crowding and facial divergence [47, 48]. Increased divergence might be expected to increase the risk of malalignment due to associated 1) increases in lower incisor eruption [49, 50], 2) retroclination of the lower incisors, and 3) less bone and less dense bone surrounding the teeth.

5.4.2 Eruption problems associated with space loss

Although not as important as some believe, tooth size is related to crowding. The mesiodistal size of the incisors has been correlated to crowding [50]. Larger incisors are found among individuals with Class I malocclusion than among those with normal occlusion [51, 52]. Agenter et al. [53] showed that the crown dimensions (mesiodistal and buccolingual) of subjects with crowding are consistently larger than in subjects with normal occlusion. Importantly, the statistically significant associations reported by these studies have been consistently low, usually explaining less than 10% of the variation.

There have also been several studies that have linked arch size to crowding, with inverse relationships reported for arch width, arch depth, and arch perimeter [54, 55], suggesting that individuals with smaller arches have greater amounts of crowding. These associations should be interpreted with caution because, as previously emphasized, the teeth of individuals who exhibit crowding move mesially into a narrower part of the arch, which necessarily decreases arch dimensions. In other words, the relationship between jaw size and crowding should not be based on dental arch dimensions. However, this does not mean that there is no relationship between jaw size and crowding. Crowding has been related to maxillary apical base size but not to mandibular apical base size, and the relationship is weak [56]. Crowding and irregularities should be also expected if the basal arch form is too small to house the teeth. For example, maxillary synostosis seen in individuals with Apert and Crouzon syndromes results in smaller jaw size and causes substantial crowding and ectopic eruption of teeth.

Space loss and associated mesial tooth movements provide another explanation for early crowding. Early loss of leeway space before the permanent premolars and canines emerge can substantially increase the risk of crowding. It is generally thought that greater space will be lost with the premature loss of the second primary molar than with the premature loss of the other deciduous teeth [57]. Longitudinal evaluations of 6-to-12-year-old children show that severe caries or premature exfoliation of the deciduous molars result in substantial space loss over time [38]. In the mandible, early loss of the first and second primary molars results in 2.2 and 4.2 mm of space loss, respectively; 3.5 mm of space loss was reported for children who prematurely lost both the first and second primary molars. Space loss increased more or less regularly from 6 years of age to 12 years. In the maxilla, individuals who lost their second primary molars or both primary molars exhibited 2.9 and 3.9 mm of space loss at 12 years of age. The vast majority of the space loss was taken up by mesial migration of the posterior teeth. There also appears to be an association between the sequence of eruption and crowding. This occurs because the use of Leeway space depends in part on the posterior eruption sequence [58]. In the mandible, the canines usually erupt before the first premolars, and this is the favorable sequence. The most unfavorable eruption sequences in the mandible are those in which the premolars erupt before the canines or when the second molars erupt before the canines and premolars [59]. Recently, Lange [60] found substantially less crowding (≈2.5 mm) among untreated subjects who had left and right 345 eruption sequences, than among those who had left and right 435 eruption sequences.

5.4.3 Contact displacements associated with relapse and tooth movements

Teeth put in positions of disequilibrium will move and crowding often results. This is why increasing mandibular arch length during the mixed dentition to gain the space needed to resolve crowding results in unacceptable levels of relapse [61]. Treatment increases in intercanine width, especially in the permanent dentition, also put the teeth in disequilibrium. Patients with greater increases in intercanine width during treatment show greater posttreatment increases in crowding [46, 62].

Anteriorly directed forces on the teeth can cause contacts to slip and thereby contribute to malalignment. Due to their axial inclination, the posterior teeth tip forward during occlusal loading, producing an anterior component of biting force. When biting down on the posterior teeth, the anterior components of force decrease progressively from the posterior to the anterior teeth, even crossing to the other side of the arch [63]. Interestingly, the anterior component of biting force is greater in subjects with greater amounts of incisor irregularity, as demonstrated in both untreated subjects [64] and patients followed 3y 5m postretention [65]. This suggests that bone quality and quantity around the teeth are important mitigants of malalignments.

Anything that takes up arch space has the potential to move the teeth and cause the contacts to slip. For example, the teeth can be forced anteriorly by restorations, which dentists are taught to make "tight." This explains why orthodontic patients who received posttreatment interproximal restorations exhibit significantly greater increases in incisor irregularity and crowding than individuals who did not have restorations over the same 15y 6 m observation period [2].

While growth generally helps the orthodontist, it represents perhaps the most important risk factor for the development of crowding. The relationships between vertical growth, compensatory eruption, and malalignment were first established in a long-term follow-up study comparing 40 stable (incisor irregularity $\Delta < 1$ mm) to 33 unstable (incisor irregularity $\Delta > 2$ mm) Class I extraction patients [42]. While the anterior displacement of the mandible and mesial tooth movements did not differ between groups, the inferior displacement of the mandible and superior eruption of the mandibular incisors were both significantly greater in the unstable group. Facial height increases and associated lower incisor eruption were also both significantly related to the development of malaligned teeth in subjects who were followed 13y 7m years posttreatment as well as in untreated subjects followed between 14y 3m and 23y 2m [49]. This explains why growing adolescents are at significantly greater risk of posttreatment crowding than adults [66]. More recently, Goldberg et al. [46] again showed that greater vertical growth and greater incisor eruption were both related to greater posttreatment mandibular crowding. Greater amounts of vertical growth require greater eruption to compensate for the vertical space created, and eruption decreases the likelihood that the contacts between the anterior teeth will be maintained, thereby increasing the risk of crowding.

Finally, any disruptions of dentoalveolar equilibrium that cause movements of the teeth, which in turn cause contract displacements, might be expected to produce malalignments. Teeth move to compensate when the competing forces placed upon them change. Onlays as small as 2 mm cemented onto premolars can disrupt a tooth's equilibrium, causing movements similar to those produced by orthodontic appliances [29]. Any differential force, even if it is small, can cause tooth movements if it is applied over sufficiently long periods. Importantly, teeth can have more than one position of equilibrium. In addition to the intrinsic forces of the soft tissues, extrinsic forces (e.g. habits, orthodontic appliances, and so on), forces from dental occlusion, and forces from the periodontal membrane must also be considered to understand the changes in tooth position [67]. Teeth are genetically adapted to be able to move. An extensive review of dentoalveolar compensations and malalignments in treated and untreated cases was recently provided [68].

References

1. Harris EF, Vaden JL, Williams RA. Lower incisor space analysis: a contrast of methods. *Am J Orthod Dentofacial Orthop* 1987;**92**(5):375–80.
2. Myser SA, Campbell PM, Boley J, Buschang PH. Long-term stability: post-retention changes of the mandibular anterior teeth. *Am J Orthod Dentofacial Orthop* 2013;**144**(3):420–9.
3. Peck H, Peck S. An index for assessing tooth shape deviations as applied to the mandibular incisors. *Am J Orthod* 1972;**61**(4):384–401.
4. Staley RN, Shelly TH, Martin JF. Prediction of lower canine and premolar widths in the mixed dentition. *Am J Orthod* 1979;**76**(3):300–9.
5. Staley RN, Hu P, Hoag JF, Shelly TF. Prediction of the combined right and left canine and premolar widths in both arches of the mixed dentition. *Pediatr Dent* 1983;**5**(1):57–60.
6. Gardner RB. A comparison of four methods of predicting arch length. *Am J Orthod* 1979;**75**(4):387–98.
7. Hixon EH, Oldfather RE. Estimation of the sizes of unerupted cuspid and bicuspid teeth. *Angle Orthod* 1958;**28**(4):236–40.
8. Staley RN, Kerber PE. A revision of the Hixon and Oldfather mixed prediction method. *Am J Orthod* 1980;**78**(3):296–302.
9. Kelly JE, Sanchez M, Van Kirk LE. *An assessment of occlusion of teeth of children.* DHEW publication no 74-1612. Washington, DC: National Center for Health Statistics, 1973.

10 Proffit WR, Fields HW Jr, Moray LJ. Prevalence of malocclusion and orthodontic treatment need in the United States: estimates from the NHANES III survey. *Int J Adult Orthodon Orthognath Surg* 1998;**13**(2):97–106.

11 Foster TD, Hamilton MC, Lavelle CLB. A study of dental arch crowding in four age groups. *Dent Pract* 1972;**21**(1):9–12.

12 Moorrees CFA, Chadha JM. Available space for the incisors during dental development – A growth study based on physiologic age. *Angle Orthod* 1965;**35**(1):12–22.

13 Warren JJ, Bishara SE, Yonezu T. Tooth size-arch length relationships in the deciduous dentition: a comparison between contemporary and historical samples. *Am J Orthod Dentofacial Orthop* 2003;**123**(6):614–9.

14 Leighton BC. The early signs of malocclusion. *Eur J Orthod* 2007;**29**:i89–95.

15 Baume L. Physiological tooth migration and its significance for the development of occlusion, III. The biogenesis of the successional dentition. *J Dent Res* 1950;**29**(3):338–48.

16 Moorrees CFA. *The dentition of the growing child*. Cambridge, MA: Harvard University Press, 1959.

17 Thilander B. Dentoalveolar development in subjects with normal occlusion. A longitudinal study between the ages of 5 and 31 years. *Eur J Orthod* 2009;**31**(2):109–20.

18 Giles NB, Knott VB, Meredith HV. Increase in intraoral height of selected permanent teeth during the quadrennium following gingival emergence. *Angle Orthod* 1963;**33**(2):195–206.

19 Moyers RE, Van Der Linden FPGM, Riolo ML, McNamara JA. *Standards of human occlusal development*. Monograph #5. Craniofacial growth series. Ann Arbor, MI: Center for Human Growth and Development, The University of Michigan, 1976.

20 Sinclair PM, Little RM. Maturation of untreated normal occlusions. *Am J Orthod* 1983;**83**(2):114–23.

21 Lundy HJ, Richardson ME. Developmental changes in alignment of the lower labial segment. *Br J Orthod* 1995;**22**(4):339–45.

22 Bishara SE, Jakobsen JR, Treder JE, Stasi MJ. Changes in the maxillary and mandibular tooth size-arch length relationship from early adolescence to early adulthood. A longitudinal study. *Am J Orthod Dentofacial Orthop* 1989;**95**(1):46–59.

23 Bishara SE, Treder JE, Damon P, Olsen M. Changes in the dental arches and dentition between 25 and 45 years of age. *Angle Orthod* 1996;**66**(6):417–22.

24 Brunelle JA, Bhat M, Lipton JA. Prevalence and distribution of selected occlusal characteristics in the US population, 1988-1991. *J Dent Res* 1996;**75**(2 suppl): 706–13.

25 Asiri SN, Tadlock LP, Buschang PH. The prevalence of clinically meaningful malocclusion among US adults. *Orthod Craniofac Res* 2019;**22**(4):321–8.

26 Richardson ME. A review of changes in lower arch alignment from seven to fifty years. *Semin Orthod* 1999;**5**(3):151–9.

27 Driscoll-Gilliland J, Buschang PH, Behrents RG. An evaluation of growth and stability in untreated and treated subjects. *Am J Orthod Dentofacial Orthop* 2001;**120**(6):588–97.

28 Vaden JL, Harris EF, Gardner RI. Relapse revisited. *Am J Orthod Dentofacial Orthop* 1997;**111**(5):543–53.

29 Weinstein S, Haack DC, Morris LY, et al. On an equilibrium theory of tooth position. *Angle Orthod* 1963;**33**(1):1–26.

30 Solow B. The dentoalveolar compensatory mechanism: background and clinical implications. *Br J Orthod* 1980;**7**(3):145–61.

31 Björk A, Skieller V. Growth of the maxillary in three dimensions as revealed radiographically by the implant methods. *Br J Orthod* 1977;**4**(2):53–64.

32 McWhorter K. A longitudinal study of horizontal and vertical tooth movements during adolescence (ages 10 to 15). Master's Thesis, Baylor University, 1992.

33. Craig R. Posteruptive tooth movement during childhood. Master's Thesis, Baylor University, 1995.
34. Liu SS, Buschang PH. How does tooth eruption relate to vertical mandibular growth displacement? *Am J Orthod Dentofacial Orthop* 2011;**139**(6):745–51.
35. Sicher H. The biology of attrition. *Oral Surg Oral Med Oral Pathol* 1953;**6**(3):406–12.
36. Weinmann JP, Sicher H. *Bone and bones*. 2nd edn. St Louis, MO: Mosby, 1955.
37. Schneiderman ED. A longitudinal cephalometric study of incisor supra-eruption in young and adult rhesus monkeys (*Macaca mulatta*). *Arch Oral Biol* 1989;**34**(2):137–41.
38. Northway W, Wainright RL, Demirjian A. Effects of premature loss of deciduous molars. *Angle Orthod* 1984;**54**(4):295–329.
39. Papandreas SG, Buschang PH, Alexander RG, et al. Physiological drift of the mandibular dentition following first premolar extractions. *Angle Orthod* 1993;**63**(2):127–34.
40. Ihlow D, Kubein-Meesenburg D, Fanghänel J, et al. Biomechanics of the dental arch and incisal crowding. *J Orofac Orthop* 2004;**65**(1):5–12.
41. Stroud JL, English J, Buschang PH. Enamel thickness of the posterior dentition: its implications for nonextraction treatment. *Angle Orthod* 1998;**68**(2):141–6.
42. Alexander JM. A comparative study of orthodontic stability in Class I extraction cases. Master's Thesis, Baylor University, 1996.
43. Stubley R. The influence of transseptal fibers on incisor position and diastema formation. *Am J Orthod* 1976;**70**(6):645–62.
44. Moss JP, Picton DC. Short-term changes in the mesiodistal position of teeth following removal of approximal contacts in the monkey *Macaca fascicularis*. *Arch Oral Biol* 1982;**27**(3):273–8.
45. Nanci A. *Ten Cate's oral histology: development, structure and function*. 7th edn. St Louis, MO: Elsevier, Mosby, 2007, p. 275. 2008.
46. Goldberg AI, Behrents RG, Oliver DR, Buschang PH. Facial divergence and mandibular crowding in treated subjects. *Angle Orthod* 2013;**83**(3):381–8.
47. Leighton BC, Hunter WS. Relationship between lower arch spacing/crowding and facial height and depth. *Am J Orthod* 1982;**82**(5):418–25.
48. Richardson ME. Late lower arch crowding. The role of facial morphology. *Angle Orthod* 1986;**56**(3):244–54.
49. Bondevik O. Changes in occlusion between 23 and 34 years. *Angle Orthod* 1998;**68**(1):75–80.
50. Fastlicht J. Crowding of mandibular incisors. *Am J Orthod* 1970;**58**(2):156–63.
51. Norderval K, Wisth PJ, Böe OE. Mandibular anterior crowding in relation to tooth size and craniofacial morphology. *Scand J Dent Res* 1975;**83**(5):267–73.
52. Doris JM, Bernard BW, Kuftinec MM, Stom D. A biometric study of tooth size and dental crowding. *Am J Orthod* 1981;**79**(3):326–36.
53. Agenter MK, Harris EF, Blair RN. Influence of tooth crown size on malocclusion. *Am J Orthod Dentofacial Orthod* 2009;**136**(6):795–804.
54. Sampson WJ, Richards LC. Prediction of mandibular incisor and canine crowding changes in the mixed dentition. *Am J Orthod* 1985;**88**(1):47–63.
55. Howe RP, McNamara JA Jr, O'Connor KA. An examination of dental crowding and its relationship to tooth size and arch dimension. *Am J Orthod* 1983;**83**(5):363–73.
56. Crossley AM, Campbell PM, Tadlock LP, et al. Is there a relationship between dental crowding and the size and the maxillary and mandibular apical base? *Angle Orthod* 2020;**90**(2):216–23.
57. Hinrichsen CFL. Space maintenance in pedodontics. *Aust Dent* 1962;**7**(6):451–6.
58. Moorrees CF, Gron AM, Lebret LM, et al. Growth studies of the dentition: a review. *Am J Orthod* 1969;**55**(6):600–16.
59. Lo R, Moyers RE. Studies in the etiology and prevention of malocclusion: I. The sequence

of eruption of the permanent dentition. *Am J Orthod* 1953;**39**(6):460–7.
60 Lange GM. Correlations of sequence of eruption and crowding. Saint Louis University Master's Thesis, St. Louis, MO, 2011.
61 Little RM, Riedel RA, Stein A. Mandibular arch length increase during the mixed dentition: postretention evaluation of stability and relapse. *Am J Orthod Dentofacial Orthop* 1990;**97**(5):393–404.
62 Årtun J, Garol JD, Little RM. Long-term stability of mandibular incisors following successful treatment of Class II, Division 1, malocclusion. *Angle Orthod* 1996;**66**(3):229–38.
63 Southard TE, Behrents RG, Tolley EA. The anterior component of occlusal force. Part 1. Measurement and distribution. *Am J Orthod Dentofacial Orthop* 1989;**96**(6):493–500.
64 Southard TE, Behrents RG, Tolley EA. The anterior component of occlusal force. Part 2. Relationship with dental malalignment. *Am J Orthod Dentofacial Orthop* 1990;**97**(1):41–4.
65 Acar A, Alcan T, Erverdi N. Evaluation of the relationship between the anterior component of occlusal force and post-retention crowding. *Am J Orthod Dentofacial Orthop* 2002;**122**(4):366–70.
66 Park H, Boley JC, Alexander RA, Buschang PH. Age-related long-term post-treatment occlusal and arch changes. *Angle Orthod* 2010;**80**(2):247–53.
67 Proffit WR. Equilibrium theory revisited: factors influencing position of the teeth. *Angle Orthod* 1978;**48**(3):175–86.
68 Buschang PH. Class I malocclusion – The development and etiology of mandibular malalignments. *Semin Orthod* 2014;**20**(1):3–15.
69 Eveleth PB, Tanner JM. *Worldwide variation in human growth*. 2nd edn. Cambridge: Cambridge University Press, 1990.
70 Vargo J, Buschang PH, Boley J, et al. Treatment effects and short-term relapse of maxillomandibular expansion during the early to mid mixed dentition. *Am J Orthod Dentofacial Orthop* 2007;**131**(4):456–63.
71 O'Donnell S, Nanda RS, Ghosh J. Perioral forces and dental changes resulting from mandibular lip bumper treatment. *Am J Orthod Dentofacial Orthop* 1998;**113**(3):247–55.
72 Davidovitch M, McInnis D, Lindauer SJ. The effects of lip bumper therapy in the mixed dentition. *Am J Orthod Dentofacial Orthop* 1997;**111**(1):52–8.
73 Werner SP, Shivapuja PK, Harris EF. Skeletodental changes in the adolescent accruing from use of the lip bumper. *Angle Orthod* 1994;**64**(1):13–22.
74 Nevant CT, Buschang PH, Alexander RG, Steffen JM. Lip bumper therapy for gaining arch length. *Am J Orthod Dentofacial Orthop* 1991;**100**(4):30–6.

5.2

Section II: Intercepting developing Class I problems
Eustáquio A. Araújo, DDS, MDS

Center for Advanced Dental Education, Saint Louis University, St. Louis, MO, USA

In the first section of this chapter, Peter Buschang presented a thorough review of the development and etiology of the Class I malocclusion. A systematic revision of the development of the occlusion is also presented in Chapter 2.

Although individuals with Class I malocclusion have normal molar relationships, many other abnormalities can be found. For didactic purposes, we will classify them as *intraarch* and *interarch* deviations, to describe problems within the arches and between the arches, respectively.

Among the intraarch deviations, we highlight space issues (spacing and crowding), rotations, malposed teeth, tooth formation anomalies, number of teeth, impactions, and alterations in the curve of Spee. In Chapter 8, a description of possible intraarch eruption deviations is presented and documented.

As for the interarch deviations, we subdivide the definitions into three dimensions: anteroposterior, transverse, and vertical. In Class I malocclusions, anteroposterior deviation may include an anterior dental crossbite (Figure 5.13).

The most common interarch deviation in Class I is related to the transverse dimension, as unilateral or bilateral crossbites are frequently detected (Figure 5.14).

In the vertical dimension, it is also common to find open bites normally associated with a tongue thrust or deleterious habits (see Chapter 8). Deep bites, although not so frequently found, are also possible. Figure 5.15 illustrates vertical deviations.

5.5 Tooth size arch length discrepancy (TSALD)

The primary clinical concern is the malalignment of the teeth, particularly when related to the anterior teeth. This chapter will concentrate on the management of arch development.

Besides all the variables presented in the previous section by Peter Buschang, other facts must be remembered: growth is not capable of contributing with a great increase in the perimeter of the arches [1, 2]; the "leeway space or E space" – if not kept – will naturally decrease arch perimeter [3, 4]; although transverse increase in the dental arches occur after the transition of the incisors it does not account for a major natural gain [5–7]; the mandibular incisors tend to upright during adolescence due to the differential growth of the maxilla and mandible [8]; a continuous mesial drifting of teeth occurs throughout life [9, 10]. The natural adjustment of the Class I relationship happens through a combination of the early mesial shift, the late mesial shift, and growth [11].

Recognizing and Correcting Developing Malocclusions: A Problem-Oriented Approach to Orthodontics, Second Edition. Edited by Eustáquio A. Araújo and Peter H. Buschang.
© 2025 John Wiley & Sons, Inc. Published 2025 by John Wiley & Sons, Inc.

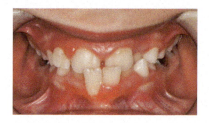

Figure 5.13 Anterior crossbite affecting the mandibular anterior arch and its periodontal health.

5.6 The assessment of crowding in the mixed dentition

The hybrid composition of a mixed dentition, with permanent and deciduous teeth in the dental arches at the same moment, implicates assessing tooth size arch length discrepancy (TSALD) through prediction equations and/or radiographic formulas. The most common analyses are Nance [4], Tanaka–Johnston [12], Moyers [13], and Hixon–Oldfather [14]. A study comparing the four concluded that the Hixon–Oldfather would be the most accurate one [13]. However, because of its simplicity, the Tanaka–Johnston analysis seems to be the most frequently used. The formulae for the maxillary and mandibular arch are, respectively:

$$\sum \frac{\overline{2,1|1,2}}{2} + 11 = \emptyset \overline{3,4,5}$$

$$\sum \frac{\overline{2,1|1,2}}{2} + 10.5 = \emptyset \overline{3,4,5}$$

With those principles in mind, our text will classify and study TSALD in three categories: zero to minor, small to moderate, and severe.

5.6.1 Zero to minor TSALD

Even when the irregularity is close to zero, monitoring the development of the occlusion is recommended. Some small irregularities normally found in the transition of the deciduous to mixed and permanent dentitions are considered normal. Some events that occur during this transition must be closely

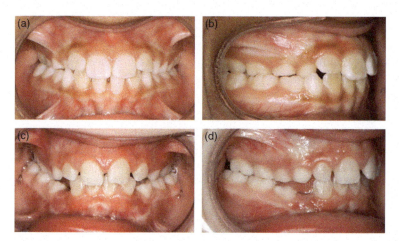

Figure 5.14 (a, b) Unilateral crossbite in the mixed dentition. Notice that the mandibular midline is slightly shifted to the right, indicating a possible functional shift. (c, d) Bilateral posterior crossbite.

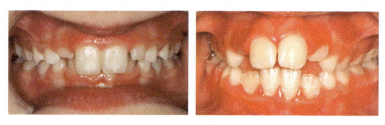

Figure 5.15 Severe dental deep bite on the left and developing dental open bite on the right.

monitored and in case of any suspicious space loss the clinician must interfere.

Unwanted mesial tooth migration may take place and it can be associated with early loss of deciduous molars and/or with severe caries. Another possibility of reducing arch length (AL) and perimeter is related to the early loss of mandibular canines. A retro-inclination or uprighting of the mandibular incisors is likely to occur as previously reported [14–16].

The use of a lower lingual holding appliance (LLHA) is the safest way to preserve and control mandibular spaces [17–20] as demonstrated in Figure 5.16.

For the maxilla, a Nance button or a transpalatal arch are frequently recommended to preserve the space generated from the leeway space as well as maintain space after an untimely loss of deciduous molars and/or extensive caries as shown in Figure 5.17 [17, 21].

5.6.2 Small to moderate TSALD

5.6.2.1 Taking advantage of the transitional dentition

During the transition between the primary and the permanent dentition, many changes occur in the dental arches. It is important to highlight the fact that the amount of change within the arches is directly correlated to the type of the deciduous dentition as classified by Baume [22, 23] with skeletal growth also playing a role as presented by Tsourakis [11].

The adjustment of the occlusion, from deciduous to permanent, can be explained by an early mesial shift, a late mesial shift, and some skeletal growth.

The deciduous dentition was classified by Baume as Type I, with interdental spaces, and Type II, without interdental spaces. One may also refer to them as "open" and "closed" dentition, respectively. Baume's Type I and Type II are shown in Figure 5.18.

In patients with a spaced primary dentition, Type I, and a straight terminal plane, with the eruption of the permanent mandibular first molars at approximately 6 years of age, the primary molars move mesially, closing the space distal to the primary cuspids, converting the straight terminal plane to a mesial step relationship, reducing AL (arch length) in the mandibular dentition, and allowing the establishment of a Class I molar relationship. This is referred to as the "early mesial shift" (Figure 5.19) [22, 23].

In patients with a closed primary dentition, Type II, and a straight terminal plane, the

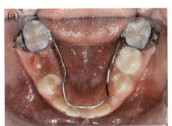
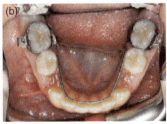
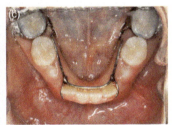

Figure 5.16 (a) A straight lower lingual holding arch (LLHA), (b) a LLHA with adjustment loops, and (c) soldered spurs to hold the incisors together.

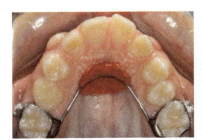
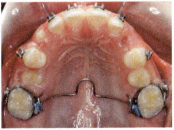

Figure 5.17 Left a Nance button and on the right a removable TPA.

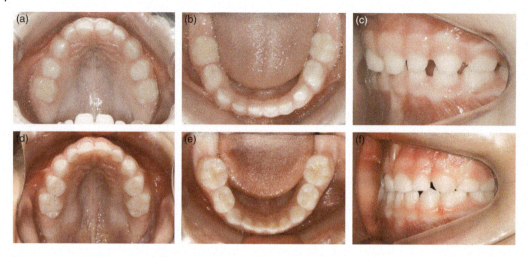

Figure 5.18 (a–c) Type I, open dentition and bottom. (d–f) Type II, closed dentition.

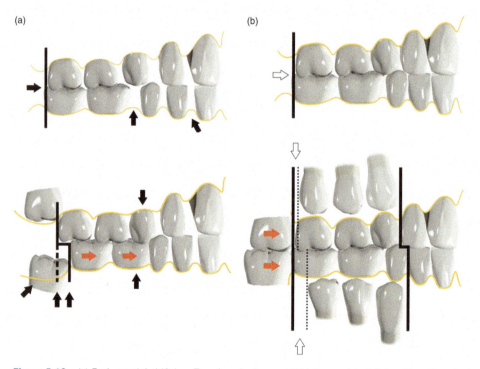

Figure 5.19 (a) Early mesial shift in a Type I occlusion and (b) late mesial shift in a Type II occlusion (Dale [24]/JPO, Inc.).

permanent maxillary and mandibular first molars emerge into a cusp-to-cusp relationship simply because there are no spaces to be closed. The Class I relationship is obtained when the primary second molars are exfoliated, and the first mandibular molars migrate mesially into the space provided by the difference in the mesiodistal dimensions of the deciduous second molars and the permanent second bicuspid known as the leeway space or E-space. This, again, reduces AL, converts the straight terminal plane to a mesial step, and provides for a Class I relationship of the permanent first molars. This has been referred to as the "late mesial shift" [22, 23] (Figure 5.19).

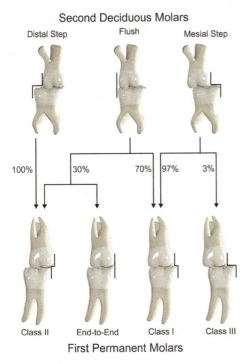

Figure 5.20 Possible adjustments from deciduous to mixed dentition (Arya et al. [25]/with permission of Elsevier).

The terminal plane, dictated by the distal relationship of the second maxillary and mandibular molars, determines tendencies and suggests possible future permanent molar relationships. The terminal planes that can be observed are flush, distal, and mesial, as illustrated in Figure 5.20, which represents the possible occlusal adjustments from deciduous to permanent dentition as described by Arya et al. [25].

5.6.3 Gaining spaces in the dental arches

5.6.3.1 The importance of the leeway space/E space

It is important, at this point, to open a parenthesis to describe the importance of the leeway space/E space. According to Gianelly, a well-done space control – along with growth changes – provides adequate space to resolve a considerable number of Class I crowded cases [18]. The author is responsible for the terminology "E" space considering his findings that the difference between mandibular C + D and 3 + 4 is basically zero. Thus, the difference – leeway space – relates only to the difference between mandibular E and 5.

Going back in history, in the 18th century, more precisely in 1771, a Scottish anatomist John Hunter, in his text *Natural History of the Human Teeth*, provided a view of the changes in dentition [26]. Without referring to the dimensional changes between the deciduous posterior teeth and their succedanea as "the leeway space," the author was able to precisely express it in a vivid illustration (Figure 5.21a).

One topic of interest that has been studied extensively in the orthodontic community is the benefit of excess space present during the mixed dentition due to a difference in size of the primary mandibular second molar and its successor, the permanent mandibular second premolar. Accurate estimation of this "E" space can give insight to the difference between the space available in the primary dentition and the space needed in the permanent dentition for proper alignment of teeth into the arches.

In master thesis projects at Saint Louis University, Lee [27] attempted to compare the mesial-distal size of the mandibular Es and compare them with mandibular second premolars. The study aimed to evaluate possible differences in the three malocclusion groups. Although the conclusion was that no significant differences were present when comparing the proportion of the Es and the 5s, in different malocclusions, a mathematical formula was created and later tested by Allbritton [28].

$P2 = 0.478(E) + 2.492$

$P2$ = mediodistal width of mandibular permanent second premolar

E = mesiodistal width of mandibular primary second molar

Assuming the mesiodistal size of the E as 10 mm, and applying the formula, the mesiodistal size of the 5 can be found: $P2 = (0.478 \times 10\,\text{mm}) = 4.78 + 2.49 = 7.272$.

Knowing ahead of time the mesiodistal sizes of the E and predicting the size of the 5, the amount of the E space can be found and added to our diagnosis [10 mm − 7.272 = 2.728]. It implies that the E space conservatively can be calculated as approximately 25% of the

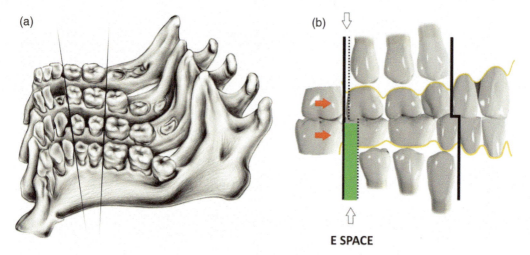

Figure 5.21 (a) Representation of the changes of dentition from deciduous to permanent now known as the leeway or the E-space (Hunter [26]/J. Johnson/Public Domain). (b) Proportion of the leeway space compared to the M-D size of the mandibular second deciduous molars.

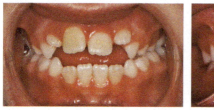 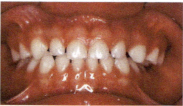

Figure 5.22 Lingual (left) and buccal (right) crossbites.

mesiodistal distance of the mandibular "*E*." Figure 5.21b.

5.6.3.2 Etiology of maxillary transverse deficiency

Maxillary constriction can stem from genetics, developmental, environmental, and even iatrogenic factors [29, 30]. Developmental issues such as mouth breathing, which can be the result of a compromised airway, or habits such as digit sucking, which can shape the maxillary arch in a manner contrary to the normally expected one. The changes in the maxillary transverse dimension may initiate a series of events leading to a high palatal vault and/or an anterior open bite, as shown in Figures 5.14 and 5.15.

In a normal occlusion, the lower dentition is expected to be capped by the upper dentition. It is important to note that in some instances, the dental arches may also be somewhat constricted but not necessarily in crossbite. Lingual crossbite is the term used when the lower teeth are outside the upper teeth upon biting. Unilateral crossbites are more prevalent than bilateral [31]. When the mandibular buccal segments fall inside the maxillary arch, unilaterally, or bilaterally, it is defined as a buccal crossbite, also known as the Brodie Syndrome. Figures 5.15 and 5.22 demonstrates examples of lingual and buccal crossbites.

Posterior crossbites may develop when there is a narrowing of the maxillary arch, premature contacts on closing – normally the deciduous canines – resulting in a shift of the mandible to the side and occasionally forward. It will typically yield a lingual crossbite on the side of the shift, and apparent normal occlusion on the other side. Profit points out that the condyle is not seated on the "normal side" [32]. This situation demands maxillary dental and/or skeletal expansion, but if it is not corrected, the jaws may grow to accommodate the shift. A differential diagnosis must be made to identify if it is a skeletal, dental, or functional crossbite.

Environmental factors can also be the cause of maxillary constriction. Changes in breathing patterns can cause crossbites in the posterior teeth, as reported in animal studies [33]. Patients with severe allergies or respiratory problems may also develop a constricted, V-shaped maxillary arch [34]. The most accepted explanation for maxillary transverse deficiency, however, is multifactorial, consisting of skeletal, dentoalveolar, environmental, and functional aspects each playing a role [25, 30, 33].

5.6.3.3 Maxillary expansion and headgear

When a reduction in the maxillary transverse dimension is observed, with or without a crossbite being diagnosed, a common way to intervene and correct this discrepancy is the use of maxillary expansion. The procedure can be done with either fixed or removable appliances. As mentioned in Chapter 2, the maturity, compliance, and behavior of the young patients must be assessed in order to select the proper way to approach the problem. When necessary, the use of headgears not only helps in the adjustment of the anteroposterior relationships but they also have a major impact on the transverse dimension outcome.

Much research has been done on the topic of maxillary expansion over the years. One of the milestone papers on expansion was written by Haas in 1961, as he reintroduced the treatment into orthodontics. Maxillary expansion had been discredited in the early to mid-1900s. Haas found that dental and skeletal changes were associated with maxillary expansion, including widening of the nose and opening of the bite as the mandible rotated down and back [35, 36]. Compilations of papers discussing expansion therapy have been arranged to produce a meta-analysis of the immediate effects of rapid maxillary expansion. It has been reported that transverse changes are mostly caused by dental tipping/expansion rather than true skeletal expansion, and that vertical and A-P changes associated with expansion are mostly transitory [37–39]. Skeletal expansion shows to be more stable when done at an earlier age. As for the slow versus rapid expansion, the literature still lacks the evidence of the advantages and disadvantages related to each of the procedures. There is little evidence-based literature endorsing rapid expansion over slow expansion or vice versa [32, 37].

In the 1960s, rapid expansion was recommended because orthodontists thought that rapid separation of the suture would lead to greater skeletal changes. Over time, however, the skeletal change relapses and dental movement amounts to 50% of the transverse dimension change. With slow expansion, the change is gradual. The dental and skeletal changes are achieved at about the same rate. With slow expansion, skeletal changes are slower at first, but after 10 weeks of treatment, the slow and rapid methods are comparable in dental and skeletal effects [32, 35, 36].

In conclusion, unless there is a great need to accelerate the treatment outcome, a slow to moderate rate of expansion of the maxillary arch is recommended during the late deciduous dentition and/or mixed dentition. A quarter of a millimeter of expansion a day is adequate to obtain stable and consistent results. In younger patients – deciduous dentition – we recommend the activation every other day. More important than the expansion is the length of time for which the clinician must stabilize the expander for a secure retention. Our protocol calls for at least 16 weeks of retention. When possible we recommend up to 6 months of stabilization.

Patient 1
This case report describes the orthodontic management of moderately crowded arches in a Class I developing occlusion with an excellent facial balance. The family reported concerns from the general dentist that crowding was an issue, and this 10-year-old boy

was brought to our clinic for evaluation. After all records were evaluated, it was decided to place a Nance button in the maxillary arch and a lower lingual holding arch in the mandible. The patient was put on observation, and 2 years later, the Class I occlusion was normal, perhaps requiring minimum if any intervention (Figures 5.23–5.25).

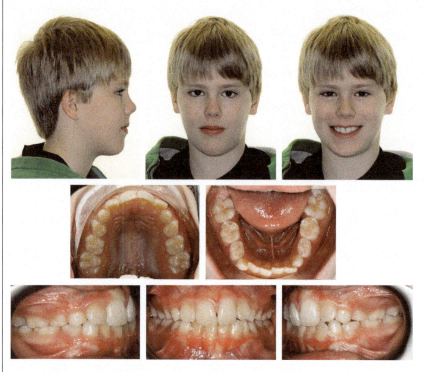

Figure 5.23 Patient One Initial Records.

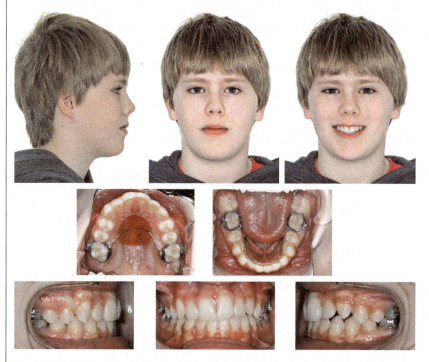

Figure 5.24 Nance Button and Lower Lingual Holding Arch.

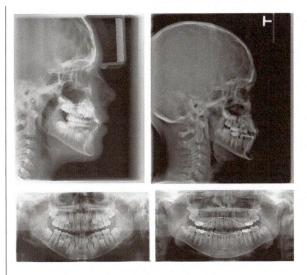

	Norms	Pre	Post
SNA	82	82.9	84.0
SNB	80	80.4	81.5
ANB	2	2.5	2.5
WITS	−1.0	−2.1	−4.9
FMA	25	29.9	28.3
SN-GoGn	32	35.1	29.5
U1-SN	105	106.0	100.7
IMPA	95	84.8	83.6

Figure 5.25 Patient One Initial and Final Records.

Patient 2

This 9-year-old girl was brought to our clinic for evaluation as the family was concerned about the difference between the right and left sides of the maxillary arch (Figure 5.26). A simple Hawley appliance with an expansion screw and a finger spring was placed to correct

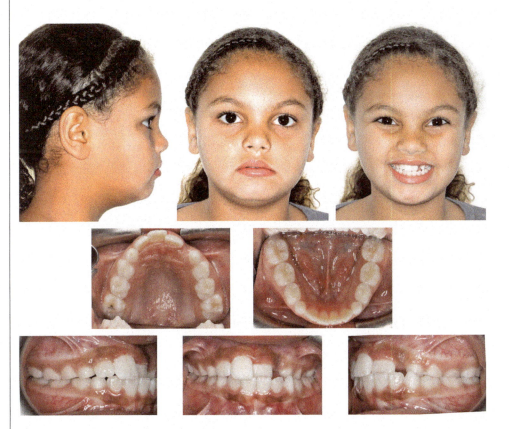

Figure 5.26 Patient Two Initial Records.

the maxillary left central in crossbite. The appliance was transversely expanded twice a week and the finger spring activated at the appointments. The procedure was successful, but the maxillary left lateral also erupted in crossbite. A two-by-four was placed, and the correction took place in a short amount of time (Figure 5.27). The total treatment was around 12 months. Figure 5.28 shows the patient cephalometric data and panoramic X-rays.

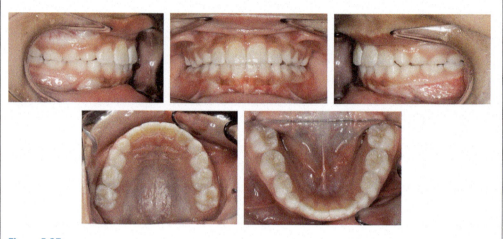

Figure 5.27

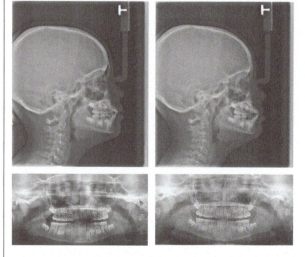

	Norms	Pre	Post
SNA	82	77.7	84.7
SNB	80	778.1	81.1
ANB	2	−0.4	3.6
WITS	−1.0	−2.0	0.5
FMA	25	9.9	10.9
SN-GoGn	32	24.4	21.8
U1-SN	105	112.0	117.2
IMPA	95	105.2	104.3

Figure 5.28

5.6 The assessment of crowding in the mixed dentition

Patient 3

This 8y 2m boy was referred to our clinic for the evaluation of his anterior crossbite (Figure 5.29). Initially, it was believed that he would be developing a Class III malocclusion. After thorough evaluation, including family history and functional diagnosis [centric relation (CR)] vs. centric occlusion (CO)] as described in Chapter 7, the patient initiated his treatment with a rapid maxillary expander (RME) and a face mask (Figure 5.30). The anterior crossbite was rapidly corrected and the face mask was interrupted after

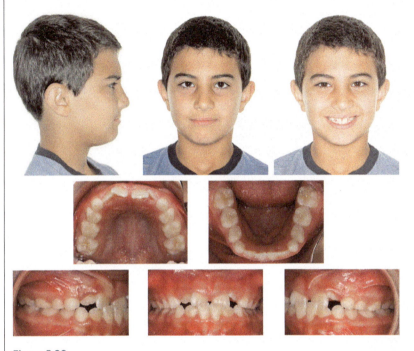

Figure 5.29

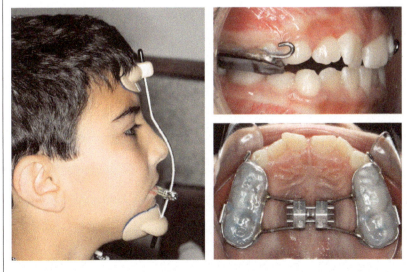

Figure 5.30

three months. A two-by-four was placed to align the teeth and the expander was removed (Figure 5.31). At the age of 9, the patient was put in retention and observation. The occlusion is developing well and will be reevaluated for the necessity or not of a phase II. The cephalometric data can be seen in Figure 5.32 and the retention observation in Figure 5.33.

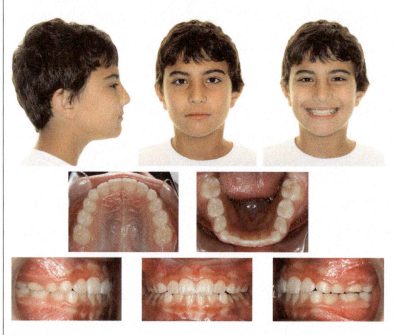

Figure 5.31

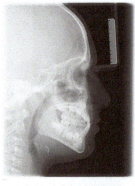

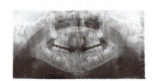

	Norms	Pre	Post
SNA	82	79.4	82.2
SNB	80	78.1	78.6
ANB	2	1.3	3.6
WITS	−1.0	−1.6	0.1
FMA	25	28.3	30.9
SN-GoGn	32	30.7	31.0
U1-SN	105	102.1	103.7
IMPA	95	93.1	87.8

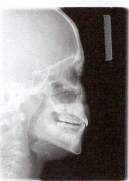

Figure 5.32

5.6 The assessment of crowding in the mixed dentition | 79

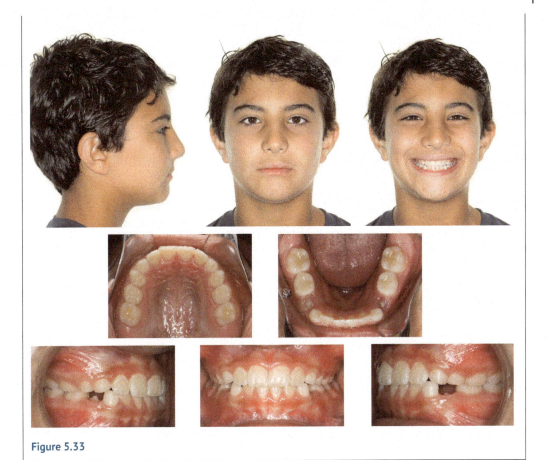

Figure 5.33

Patient 4

This 9-year-old girl presented with a unilateral crossbite (Figure 5.34). A mini expander was recommended and placed, following the protocol of one turn of activation a day (Figure 5.35). After the expansion and correction of the crossbite, the patient was given a rest period of 6 weeks, time required for the midpalatal suture to restructure. The expander was left in place for approximately 16–20 weeks. Six weeks after the interruption of the maxillary expansion, a two-by-four was placed, and the alignment of the incisors took place in a short amount of time (Figure 5.36). The illustrations on Figures 5.37 show the final outcome of phase I and the retainer recommended for mixed dentition patients. The data is presented on Figure 5.38.

5.2 Section II: Intercepting developing Class I problems

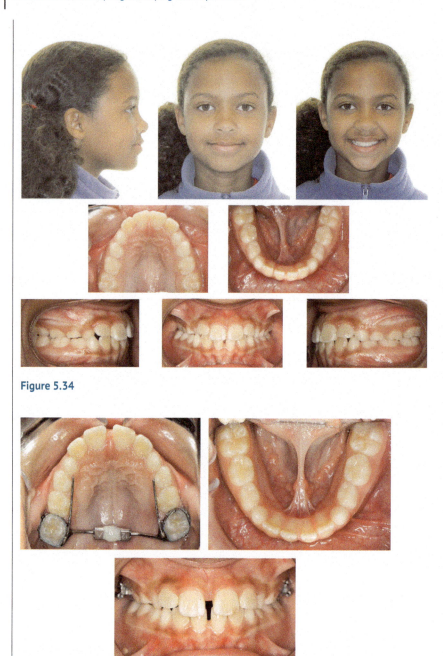

Figure 5.34

Figure 5.35

5.6 The assessment of crowding in the mixed dentition | 81

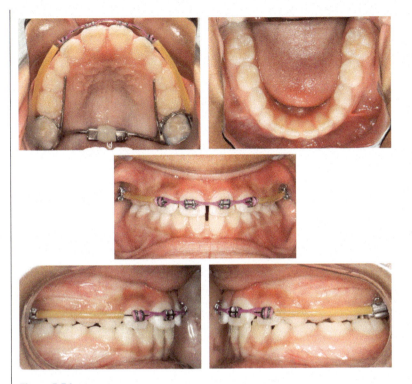

Figure 5.36

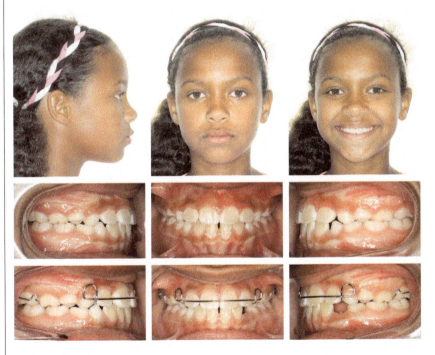

Figure 5.37

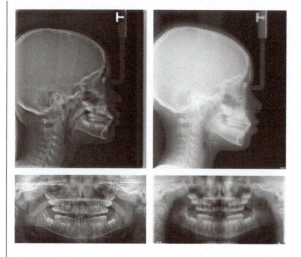

	Norms	Pre	Post
SNA	82	81.9	80.8
SNB	80	79.0	76.9
ANB	2	2.9	4.0
WITS	−1.0	−1.9	−1.0
FMA	25	22.0	21.5
SN-GoGn	32	30.7	32.9
U1-SN	105	11.4	107.0
IMPA	95	92.9	96.0

Figure 5.38

Patient 5

This 9-year-old boy presented with a unilateral functional crossbite (Figure 5.39). CO and CR bites are shown in Figures 5.39e and 5.39g. After the maxillary expansion was completed, he was placed in observation. There was minimum intervention and a positive result. The final images are shown in Figure 5.40.

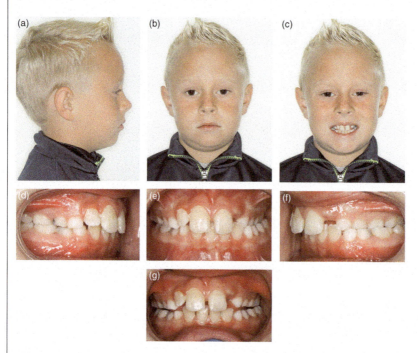

Figure 5.39

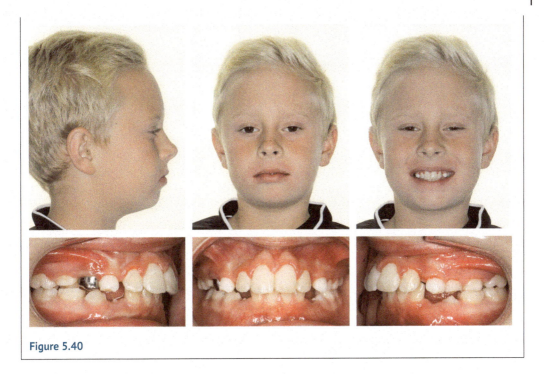

Figure 5.40

5.6.3.4 Gaining space in the mandibular arch

Gaining space in the mandibular arch during the transitional dentition can be done transversely or by anteroposterior expansion. In the transverse dimension, the lip bumper has been accepted as an appliance capable of providing stable results [40]. The concept behind this appliance is that by keeping the musculature of the lower lip and cheeks away from the mandibular teeth, the equilibrium between the external and internal musculature pressure is broken and the tongue is able to expand the mandibular arch. Also, the pressure of the lower lip against the lip bumper during swallowing is transmitted directly to the lower molars [41], which results in a slight distalization and distal tipping of the molars leading to an increase in AL (Figure 5.41).

The lip bumper can be positioned at different levels in relation to the incisor crowns – at the incisal third, middle third or gingival third of the incisor crowns [42]. If placed at the incisal third, the lower lip will lift the lip bumper, creating an uprighting force at the molars. When placed in the middle third, depending on the desired effect, the lip is kept away from

Figure 5.41 Biomechanics of the lip bumper.

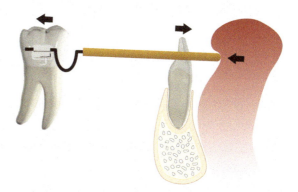

the incisors allowing them to translate labially. When placed at the gingival third or low in the vestibule, the lip goes over the bumper contacting the incisors and minimizing incisor movement [42, 43].

In one of the early studies on the effect of the lip bumper, it was used in patients who had strong mentalis habits in order to keep the lower lip away from the teeth. As a side effect, it was noticed that AL in these patients increased. This observation led to a study of 25 patients utilizing cephalometrics, and the conclusion was that the increase in AL could be attributed to the distal movement and uprighting of the molars more so than the labial movement of the incisors. It was also observed that, when effective, the mandibular arch usually leveled off well [41].

5.6.3.5 Arch dimensions changes

Lip bumpers are able to produce significant changes in arch dimensions. There is ample evidence of these changes in the literature, both in research and in the review of the literature [40]. Figures 5.41–5.44 bring together some of the most important studies and their results. These studies are considered important contributions to the orthodontic literature [44–54].

5.6.3.6 Arch length and mandibular molar/MP

The effect of lip bumper therapy on AL and mandibular first molar in relation to the mandibular plane – L6/MP can be seen in Figure 5.42.

5.6.3.7 Arch length and mandibular incisors/MP

The effect of lip bumper therapy on AL and mandibular incisors in relation to the mandibular plane (IMPA) can be seen in Figure 5.43.

5.6.3.8 Transverse changes

The effect of lip bumper therapy on transverse arch dimensions at the intercanine and intermolar levels can be seen in Figure 5.44.

5.6.3.9 Incisor irregularity changes

Figure 5.45 shows changes in mandibular incisors irregularity following lip bumper therapy. These changes are due to the increase in the transverse dimension as well as the relationship of the mandibular molars and incisors to the mandibular plane.

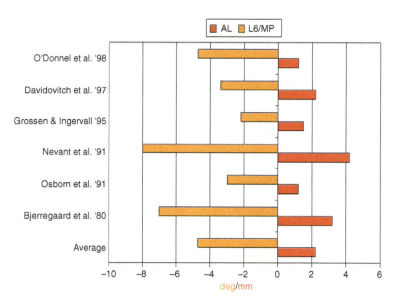

Figure 5.42 Effect of the lip bumper on arch length and mandibular molar in relation to the mandibular plane.

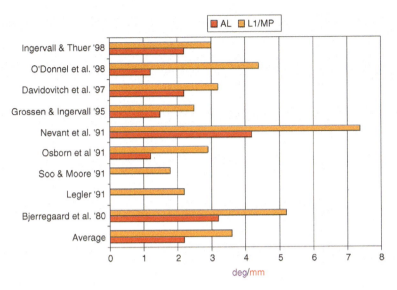

Figure 5.43 Effect of lip bumper therapy on arch length and mandibular incisors in relation to the mandibular plane.

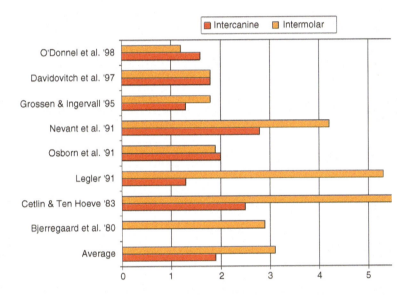

Figure 5.44 The effect of lip bumper therapy on transverse arch dimensions at the intercanine and intermolar levels.

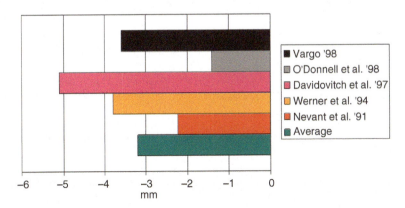

Figure 5.45 The effect of lip bumper therapy on the irregularity index.

5.6.3.10 The Schwarz appliance

Another popular appliance to improve maxillary and mandibular arch development is the Schwarz appliance [55–59]. This mandibular appliance has been used, and it is intended to improve transverse dental expansion. It is constructed with an activation screw and in general is fabricated with posterior clasps and no labial bow. If additional retention is necessary, a labial bow may be added although it will possibly inhibit the response of the incisors to transverse activation. Although it may be considered an effective therapy, expansion with the Schwarz appliance requires good compliance (Figure 5.46).

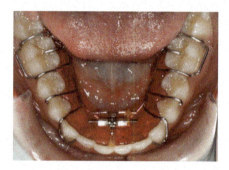

Figure 5.46 The Schwarz appliance.

5.6.3.11 Two-by-four fixed therapy

The 2×4 appliance comprises bonds on the maxillary incisors, bands or bonds on the first permanent maxillary molars, and a continuous archwire. The appliance is normally used in the mixed dentition, mainly to achieve a good alignment of the incisors, and to correct anterior crossbites and other irregularities. As mentioned in Chapter 2, this type of treatment must be implemented only when it is absolutely necessary. Some irregularity such as that observed in the "ugly duckling" stage is part of a normal development of the occlusion. This appliance offers advantages over alternative techniques as it provides good control of anterior tooth position, is well tolerated, requires no adjustment by the patient, and allows accurate and rapid positioning of the teeth [60]. It is recommended to carefully examine the relationship of the roots of the maxillary lateral incisors to the erupting canines. In many instances, the changes in root angulations may be iatrogenic. Proper bracket angulation helps to avoid damage to the lateral incisor roots. Illustrations of the 2×4 treatment can be found in the case presentations anteriorly described.

Patient 6

The patient was referred to our clinic to be evaluated for a possible intervention. At the time, she was 10y 2m old, in the mixed dentition stage, with all first molars and incisors erupted. The molars were in a Class I relation, but the incisors had a clear indication of a Class II, Div 2 malocclusion, severe deep bite, uprighted incisors, and crowding (Figure 5.47). A phase I intervention was recommended with the indication for a maxillary two-by-four (Figure 5.48) and a mandibular lip bumper. At the end of phase I, the patient showed excellent alignment. Figure 5.49 shows the sequence of lip-bumper-only therapy at different stages of development. Retention was done with a Hawley with a bite plate (Figure 5.50). The second phase with fixed appliances was not complex, and the patient presents a stable occlusion (Figure 5.51).

5.6 The assessment of crowding in the mixed dentition | 87

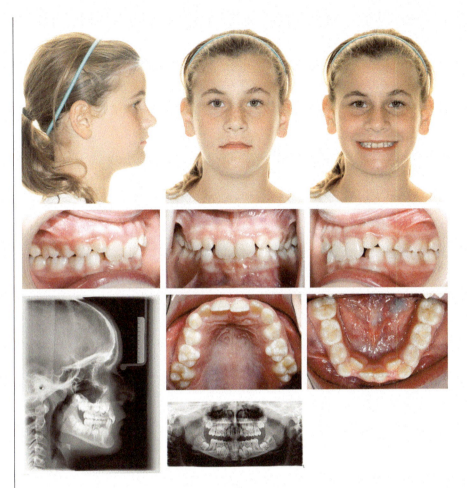

Figure 5.47

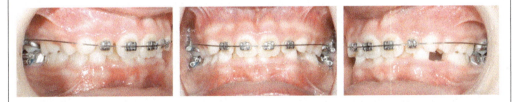

Figure 5.48

5.2 Section II: Intercepting developing Class I problems

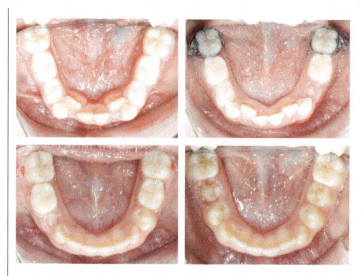

Figure 5.49

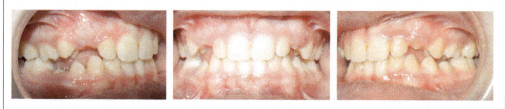

Figure 5.50

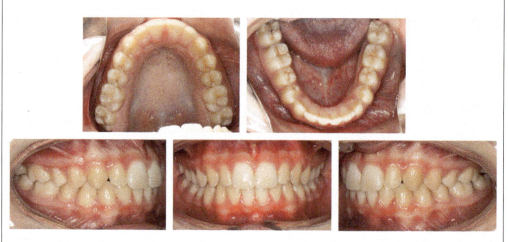

Figure 5.51

5.6 The assessment of crowding in the mixed dentition

Patient 7

This 10y 2m boy presented with a dental Class II, Div 1 severe deep bite, large overjet, chipped maxillary incisor, and a desire to have his teeth fixed. His frontal smile clearly shows the protrusion and the reason he wanted to be treated (Figure 5.52). A maxillary expansion followed by a two-by-four was recommended, together with a mandibular lip bumper (Figure 5.53). The family accepted the treatment, which took less than a year. The lip bumper effectiveness is shown in Figure 5.54. Upon evaluation, it was recommended not to interrupt the treatment since the permanent teeth were coming in fast. The patient was put in active observation until full appliances could be placed.

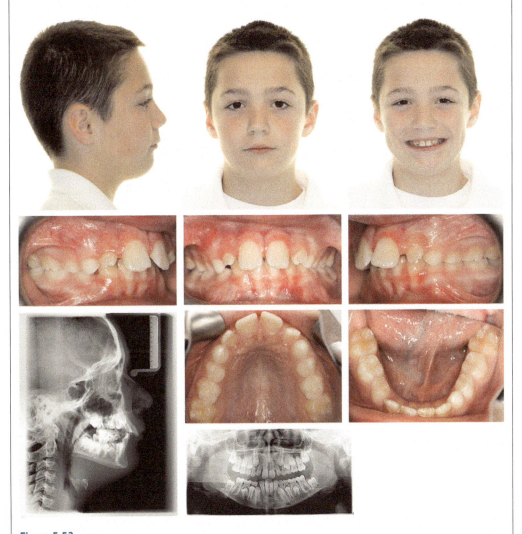

Figure 5.52

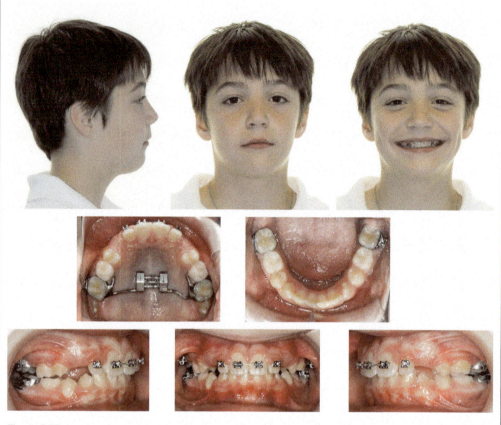

Figure 5.53

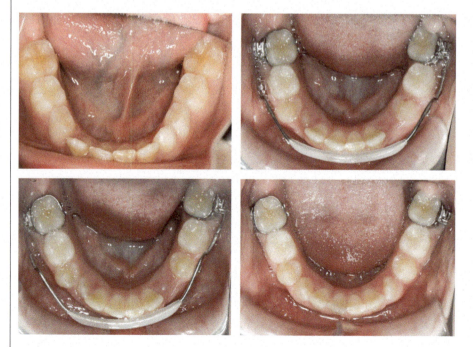

Figure 5.54

5.6 The assessment of crowding in the mixed dentition | 91

Patient 8

This 5y 6m boy was brought to our clinic to be evaluated. His mother was concerned about his bite and wanted to find out if it was the correct time to intervene. After examining the patient and his records, the diagnosis was of a unilateral Brodie (buccal) bite (Figure 5.55). The proposed treatment plan was to insert a lip bumper and expand it progressively (Figure 5.56). On the maxillary arch, the recommendation was an Essix to eliminate any occlusal interference that would probably delay the correction (Figure 5.57). In a short time, the Brodie bite was corrected and an HLLA was placed in retention. Figure 5.58 shows the patient at a more advanced and stable dental age.

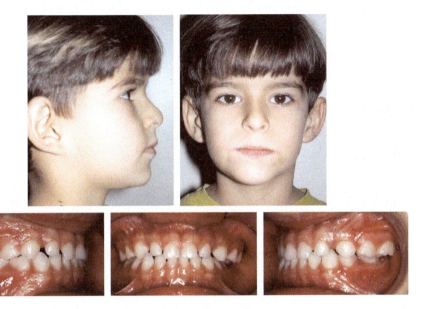

Figure 5.55

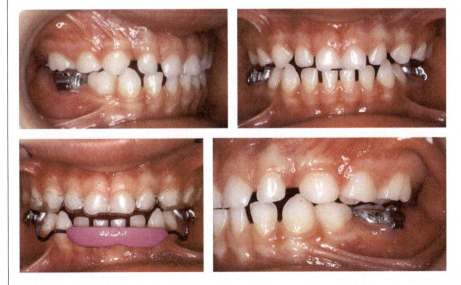

Figure 5.56

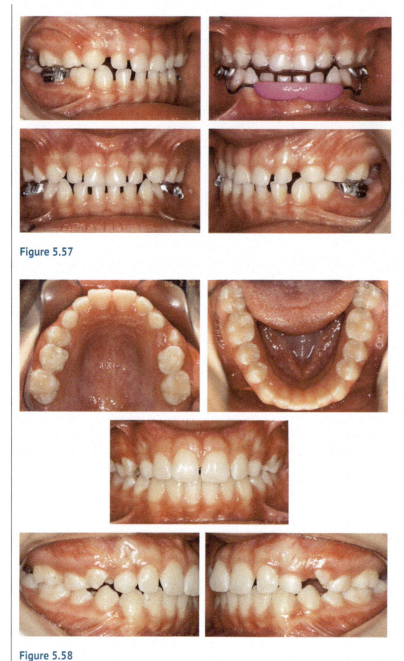

Figure 5.57

Figure 5.58

5.6.4 Severe TSALD: fundamentals of serial extraction

Malocclusions with crowding over 8–10 mm must be considered severe and normally require a more comprehensive treatment plan.

Applying the fundamentals of interception – efficacy and efficiency – in cases that fall in this category is rather difficult. Considering that efficiency can be stated as obtaining the best result possible in the shortest amount of time, early extractions of deciduous and permanent teeth as preconized in a serial extraction (SE) protocol would not fit the principle of efficiency. The procedure can be followed with excellent results, but it is long and requires patience and understanding from patients and families.

SE has been used to describe the timely removal of deciduous and permanent teeth in the mixed dentition. Robert Bunon [61], in 1743, was the first to utilize extractions in the mixed dentition to improve occlusion in the permanent dentition, advocating extractions of the deciduous canines followed by the extractions of the premolars. Later, other prominent authors recommended the procedure [62, 63].

The term SE was introduced by Kjellgren around 1950 [64], and it comprises the extractions of certain deciduous and later some permanent teeth. Hotz [65] objected to the term SE and named the procedure "active supervision of the eruption of the teeth by extraction," changing it later to "active supervision of dental eruption or guidance of eruption." In 1970, the same author, in an the article "Guidance of eruption versus serial extractions," regards "SE" as an incorrect, misleading and perhaps even dangerous term [66].

The term SE has been widely adopted instead of progressive eruption or guidance of eruption [67–79]. Few studies are reported on the effects of SE on the occlusion. Araújo [16] conducted a prospective study and analyzed the behavior of the dental arches and the occlusion up to 1 year after the extraction of the first premolars.

5.6.5 Indications and contraindications for serial extraction (SE) [16]

A comprehensive examination must be completed for each patient. Prior to the initiation of SE procedures, accurate records of the patient must be gathered. These records normally include casts, panoramic radiograph, cephalogram, and extraoral and intraoral photographs. All of these records have a purpose and must be used to determine the facial, skeletal, and dental components of the malocclusion.

The following may serve as guidelines that could impact implementation of SE.

1) **Facial type and balance:** The procedure is indicated for patients with a Class I crowded occlusion. Good facial balance is usually found in patients who have Class I malocclusions. The SE procedure seems to work best when the face has balance or is, at best, mildly protruded. Note that in severe bialveolar protrusion, SE has to be reevaluated, since the extraction spaces should be conserved for maximum reduction of the protrusion.

2) **Skeletal imbalance:** It is important to state that SE is not capable of correcting a skeletal – Class II or III – malocclusion. Attempting to use it for the developing Class II or III malocclusion is generally not prudent.

3) **AL or tooth size deficiency:** In the past, SE was often considered for deficiencies of about 7 mm [76]. With the evolution of orthodontic diagnosis and techniques – bonding, interproximal reduction, reduction of interproximal decay, and use of leeway space – the new recommendation is for 10+ mm of crowding [80].

   Items 4–8 are other diagnostic considerations for SE:

4) **Premature loss of one or more deciduous canines and midline shift:** One of the first signs of lack of space for erupting permanent incisors is the early loss of, or displacement of, deciduous canines. It is common to observe an early midline deviation.

5) **Impacted or ectopically displaced lateral incisors:** Permanent lateral incisors rarely become impacted or ankylosed. When they do not displace the deciduous canines during eruption, they may deviate from their natural path of eruption.

6) **Gingival recession and alveolar destruction:** Excessive crowding of the erupting incisors can cause periodontal problems such as gingival recession and sometimes even the dehiscence of gingival tissues.

7) **Loss of space due to ectopic eruption of molars:** Both maxillary and mandibular molars may erupt ectopically, assuming an excessive mesial direction of eruption and reducing the space for the permanent teeth.
8) **Ankylosis of deciduous molars followed by space loss:** The normal vertical development of alveolar bone can be compromised by ankylosis of deciduous molars. The initial stages of ankylosis may not create problems, but as soon as the development of the permanent teeth advances with growth, tipping of the permanent teeth adjacent to the ankylosed deciduous tooth and subsequent loss of space can be observed.

It is important to reinforce some instances in which SE may not be indicated: mild crowding, congenitally missing teeth, skeletal Class IIs and Class IIIs, large midline diastemas, deep overbite, retroclined anterior teeth mainly the mandibular ones, and lack of knowledge of the fundamentals involved with it.

There is a stage of the procedure that may bring euphoria to patients and families and that is represented by the natural alignment of the anterior teeth. Many tend to believe that everything is working really well and then disappear from the clinician's control. A detailed informed consent with the consequences of not following each step of the procedure, including regular 4–6 monthly visits has to be emphasized.

5.6.5.1 Additional important fundamentals in serial extraction

1) Changes in the Dental Arches.
   The natural development of the dental arches decreases arch depth and perimeter.
2) Sequence of Eruption.
   One of the most extensive studies of eruption patterns of the permanent teeth was done in 1963 by Lo and Moyers [81]. It was found that the most common sequence of eruption in the maxilla is 6, 1, 2, 4, 5, 3, 7. This sequence occurred in approximately 48% of the patients studied. The above described maxillary eruption pattern is considered favorable to SE. An immediate conclusion is that SE in the maxilla may not represent a problem for the orthodontist since the eruption pattern is normally very favorable. Conversely, in the mandible, the most frequent sequence of eruption of the permanent teeth found was 6, 1, 2, 3, 4, 5, 7. This sequence occurred 46% of the time [82, 83]. In the vast majority of patients, the permanent mandibular canines erupt prior to the permanent first premolars. This pattern complicates the SE procedure. Special decisions are required to determine the extraction sequence.
3) Factors Influencing Timing of Eruption.
   The emergence of a tooth into the oral cavity occurs when ⅔ to ¾ of the root is developed [84, 85], but this timing of emergence can be affected by many variables. Tooth emergence or dental age must be well understood [84, 86]. Dental age is defined by the stage of root development. Another variable that must be considered is how height and body weight might affect tooth emergence; taller and heavier children tend to have earlier eruption of permanent teeth [87]. A dichotomy is also observed in relation to gender: girls normally have earlier eruption. Girls have more advanced deciduous root resorption, but boys and girls coincide in early developmental stages of root formation [88]. In girls, however, crown formation is completed first. All these studies concluded that girls tend to have earlier eruption, especially of the mandibular permanent canines.

One of the most important questions to be answered when a SE procedure is to be considered is how the extraction of the deciduous teeth will impact the eruption of their successors. Extraction of a deciduous tooth causes an immediate acceleration in the eruption of its permanent successor [85]. However, if the deciduous extraction occurs in the early stages of permanent tooth root formation, the initial spurt can be followed by delayed eruption.

Other possible factors that may cause early emergence of a permanent tooth are abscesses of a predecessor deciduous tooth as well as caries of the deciduous tooth. A longitudinal observation concluded 1) the extraction of a deciduous molar, when the underlying premolar is well on in root formation, results in accelerated eruption of the premolar, and 2) the early loss of the deciduous second molar may result in impaction of the second premolar due to mesial drift of the permanent first molar [85]. A similar study concluded that the primary teeth should be maintained in a healthy condition in order to permit normal eruption of the succedaneous teeth, and that premature deciduous tooth extractions may result in a high degree of impaction of permanent teeth [89]. Other practical but important information are 1) deciduous canines should not be removed before the permanent canine has attained half of its root length, 2) deciduous molars should not be removed before the root of the permanent first premolar is over half formed, and 3) if the first premolar is close to the alveolar crest, its root should be at least partially developed before the extraction of the deciduous molar that covers it is performed [90].

4) Path of Eruption.

The path of eruption of permanent teeth is another factor that must be observed prior to SE procedures. Malpositioned developing teeth may require a change in the sequence of extractions.

5) Surgical Skill in the Extractions.

Extraction must be performed with skill and ability. Each extraction, as well as any other procedure, must be done carefully. Some professionals may opt for the enucleation of the mandibular first premolars to ensure that the canines do not erupt before the premolars. This procedure requires the child to have only one surgical procedure and it is normally done with sedation. During any extraction and/or enucleation, the dentist/oral surgeon should be aware of the fact that neither the buccal nor the lingual supporting bone should be disturbed. Destruction of bone in either area may cause a permanent defect and exponentially increase the difficulty of extraction space closure. After being involved with hundreds of SE cases, we have abandoned enucleation as a resource, since it may cause iatrogenic damage.

5.6.5.2 Sequence and timing of extractions

When all conditions are "favorable," as the drawings of Figure 5.59 illustrate, a classic SE procedure works to perfection. The benefit of initiating and completing SE may certainly outweigh the burden. The patient is ultimately well served. Guidelines for SE sequences are well described in the literature [24, 91, 92].

Step 1. Extract the deciduous canines to allow physiologic self-alignment of the incisors.

Step 2. Extract the deciduous first molars to expedite and accelerate the eruption of the first premolars. Sometimes, both the deciduous canines and the first deciduous molars can be removed simultaneously to minimize surgical procedures.

Step 3. Extract the erupted first premolars to allow a more favorable distal eruption of the canines.

Step 4. Allow the eruption of the canines and the second premolars.

5.6.5.3 Alternative extraction sequences

There are occasions on which the sequence of eruption in the mandibular arch is not favorable. The mandibular permanent canines, in this scenario, are at the same level as, or ahead of, the mandibular first premolars. A possible solution to avoid enucleation of the first premolars is the extraction sequence that is illustrated in Figure 5.60.

Step 1. Extract the first deciduous molars.

Step 2. Extract the deciduous maxillary canines, if present. Insert an LLHA and extract the deciduous mandibular second molars.

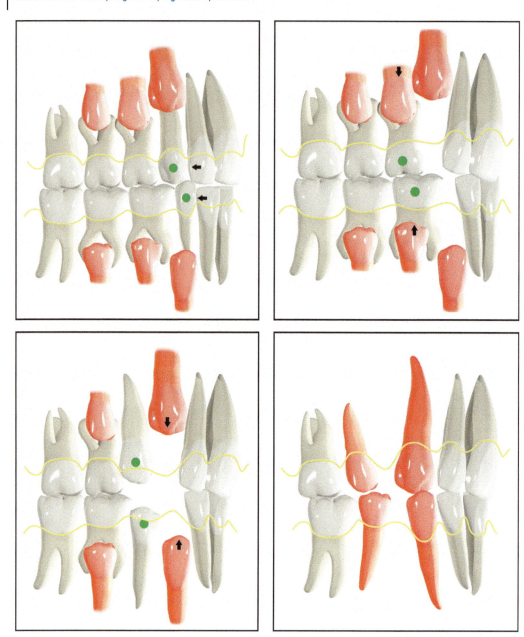

Figure 5.59 Representation of the classic serial extraction sequence when the sequence of eruption is favorable.

The maxillary first premolars must also be monitored for extraction.

Step 3. Extract the mandibular first premolars – and the maxillary second deciduous molars, if indicated.

Step 4. Eruption of the canines and premolars.

The cases of patients 9 and 10 illustrate the two scenarios described above.

5.6 The assessment of crowding in the mixed dentition | 97

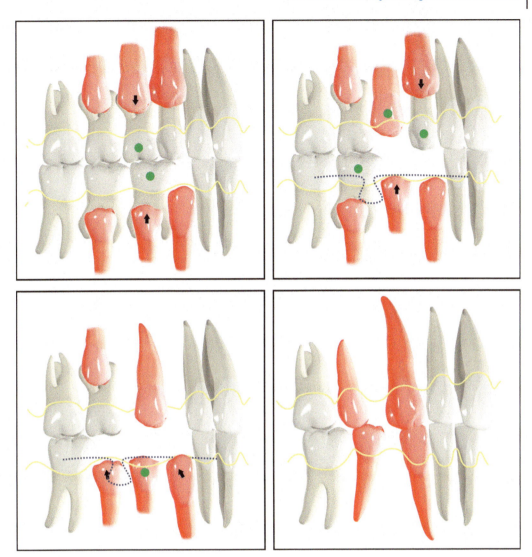

Figure 5.60 Alternative extraction sequence: in cases in which the mandibular canines are at the same level or ahead of the premolars and enucleation has not been part of our protocol. A LLHA is placed, and the extractions of the second deciduous molars followed by the extraction of the first premolars are recommended.

Patient 9
This 7-year-old boy presented with extreme crowding, a good balanced profile, and an appropriate sequence of eruption, suggesting an ideal case for a classic SE (Figure 5.61). The procedure was implemented with the extractions of Ds followed by 4s, and it was successful (Figures 5.62 and 5.63). The retention pictures after 1 year of full braces show the success of the procedure (Figure 5.64).

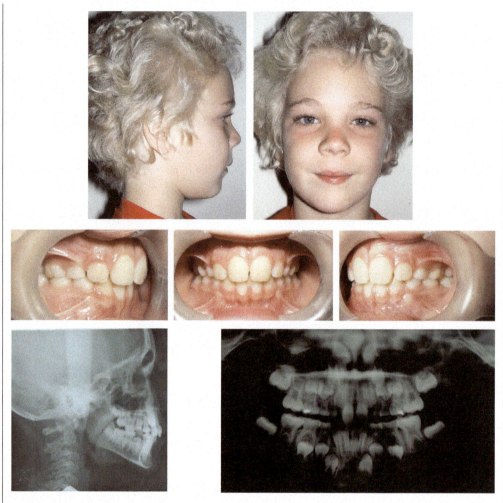

Figure 5.61

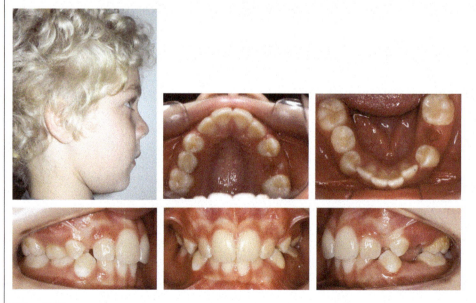

Figure 5.62

5.6 The assessment of crowding in the mixed dentition | 99

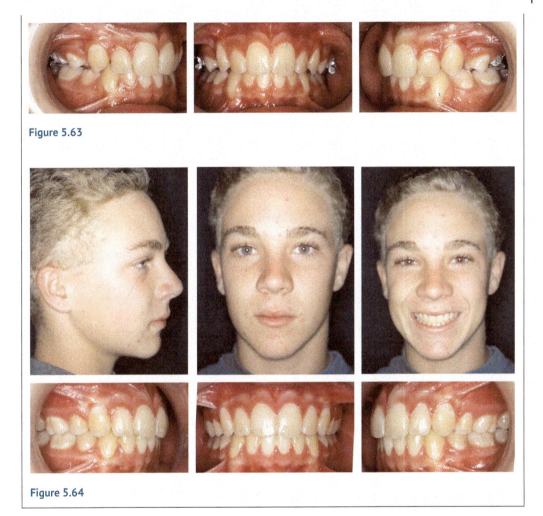

Figure 5.63

Figure 5.64

Patient 10

The initial evaluation of this 10y 3m girl showed that she had balanced facial features but no spaces for all her permanent teeth (Figure 5.65). Although she was slightly Class II, the treatment plan presented to the family was of an alternative SE. The sequence of eruption of the mandibular teeth required an alternative approach to avoid enucleation of the first premolars (Figures 5.66–5.68). An LLHA was introduced before the removal of the mandibular Es. To control the Class II tendency, the patient was asked to wear a high-pull headgear. The sequence of extraction can be followed in the photo sequence. Figure 5.69 shows the patient in Class I molar and well-controlled mandibular and maxillary arches. Full bonding is expected in the near future to establish a good final occlusion.

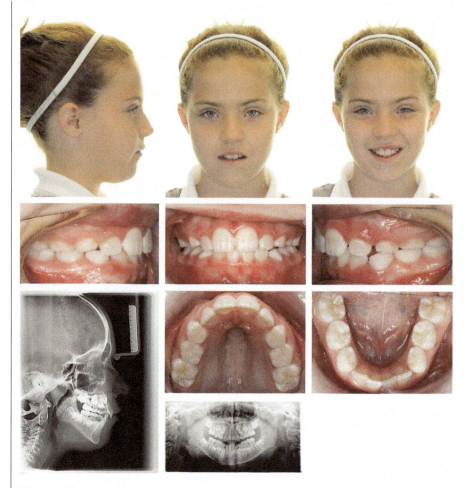

Figure 5.65

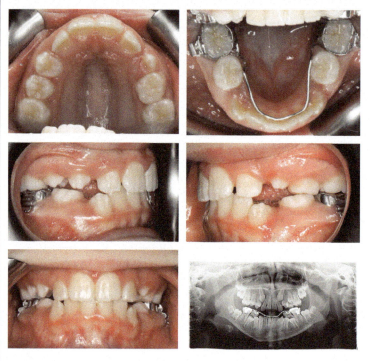

Figure 5.66

5.6 The assessment of crowding in the mixed dentition | 101

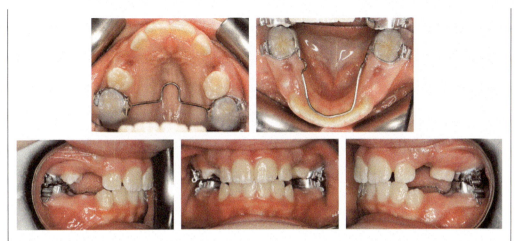

Figure 5.67

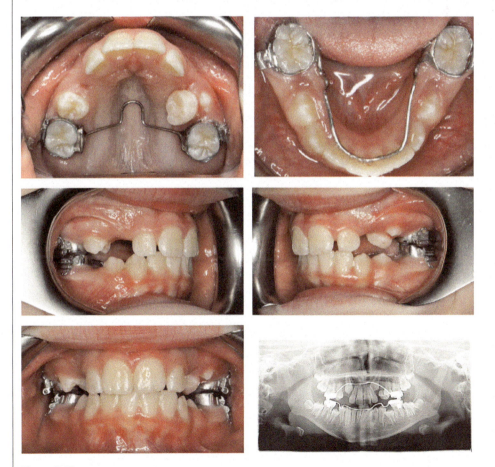

Figure 5.68

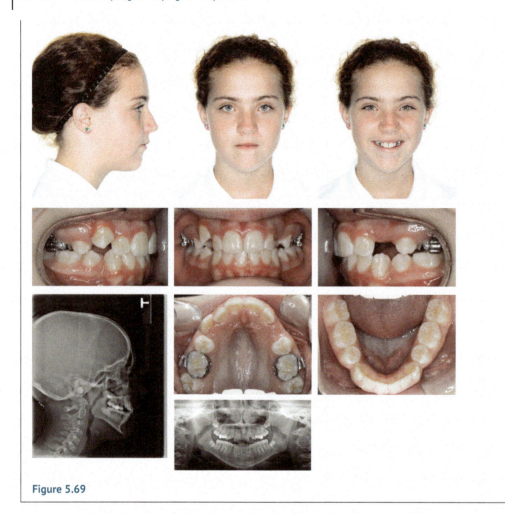

Figure 5.69

References

1 Enlow, D.H. (1975). *Handbook of facial growth*, 2nd edn., 423. Philadelphia, PA: WB Saunders.
2 Enlow, D.H. and Harris, D.B. (1964). A study of the postnatal growth of the human mandible. *Am J Orthod* **50**: 25–50.
3 Moyers, R.E., van der Linden, F.P.G.M., Riolo, M.I., and McNamara, J.A. (1976). *Standards of human occlusal development*. Ann Arbor, MI: University of Michigan Press.
4 Nance, H.N. (1947 Apr). The limitations of orthodontic treatment; mixed dentition diagnosis and treatment. *Am J Orthod* **33**(4): 177–223.
5 Sillman, J.H. (1964). Dimensional changes of the dental arches: longitudinal study from birth to 25 years. *Am J Orthod* **50**: 824–842.
6 Moorrees, C.F. and Reed, R.B. (1965 Feb). Changes in dental arch dimensions expressed on the basis of tooth eruption as a measure of biologic age. *J Dent Res* **44**: 129–141.
7 Moorrees, C. (1958). Growth changes of the dental Arches: a longitudinal study. *J Can DA* **24**: 449–457.
8 Bjork, A. (1963; Feb). Variations in the growth pattern of the human mandible: longitudinal radiographic study by the implant method. *J Dent Res* **42**(1, Pt 2): 400–411.

9 Southard, T.E., Behrents, R.G., and Tolley, E.A. (1989 Dec). The anterior component of occlusal force. Part 1. Measurement and distribution. *Am J Orthod Dentofacial Orthop* **96**(6): 493–500.

10 Southard, T.E., Behrents, R.G., and Tolley, E.A. (1990 Jan). The anterior component of occlusal force. Part 2. Relationship with dental malalignment. *Am J Orthod Dentofacial Orthop* **97**(1): 41–44.

11 Tsourakis AK. Dental and skeletal contributions to molar occlusal development. Master's Thesis, St. Louis, MO, Saint Louis University, 2012.

12 Tanaka, M.M. and Johnston, L.E. (1974 Apr). The prediction of the size of unerupted canines and premolars in a contemporary orthodontic population. *J Am Dent Assoc* **88**(4): 798–801.

13 Moyers, R.E. (1988). *Handbook of orthodontics*, 4th edn., 235–239. Chicago, IL: Year Book Medical Publishers.

14 Hixon, E. and Oldfather, R. (1958). Estimation of the sizes of unerupted cuspid and bicuspid teeth. *Angle Orthod* **28**: 236–240.

15 Ovens, P. (1976 Mar). Modified serial extraction. *Ariz Dent J* **22**(1): 30–31.

16 Araújo, E.A. (1981). *The effect of serial extraction on Class I malocclusions: a one year report on the behavior of the incisors and canines*. Pittsburgh, PA: University of Pittsburgh.

17 Simon, T., Nwabueze, I., Oueis, H., and Stenger, J. (2012 Jan). Space maintenance in the primary and mixed dentitions. *J Mich Dent Assoc* **94**(1): 38–40.

18 Owais, A.I., Rousan, M.E., Badran, S.A., and Abu Alhija, E.S. (2011 Feb). Effectiveness of a lower lingual arch as a space holding device. *Eur J Orthod* **33**(1): 37–42.

19 Gianelly, A.A. (1994). Crowding: timing of treatment. *Angle Orthod* **64**(6): 415–418.

20 Viglianisi, A. (2010 Oct). Effects of lingual arch used as space maintainer on mandibular arch dimension: a systematic review. *Am J Orthod Dentofacial Orthop* **138**(4): 382.e1–382.e4; discussion 382–3.

21 Stivaros, N., Lowe, C., Dandy, N. et al. (2010 Apr). A randomized clinical trial to compare the Goshgarian and Nance palatal arch. *Eur J Orthod* **32**(2): 171–176.

22 Baume, L.J. (1950 Apr). Physiological tooth migration and its significance for the development of occlusion. I. The biogenetic course of the deciduous dentition. *J Dent Res* **29**(2): 123–132.

23 Baume, L.J. (1950 Jun). Physiological tooth migration and its significance for the development of occlusion; the biogenesis of accessional dentition. *J Dent Res* **29**(3): 331–337.

24 Dale, J.G., Brandt, S., and Jack, G. (1976 Jan). Dale on serial extraction. *J Clin Orthod* **10**(1): 44–60.

25 Arya, B.S., Savara, B.S., and Thomas, D.R. (1973 Jun). Prediction of first molar occlusion. *Am J Orthod* **63**(6): 610–621.

26 Hunter, J. (1771). *The natural history of the human teeth*. London: J. Johnson.

27 Lee JL. Comparison of E-space among different skeletal groups. Master's Thesis,. St. Louis, MO, Saint Louis University, 2015.

28 Allbritton EE. Prediction of the mesiodistal width of the unerupted mandibular second premolar and mandibular e-space. Master's Thesis, St. Louis, MO, Saint Louis University, 2018.

29 Betts, N.J., Vanarsdall, R.L., Barber, H.D. et al. (1995). Diagnosis and treatment of transverse maxillary deficiency. *Int J Adult Orthodon Orthognath Surg* **10**(2): 75–96.

30 Da Silva Filho, O.G., Montes, L.A., and Torelly, L.F. (1995 Mar). Rapid maxillary expansion in the deciduous and mixed dentition evaluated through posteroanterior cephalometric analysis. *Am J Orthod Dentofacial Orthop* **107**(3): 268–275.

31 Da Silva, F.O.G., Santamaria, M., and Capelozza, F.L. (2007). Epidemiology of posterior crossbite in the primary dentition. *J Clin Pediatr Dent* **32**(1): 73–78.

32 Proffit, W.R., Fields, H.W., and Sarver, D.M. (2007). *Contemporary orthodontics*, 4th edn. St. Louis, MO: Mosby, Inc.

33 Harvold, E.P., Chierici, G., and Vargervik, K. (1972 Jan). Experiments on the development of dental malocclusions. *Am J Orthod* **61**(1): 38–44.

34 Gungor, A.Y. and Turkkahraman, H. (2009 Jul). Effects of airway problems on maxillary growth: a review. *Eur J Dent* **3**(3): 250–254.

35 Haas, A.J. (1970 Mar). Palatal expansion: just the beginning of dentofacial orthopedics. *Am J Orthod* **57**(3): 219–255.

36 Haas, A.J. (1965 Jul). The treatment of maxillary deficiency by opening the mid-palatal suture. *Angle Orthod* **35**:200–217.

37 Lagravere, M.O., Major, P.W., and Flores-Mir, C. (2005 Nov). Long-term skeletal changes with rapid maxillary expansion: a systematic review. *Angle Orthod* **75**(6): 1046–1052.

38 Lagravère, M.O., Heo, G., Major, P.W., and Flores-Mir, C. (2006 Jan). Meta-analysis of immediate changes with rapid maxillary expansion treatment. *J Am Dent Assoc* **137**(1): 44–53.

39 Garib, D.G., Henriques, J.F.C., Carvalho, P.E.G., and Gomes, S.C. (2007 May). Longitudinal effects of rapid maxillary expansion. *Angle Orthod* **77**(3): 442–448.

40 Buschang, P.H. (2006 Apr). Maxillomandibular expansion: short-term relapse potential and long-term stability. *Am J Orthod Dentofacial Orthop* **129**(4 Suppl): S75–S79.

41 Subtelny, J.D. and Sakuda, M. (1966 Jul). Muscle function, oral malformation, and growth changes. *Am J Orthod* **52**(7): 495–517.

42 Spena, R. (2002). *Nonextraction treatment: an Atlas on cetlin mechanics*. Bohemia, NY: Dentsply GAC Int.

43 Graber, T.M., Vanarsdall, R.L., and Vig, K.W.L. (2005). *Orthodontics: current principles & techniques*. St. Louis, MO: Elsevier Mosby.

44 O'Donnell, S., Nanda, R.S., and Ghosh, J. (1998 Mar). Perioral forces and dental changes resulting from mandibular lip bumper treatment. *Am J Orthod Dentofacial Orthop* **113**(3): 247–255.

45 Davidovitch, M., McInnis, D., and Lindauer, S.J. (1997 Jan). The effects of lip bumper therapy in the mixed dentition. *Am J Orthod Dentofacial Orthop* **111**(1): 52–58.

46 Grossen, J. and Ingervall, B. (1995 Apr). The effect of a lip bumper on lower dental arch dimensions and tooth positions. *Eur J Orthod* **17**(2): 129–134.

47 Nevant, C.T., Buschang, P.H., Alexander, R.G., and Steffen, J.M. (1991 Oct). Lip bumper therapy for gaining arch length. *Am J Orthod Dentofacial Orthop* **100**(4): 330–336.

48 Osborn, W.S., Nanda, R.S., and Currier, G.F. (1991 Jun). Mandibular arch perimeter changes with lip bumper treatment. *Am J Orthod Dentofacial Orthop* **99**(6): 527–532.

49 Bjerregaard, J., Bundgaard, A.M., and Melsen, B. (1980). The effect of the mandibular lip bumper and maxillary bite plate on tooth movement, occlusion and space conditions in the lower dental arch. *Eur J Orthod* **2**(4): 257–265.

50 Ingervall, B. and Thüer, U. (1998 Oct). No effect of lip bumper therapy on the pressure from the lower lip on the lower incisors. *Eur J Orthod* **20**(5): 525–534.

51 Soo, N.D. and Moore, R.N. (1991 May). A technique for measurement of intraoral lip pressures with lip bumper therapy. *Am J Orthod Dentofacial Orthop* **99**(5): 409–417.

52 Cetlin, N.M. and Ten Hoeve, A. (1983 Jun). Nonextraction treatment. *J Clin Orthod* **17**(6): 396–413.

53 Legler LR. The effects of removable expansion appliances on the mandibular arch. Master's Thesis. Dallas, TX, Baylor College of Dentistry, 1991.

54 Vargo, J., Buschang, P.H., Boley, J.C. et al. (2007 Apr). Treatment effects and short-term relapse of maxillomandibular expansion during the early to mid mixed dentition. *Am J Orthod Dentofacial Orthop* **131**(4): 456–463.

55 Hamula, W. (1993 Feb). Modified mandibular Schwarz appliance. *J Clin Orthod* **27**(2): 89–93.

56 O'Grady, P.W., McNamara, J.A., Baccetti, T., and Franchi, L. (2006 Aug). A long-term evaluation of the mandibular Schwarz appliance and the acrylic splint expander in early mixed dentition patients. *Am J Orthod Dentofacial Orthop* **130**(2): 202–213.

57 Wendling, L.K., McNamara, J.A., Franchi, L., and Baccetti, T. (2005 Jan). A prospective study of the short-term treatment effects of the acrylic-splint rapid maxillary expander combined with the lower Schwarz appliance. *Angle Orthod* **75**(1): 7–14.

58 Motoyoshi, M., Shirai, S., Yano, S. et al. (2005 Apr). Permissible limit for mandibular expansion. *Eur J Orthod* **27**(2): 115–120.

59 Tai, K. and Park, J.H. (2010). Dental and skeletal changes in the upper and lower jaws after treatment with Schwarz appliances using cone-beam computed tomography. *J Clin Pediatr Dent* **35**(1): 111–120.

60 McKeown, H.F. and Sandler, J. (2001 Dec). The two by four appliance: a versatile appliance. *Dent Update* **28**(10): 496–500.

61 Bunon, R. (1743). *Essay sur las maladies des dents*. Paris: Briasson.

62 Fox, J. (1803). *The natural history of human teeth: to which is added an account of the diseases which affect children during the first dentition*, 6th edn. London: J. Cox.

63 Colyer, J. (1896). Discussion on the early treatment of crowded mouths. *Odont Soc Trans* **28**(2): 215–233.

64 Kjellgren, B. (1948 Jan). Serial extraction as a corrective procedure in dental orthopedic therapy. *Acta Odontol Scand* **8**(1): 17–43.

65 Hotz, R.P. (1947). Active supervision of the eruption of teeth by extraction. *Tr Eur Orthod Soc* **48**: 34–47.

66 Hotz, R.P. (1970 Jul). Guidance of eruption versus serial extraction. *Am J Orthod* **58**(1): 1–20.

67 Heath, J. (1953). The interception of malocclusion by planned serial extraction. *NZ Dent J* **49**: 77–88.

68 Dewell, B.F. (1968 Sep 15). Serial extraction; its limitations and contraindications. *Ariz Dent J* **14**(6): 14–30.

69 Dewell, B.F. (1969 Jun). Prerequisites in serial extraction. *Am J Orthod* **55**(6): 533–539.

70 Dewell, B.F. (1970 Jul). Editorial. A question of terminology: serial extraction or guidance of eruption. *Am J Orthod* **58**(1): 78–79.

71 Dewell, B.F. (1971 Dec). Precautions in serial extraction. *Am J Orthod* **60**(6): 615–618.

72 Lloyd, Z.B. (1956). Serial extraction as a treatment procedure. *Am J Orthod* **42**: 728–739.

73 Newman, G.V. (1959). The role of serial extraction in orthodontic treatment. *N J State Soc J* **31**: 8–13.

74 Tweed, C.H. (1944). Indications for the extraction of teeth in orthodontic procedure. *Am J Orthod Oral Surg* **42**: 22–45.

75 Tweed, C.H. (1963). Treatment planning and therapy in the mixed dentition. *Am J Orthod* **49**(12): 881–906.

76 Ringenberg, Q. (1964). Serial extraction: stop, look, and be certain. *Am J Orthod* **50**: 327–336.

77 Jacobs, J. (1965 Jun). Cephalometric and clinical evaluation of Class I discrepancy cases treated by serial extraction. *Am J Orthod* **51**: 401–411.

78 Graber, T.M. (1971 Dec). Serial extraction: a continuous diagnostic and decisional process. *Am J Orthod* **60**(6): 541–575.

79 Glauser, R.O. (1973 Jun). An evaluation of serial extraction among Navajo Indian children. *Am J Orthod* **63**(6): 622–632.

80 Proffit, W.R. (2006 Apr). The timing of early treatment: an overview. *Am J Orthod Dentofacial Orthop* **129**(4 Suppl): S47–S49.

81 Lo, R. and Moyers, R.E. (1953). Studies in the etiology and prevention of malocclusion: I. The sequence of eruption of the permanent dentition. *Am J Orthod* **39**(6): 460–467.

82 Nanda, R.S. (1960). Eruption of human teeth. *Am J Orthod* **46**(5): 363–378.

83 Sturdivant, J., Knott, V., and Meredith, H. (1962). Interrelations from serial data for eruption of the permanent dentition. *Angle Orthod* **32**(1): 1–13.

84 Gron, A.M. (1962 Jun). Prediction of tooth emergence. *J Dent Res* **41**: 573–585.

85 Fanning, E.A. (1962). Effect of extraction of deciduous molars on the formation and eruption of their successors. *Am J Orthod* **32**: 44–53.

86 Lamons, F.F. and Gray, S. (1958). Study of the relationship between tooth eruption age, skeletal development age, and chronological age in sixty-one Atlanta children. *Am J Orthod* **44**: 687–691.

87 Maj, G., Bassani, S., Menini, G., and Zannini, O. (1964). Studies on the eruption of permanent teeth in children with normal occlusion and with malocclusion. *Rep Congr Eur Orthod Soc* **40**: 107–130.

88 Fanning, E.A. (2008). A longitudinal study of tooth formation and root resorption. *NZ Dent J* **104**(2): 60–61.

89 Maclaughlin, J.A., Fogels, H.R., and Shiere, F.R. (1967 Sep). The influence of premature primary molar extraction on bicuspid eruption. *J Dent Child* **34**(5): 399–405.

90 Moorrees, C.F., Fanning, E.A., and Hunt, E.E. Jr. (1963 Dec). Age variation of formation stages for ten permanent teeth. *J Dent Res* **42**: 1490–1502.

91 Dale, J.G., Brandt, S., and Jack, G. (1976 Feb). Dale on serial extraction. 2. *J Clin Orthod* **10**(2): 116–136.

92 Dale, J.G., Brandt, S., and Jack, G. (1976 Mar). Dale on serial extraction. 3. *J Clin Orthod* **10**(3): 196–217.

6

Recognizing and correcting Class II malocclusions

6.1

Section I: The development, phenotypic characteristics, and etiology of Class II malocclusion

Peter H. Buschang, MA, PhD

Regents Professor Emeritus, Department of Orthodontics, Texas A&M University School of Dentistry, Dallas, TX, USA

6.1 Introduction

A Class II molar relationship, also referred to as distocclusion, occurs when the mesiobuccal cusps of the maxillary first molars occlude anterior to the mesiobuccal grooves of the mandibular first molars. Class II permanent molar relationships develop from either distal step or flush terminal plane relationships in the deciduous dentition (Figure 6.1). Young children with full distal step relations in the deciduous dentition will also have distal step relationships in the mixed and permanent dentitions. Some children with flush terminal plane relationships in the deciduous dentition will develop distal steps in the mixed dentition and Class II relationships in the permanent dentition. Most of those who start with flush terminal plane relationships will have cusp-to-cusp relationships in the early mixed dentition and some of these will have permanent Class II molar relationships. Most cusp-to-cusp relationships become Class I in the permanent dentition.

To understand the growth changes that occur, the various types of Class II malocclusions need to be distinguished. The most important distinction is between Class II, division 1 and division 2 malocclusion (Figure 6.2). Subjects with division 1 have normally inclined or proclined maxillary central incisors; those with division 2 have retroclined maxillary central incisors. Angle distinguished the two by noting that Class II division 2 subjects have "… distal occlusion of the teeth in both lateral halves of the lower dentition, indicated by the mesiodistal relations of the first permanent molars, but with retrusion instead of protrusion of the upper incisors" [1]. From a skeletal perspective, Ricketts characterized Class II division 2 subjects as having "brachyfacial patterns with resulting strong musculature. The lower facial height and mandibular arc are below the normal range, therefore the teeth are deep in the basal bone" [2].

To understand a patient's growth potential, the traditional anteroposterior (AP) categories that have been used to classify Class II patients are insufficient. Both the vertical and AP skeletal relationships must be considered. While subjects with Class II division 1 malocclusion are usually mandibular retrognathic, their vertical characteristics are, on average, similar to those of Class Is. From a treatment view, it is important to distinguish between the Class II division 1 subjects who are hypodivergent, and those who are hyperdivergent (Figure 6.3). Subjects with Class II, division 2 malocclusion are usually orthognathic and more hypodivergent than Class Is.

Class IIs usually present with functional deficits (Figure 6.4). Their masticatory performance

---

Recognizing and Correcting Developing Malocclusions: A Problem-Oriented Approach to Orthodontics,
Second Edition. Edited by Eustáquio A. Araújo and Peter H. Buschang.
© 2025 John Wiley & Sons, Inc. Published 2025 by John Wiley & Sons, Inc.

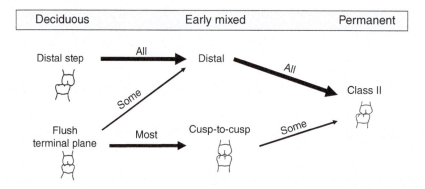

Figure 6.1 Development of Class II molar relationships between the deciduous (distal steps larger than 0.5–1.0 mm), mixed (distal relative to cusp-to-cusp), and permanent dentitions.

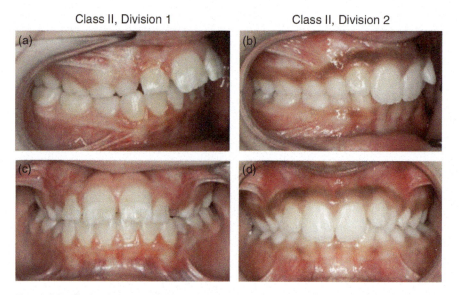

Figure 6.2 Occlusal characteristics of Class II division 1 (a & c) and Class II division 2 (b & d) malocclusions (Courtesy of Dr. Hiroshi Ueno).

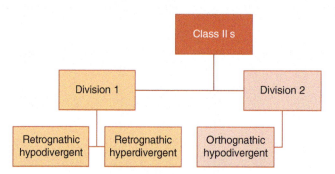

Figure 6.3 Anteroposterior and vertical skeletal characteristics of subjects with Class II division 1 and division 2 malocclusion.

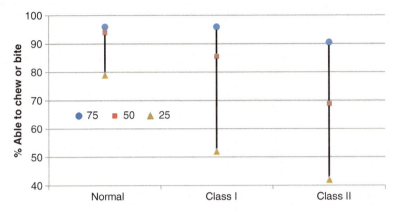

Figure 6.4 Percentages of individuals with normal occlusion, Class I malocclusion, and Class II malocclusion who are ordinarily able (0% unable; 100% very able) to chew or bite steaks, chops, or firm meats (adapted from English et al. [3]).

(i.e. ability to break down foods) has been reported to be only 60% of normal [4]. Chewed particle sizes of untreated Class IIs are approximately 15% larger than those of subjects with normal occlusion [3]. The inability of subjects with Class II malocclusion to break down foods has been directly related to the decreased areas of interdental contact and near contact [5]. Reduced areas of contact and near contact are important because they are also related to reduced bite forces, reduced occlusal support, and abnormal jaw kinematic patterns [6]. This explains why Class IIs apply less energy during mastication than Class Is [7], and why Class IIs often experience problems chewing foods [3]. The functional deficiencies are most pronounced in hyperdivergent Class IIs, who have smaller masticatory muscles and weaker bite forces than hypodivergent Class IIs [8–10].

Class IIs also require treatment to correct their aesthetic concerns. The convex profiles and retrusive chins that characterize Class IIs are among the least favored by dental professionals [11]. Excessively convex profiles have been consistently shown to be aesthetically less pleasing than straight profiles [12, 13]. Both dental professionals and lay people believe that changing a patient's profile to be straighter and less retruded significantly increases attractiveness [14]. It is not just an AP skeletal aesthetic problem. Excessive anterior lower face height is also perceived as unattractive by orthodontists and laypeople [15].

6.1.1 Prevalence

Large-scale epidemiological surveys conducted during the 1970s [16, 17] reported that bilateral Class II molar relationships decreased from approximately 20.4% in children 6–11 years of age to 14.5% among youths 12–17 years (Figure 6.5). The prevalence of Class II malocclusion was 3.8 times higher among white than black children, and 2.6 times higher among white than black youths.

More recent data collected by the NHANES III showed that the prevalence of Class II malocclusion (defined as overjet ≥ 5 mm) among the US population decreased from 22.5% among 8–11 year-olds, to 15.6% among 12–17 year-olds, and then to 13.4% among adults [18]. The prevalence of Class II malocclusion was slightly higher among blacks (16.5%) than whites (14.2%), and lowest among Mexican Americans (9.1%). Combined, the best available epidemiological data indicates that approximately 21.5% of children 6–11 and 15% of youths 12–17 years of age have bilateral Class II malocclusions.

A systematic review of 53 studies, each with sample sizes >200, showed that the worldwide

6.1 Section I: The development, phenotypic characteristics, and etiology of Class II malocclusion

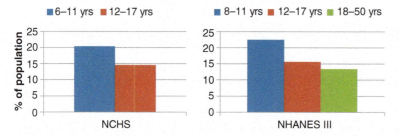

Figure 6.5 Prevalence of Class II malocclusion among US children, youths, and adults (data from the National Center of Health Statistics [15, 16] and NHANES III) [18].

prevalence of Class II malocclusion decreases from 23.1% in the mixed dentition to 19.6% in the permanent dentition [19]. There were significant differences between geographic locations, with the highest prevalence of Class II malocclusion in Europe (33.5%), followed by the Americas (15.3%), Asia (12.3%), and Africa (11.5%), respectively. Among the various racial groups, Caucasians and Africans exhibit the highest and lowest prevalences of Class II malocclusion, respectively.

While these epidemiological surveys did not evaluate Class II skeletal relationships, others have established a correspondence between Class II skeletal and Class II dental relationships. Of the 2000 cases 6–18 years of age evaluated by Beresford [20], the majority (≈70%) of Class II cases had corresponding dental and skeletal relationships. Milacic and Markovic [21] reported that approximately 75% of the mixed and early permanent dentition cases had corresponding Class IIs dental and skeletal relationships.

Approximately 2–3% of Caucasians have Class II, division 2 malocclusion. Ast et al. [22] found that 3.4% of the 1462 youths 15–18 years of age whom they evaluated had Class II division 2 malocclusion. Massler and Frankel [23] evaluated 2758 Caucasians 14–18 years of age and found that 2.7% had division 2 malocclusions; Mills [24] evaluated 1455 school children 8–17 years of age and found that 2.3% had Class II division 2 malocclusions.

6.2 Characterization of the Class II, division 2 phenotype

Most studies evaluating the morphological characteristics of Class II, division 2s have been cross-sectional (Table 6.1). They consistently report division 2s as hypodivergent, with square jaws, small gonial and mandibular plane angles (MPAs), and decreased lower anterior facial heights [26, 27, 30, 31]. The maxilla is typically

Table 6.1 Cross-sectional studies characterizing untreated Class II division 2 subjects based on comparisons against Class Is.

	Divergence	AP Mx position	AP Md position	AP dentoalveolar
Baldridge [25]	Normal	N/A	Normal	Deficient
Renfroe [26]	Hypodivergent	Orthognathic	Slight retrognathic	N/A
Wallis [27]	Hypodivergent	N/A	Slight retrognathic	Deficient
Godiawala and Joshi [28]	Hypodivergent	Orthognathic	Retrognathic (SNB)	Slightly deficient
Hitchcock [29]	Normal	Orthognathic	Retrognathic (SNB)	N/A
Karlsen [30]	Hypodivergent	N/A	Retrognathic	Deficient
Brezniak et al. [31].	Hypodivergent	Orthognathic	Slight retrognathic	Deficient

reported to be well-positioned. The mandibles of Class II, division 2s have been reported to be both normal and retrognathic [25–31]. Importantly, most studies showing retrognathic or short mandibles based their assessments on the B-point. Direct measurements of chin position indicate that the mandible is either in a normal position or only slightly retrognathic. The difference between the position of the B-point and the chin explains why the dentoalveolar component of the mandible among Class II, division 2s is deficient in length [25, 27, 30–33].

Compared to Class Is, Class II division 2 subjects exhibit substantially greater retroclination of the upper incisors, greater retroclination of the lower incisors, much larger interincisal angles, and increased overbite [28, 29, 31]. While overjet in Class II division 2 subjects has been reported to be both similar to [31] or larger [29] than overjet in Class I subjects, it is smaller than typically found among Class II division 1 subjects [34].

Two recent cross-sectional studies compared Class II, division 1s and division 2s. The division 2 subjects were shown to be substantially less convex (≈5°), more hypodivergent, and less retrognathic than division 1 subjects [34]. There were no differences in the SNA angle. The Class II division 2 cases also had more upright maxillary incisors (≈30°), more retroclined mandibular incisors (≈15°), less overjet (3.7 vs. 10.0 mm) and more overbite (6.2 vs. 4.6 mm) than the Class II division 1 subjects. Al-Khateeb and Al-Khateeb [35], who compared 293 Class II division 1s to 258 Class II division 2s, confirmed that there was no difference in AP maxillary position, but the faces of division 1 subjects were more convex, the mandibles were more retrognathic, and the lower face heights were greater than in division 2s. The interincisal angle of division 2s was almost 18° larger, due to retroclined upper (≈19°) and lower (≈6°) incisors.

When compared longitudinally, untreated Class II division 2s and untreated Class Is 6–19 years of age show relatively few skeletal differences [36]. There were no group differences in the anteroposterior positions of either the maxilla or the mandible. Between 6 and 19 years of age, the cranial base angle remained approximately 4° larger in the Class II division 2s than in Class Is. The other skeletal differences were primarily vertical (Figure 6.6). The anterior-to-posterior facial height ratio, as well as the mandibular plane and gonial angles, were already smaller among 6–7 year-old Class II division 2s than Class Is, and the differences increased over time. The interincisal angle of the Class IIs was 5° larger at 6–7 years of age, and the differences increased slightly thereafter. While upper incisor inclination (U1/SN) was similar at 6–7 years of age, the angle increased significantly more in Class Is during the full eruption of the maxillary incisors and remained larger throughout the growing years.

The anterior dentition, especially the upper anterior dentition, plays an important role in the development of Class II division 2 malocclusion. Leighton and Adams [37], who closely evaluated the upper incisors of Class II division 2 subjects, showed that they started retroclining before permanent incisor emergence, and continued retroclining during emergence and for several years thereafter. The more upright position of the upper incisors among division 2 subjects allows the mandible to overrotate. There is a negative relationship between upper incisor angulation and lower lip height, with greater coverage associated with greater incisor retroclination [38]. Subjects with Class II division 2 malocclusion have higher lip lines [33, 39]. They also have resting lip pressures that are greater on the tooth's incisal areas [39].

6.3 Characterization of the Class II division 1 phenotype

Due to approximately equal numbers of early studies showing Class II division 1 subjects as having either retrusive, orthognathic, or protrusive maxillae, McNamara [40] performed a better-controlled evaluation of 277 Class II subjects 8–10 years of age. Based on the SNA angle

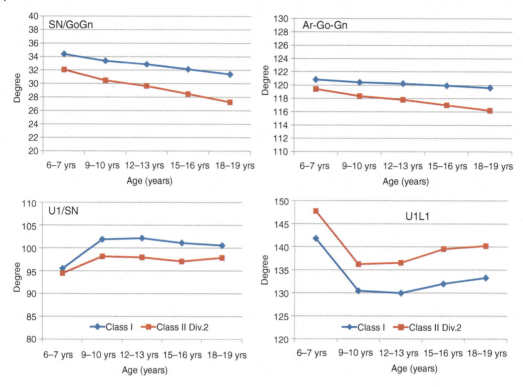

Figure 6.6 Changes in vertical skeletal relationships and incisor angulation of Class Is and Class II division 2s between 6 and 19 years of age (Barbosa et al. [36]/with permission of Elsevier).

and maxillary depth (N-A/FH), the maxilla of the Class IIs was found to be slightly retrusive. More recent studies report maxillary protrusion and retrusion among untreated Class IIs, but few show statistically significant differences between Class IIs and Class Is (Table 6.2). The two studies that classified their subjects based on the ANB angle, rather than occlusal relations, showed that the greater convexity of Class IIs was due to maxillary protrusion, rather than mandibular retrusion [44, 48]. One of them [48] also reported smaller posterior facial height among Class IIs than Class Is.

Regarding AP mandibular position, most of the early studies reviewed by McNamara reported mandibular retrusion among Class IIs. McNamara's [40] sample also showed mandibular retrusion, as does the more recent literature (Table 6.2). The vast majority of studies show statistically significant differences between Class IIs and Class Is. In other words, differences in the ANB angle between Class Is and Class IIs are primarily due to the mandible, not the maxilla.

The early literature also indicated that the maxillary incisors of Class IIs are protrusive and that the maxillary molars are in the correct or neutral position [40]. The children evaluated by McNamara [40] also had maxillary incisors that were 2–3 mm more protrusive than expected relative to the A-Pg plane, but the horizontal distance of the upper incisor to the A-point was within normal limits. Relative to the palatial plane, the upper incisors are more protrusive (>10°) in Class IIs than in Class Is [43, 49]. Both the angular and mm distance of the upper incisor to the N-A plane indicate greater protrusion among Class IIs [50].

Although not consistently evaluated, it appears that the size of the Class II maxilla, its AP position from the cranial base, and its anterior height are within the normal limits expected for Class Is (Table 6.3). In contrast,

6.3 Characterization of the Class II division 1 phenotype

Table 6.2 Literature comparing AP maxillary and mandibular positions of Class IIs and Class Is.

	SNA Amt	SNA Prob	SNB Amt	SNB Prob	ANB Amt	ANB Prob
Ngan et al. [41]	←1.2°	NS	←3.6°	Sig	N/A	N/A
Bishara [42]	→0.2°	N/A	←0.6°	NS	↑0.8°	Sig (♂ only)
Dhopatkar et al. [43]	←0.3°	NS	←2.5°	Sig	↑2.3°	Sig
Riesmeijer et al. [44]	→2.2°	Sig	←0.5°	NS	↑2.7°	Sig
Stahl et al. [45]	←0.8°	NS	←3.4°	Sig	↑2.7°	Sig
Baccetti et al. [46]	→0.3°	NS	←5.5°	Sig	↑4.0°	Sig
Jacob and Buschang [47]	←0.5°	NS	←2.5°	Sig	↑2.1°	Sig
Yoon and Chung [48]	→2.1°	Sig	←0.6°	NS	↑2.9°	Sig
Most common	→	NS	←	Sig	↑	Sig

NS, no statistically significant difference; N/A, not available; Sig, prob < 0.05.

Table 6.3 Differences (Class II minus Class I) in maxillary size and position.

	Size (ANS-PNS)	AP distance from CB	Palatal Ht
Craig [51]	NS	N/A	N/A
Menezes [49]	NS	N/A	N/A
Ngan et al. [41]	N/A	N/A	NS
Dhopatkar [43]	↑	↑	N/A
Riesmeijer et al. [44]	N/A	N/A	↑
Stahl et al. [45]	N/A	NS	NS
Baccetti et al. [46]	N/A	NS	NS
Most common	NS	NS	NS

Dhopatkar et al. [43] showed that Class IIs have longer maxilla and that ANS is positioned further from condylion than expected, which might be expected because their Class II subjects had significantly larger cranial base angles than their Class I subjects. Greater upper anterior face height among Class IIs was reported by Riesmeijer et al. [44], but the differences did not become apparent until 13–14 years of age. Others have also reported slightly greater anterior face height among Class IIs than Class Is, but the differences were not statistically significant [41, 46]. The palatal plane angle and changes in the angle are similar among Class IIs and Class Is [46].

Among the first to identify mandibular growth deficiencies, Nelson and Higley [52] showed that corpus length was up to 2.6 mm shorter in 7–10-year-old Class IIs than Class Is, and that the differences had increased slightly by 11–14 years of age. The Class II dentoalveolar complex was also shorter. More recent literature indicates that the mandibles of Class IIs are smaller than the mandibles of Class Is (Table 6.4). The differences between Classes Is and IIs are approximately twice as large for overall length than for ramus height and corpus length [47]. By late adolescence, differences in overall length range from 2 to 6 mm, whereas differences in ramus height and corpus length range from 1 to 3 and 1 to 4 mm, respectively [41, 45–47].

Most Class IIs who have been categorized based on their molar relationships are not hyperdivergent; their MPAs are slightly, but not significantly, larger (Figure 6.7). Class IIs categorized based on the ANB angle have greater lower face heights (ANS-ME) than Class Is, with differences increasing slightly between 7–14 years of age [44]. They also have

Table 6.4 Differences (Class II minus Class I) in mandibular size and position.

	Total LT (e.g. Co-Gn)	Ramus Ht	Corpus Lt	MPA	Gonial angle
Menezes [49]	↓	↓	↓	↑	N/A
Ngan et al. [41]	↓	N/A	↓	NS	NS
Bishara [42]	NS	N/A	N/A	NS	N/A
Dhopatkar et al. [43]	NS	N/A	NS	NS	N/A
Stahl et al. [45]	↓	NS	N/A	NS	NS
Riesmeijer et al. [44]	NS	N/A	↓	↑	↑
Baccetti et al. [46]	↓	↓	N/A	NS	NS
Vásquez et al. [50]	NS	NS	NS	NS	NS
Jacob and Buschang [47]	↓	NS	NS	NS	NS
Yoon and Chung [48]	↓	NS	↓	NS	NS
Most common	↓	↓	↓	NS	NS

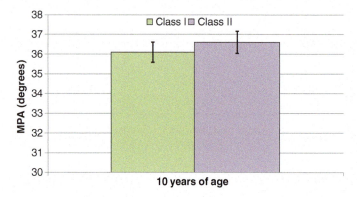

Figure 6.7 Mandibular plane angles (MPAs) of Class Is and Class IIs (Adapted from Jacob and Buschang [47]).

MPAs that are 1–2° larger and gonial angles that are 2–3° larger. The other comparison of Class Is and Class IIs that categorized its subjects based on the ANB angles reported no statistically significant differences in the MPA, posterior-to-anterior facial height ratio, or the gonial angle [48].

Lower incisor inclinations have been reported as being similar or only slightly more protrusive among Class IIs than Class Is. Relative to the A-Pg plane, the lower incisors have been reported as protrusive [45] or in normal position [40]. The lower incisor to MPA is similar to [29, 49, 53] or slightly larger for Class IIs than Class Is, but the differences were not statistically significant [43, 45].

6.3.1 Hyperdivergent vs. hypodivergent Class II division 1 malocclusion

While the MPA of Class IIs is only slightly – not significantly – larger than that of Class Is, it is clinically important to distinguish between hyperdivergent and hypodivergent Class IIs. The skeletally hypodivergent and normodivergent

Class IIs tend to have favorable growth patterns. Their ANB and MPAs decrease over time, and their mandibles undergo true forward rotation, advancing the chin almost 1 mm/yr [54]. These are the mixed dentition subjects who self-correct to Class I relationships in the permanent dentition. It is the skeletally hyperdivergent Class IIs who usually have unfavorable growth patterns. These subjects have ANB and MPAs that increase over time, their mandibles rotate forward less than expected, and their chins advance less than expected.

As reviewed by Buschang et al. [55], anterior and posterior maxillary heights of hyperdivergent Class IIs are usually similar to normal controls. Maxillary length and its AP position (based on the SNA angle) are smaller when hyperdivergent subjects are classified based on open-bite, but not when their vertical classification is skeletally based. Hyperdivergence does not affect the palatal plane angle. The review consistently showed increased anterior and posterior dentoalveolar heights among hyperdivergent subjects, indicating that the primary maxillary problems among hyperdivergent Class IIs are vertical and dentoalveolar, rather than skeletal.

The literature review also showed that the differences between untreated hyperdivergent Class IIs and control subjects are substantially more pronounced in the mandible than in the maxilla [55]. Hyperdivergent Class IIs have greater anterior face heights and shorter ramus heights. The gonial angle is consistently larger and the mandibular plane is steeper among hyperdivergent Class IIs. Posterior dentoalveolar heights appear to be more affected than anterior heights.

The transverse dimensions of hyperdivergent Class IIs are also affected. Molar widths, both in the upper and lower jaws, tend to be narrower in Class II division 1 subjects than in normal subjects [56–59]. Width differences between Class IIs and Class Is often become evident during the deciduous dentition stage of development (Figure 6.8). Hyperdivergent subjects also have taller and thinner mandibular symphyses than normo- and hypodivergent

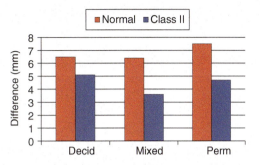

Figure 6.8 Differences in maxillary and mandibular intermolar widths of males with normal and Class II malocclusion during the deciduous (Decid), mixed, and permanent (Perm) dentition stages (Bishara et al. [57]/with permission of Elsevier).

subjects [60]. Finally, hyperdivergent subjects have thinner cortical bone, both in the maxilla and the mandible [61–63].

6.4 Developmental changes of Class IIs

From a growth perspective, it is the hyperdivergent retrognathic Class IIs that the orthodontist must be most concerned about. Compared to Class II individuals whose AP relations improve over time, those whose relations worsen show less anterior displacement of pogonion and greater posterior movements of gonion (Figure 6.9). This shows that the changes in AP skeletal relationships that occur are usually related to the vertical changes that occur. Untreated subjects whose AP relationships worsen over time also become more hyperdivergent over time [64].

Orthodontists must understand that the growth patterns of most hyperdivergent Class II patients are established early. Differences in lower facial height between deep and open-bite subjects are well established before the mixed dentition phase [65]. Individuals who have higher MPAs in the permanent dentition also have higher MPAs during the mixed dentition [66]. Bishara and Jakobsen [67] showed that 82% of adults classified as hyperdivergent were hyperdivergent when they were 5 years

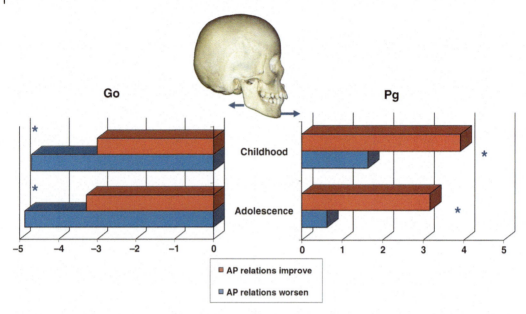

Figure 6.9 The anteroposterior changes in the position of gonion (Go) and pogonion (Pg) of females during childhood (6–10 years) and adolescence (10–15 years), based on cranial base superimposition (Adapted from Buschang and Martins [64]).

of age. Larger samples have shown that approximately 75% of 10-year-olds classified as hyperdivergent, within normal limits, or hypodivergent maintain their classifications through 15 years of age [68]. In contrast, AP discrepancies are more difficult to distinguish early [69]. Orthodontists should consider early-developing vertical and transverse discrepancies as evidence of later-developing AP discrepancies.

To be able to effectively treat hyperdivergent retrognathic Class II patients, the clinician must understand what true mandibular rotation is, when it occurs, and how it occurs. True forward or anterior rotation (a.k.a. total rotation, as described by Björk and Skieller [70]) occurs when the posterior aspect of the mandible is displaced down more than its anterior aspect (Figure 6.10). Due to the orientation of the corpus, this results in both inferior and anterior mandibular displacements. True mandibular rotation is not the same as the rotation of the mandibular plane (a.k.a. apparent rotation): true rotation is not affected by surface modeling changes, whereas the MPA is substantially affected by modeling. Most of the true rotational changes that occur are masked by the modeling changes (i.e. posterior resorption and anterior deposition) that normally occur on the lower mandibular border.

True mandibular rotation is important because it explains the divergence, the retrognathia, and the other morphological characteristics of the most problematic Class II division 1 patients. Untreated subjects who undergo backward rotation or less than average forward rotation tend to be more hyperdivergent [71]. Karlsen [30], who designed a study to evaluate this relationship, showed that 12-year-old boys with low MPAs (SN-MP ≤ 26°) exhibited significantly greater (1.6–3.5°) true forward rotation than boys with high (SN-MP ≥ 35°) MPA.

Most importantly, true mandibular rotation is the primary determinant of AP chin and AP mandibular tooth positions. True rotation is more closely associated with AP changes in chin position than condylar growth or fossa displacement; for every degree of true rotation, the chins of children and adolescents come forward 1.2 and

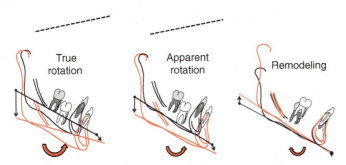

Figure 6.10 True rotation of the mandible's implant or stable structure line relative to the cranial base, apparent rotation of the lower border of the mandible relative to the cranial base, and angular remodeling of the lower mandibular border (Buschang and Jacob [71]/with permission of Elsevier).

1.4 mm, respectively [71]. Because the glenoid fossa is typically displaced back more than the condyle grows back, true rotation remains the key mechanism explaining the normal anterior repositioning of the chin and mandibular teeth [72]. True rotation is also the key to understanding AP changes in chin position of treated patients [73].

Importantly, true rotation also explains why the mandibles of hyperdivergent Class IIs are abnormally shaped (Figure 6.11). Untreated individuals whose mandibles rotate only slightly forward or backward exhibit less condylar growth, oriented in a more posterior direction than subjects who undergo greater amounts of forward rotation [74–76]. Modeling of the entire mandible is affected by its rotational pattern. Rotation affects the mandibular morphology of both untreated and treated children. Compared to untreated controls, mixed-dentition patients randomly allocated for bionator therapy had mandibles that protracted and rotated slightly backward, producing a posterior redirection of condylar growth and ramus modeling [77]. Functional appliances protract the mandible and rotate it slightly backward, and the condyles adapt by growing more posteriorly [66, 78, 79]. More posterior-directed condylar growth explains the larger gonial angles seen among hyperdivergent Class IIs. True rotation

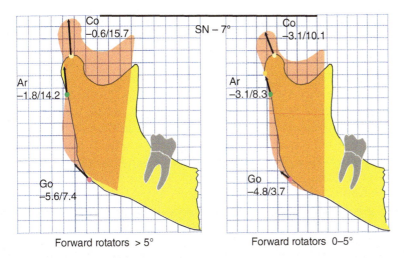

Figure 6.11 The horizontal and vertical (hor/vert) growth and modeling changes of selected landmarks in adolescents 10–15 years of age who exhibited true mandibular rotation greater and less than five degrees (Adapted from Buschang and Gandini Júnior [66]).

has also been closely related to the modeling changes that occur on the lower border of the mandible [80, 81]. Finally, less than-average amounts of true forward rotation and backward rotation are related to lower incisor retroclination, resulting in a loss of arch perimeter [74]. Backward rotators often do not develop chins because their symphyses rotate downwards, causing the incisors to retrocline and supraerupt, which in turn produces a straight, long, and narrow symphyseal morphology.

6.5 Class II developmental changes

Longitudinal studies consistently show little or no differences between Class IIs and Class Is in the AP maxillomandibular changes that occur during childhood and adolescence. Most studies have found no class differences in the ANB or Wits changes [41, 42, 44], or in the increases of SNA and SNB that occur [41, 42, 45, 47], although there are exceptions. Ngan et al. [41] showed that the Class II ANB angle decreased slightly over time due to greater decreases of SNA than SNB; the ANB angle of Class Is decreased due to greater increases of SNB than SNA. Significantly larger increases in the maxillomandibular differential have also been reported in Class Is than in Class IIs [45].

While Class Is and Class IIs generally show longitudinal decreases in mandibular divergence, the decreases tend to be somewhat greater for Class Is [42, 44]. Stahl et al. [45] showed slightly greater decreases during adolescence in the mandibular plane and gonial angles in Class Is than in Class IIs, but the differences were not statistically significant. Ngan et al. [41] showed that Class IIs develop slight vertical tendencies after 10 years of age (MPA and Y-axis increase slightly and the PFH/AFH ratio decreases slightly) while the growth pattern of Class Is becomes more horizontal. The differences between Class Is and Class IIs appear to be more pronounced for females [42, 44].

Riesmeijer et al. [44] also showed that the gonial angle (Ar-Go-Me) increases more in Class IIs than Class Is between 7 and 14 years of age. Similar growth changes in the direction of mandibular growth (Y-axis or N-S-Gn) have also been reported for Class Is and Class IIs [82]. Based on 130 subjects followed between 10 and 15 years of age, Class IIs showed only slightly greater (0.2°) decreases in the MPA than Class Is [47].

In terms of size, Class II mandibles tend to be smaller than Class I mandibles, but the growth differences are small and do not become apparent until adolescence. Ngan et al. [41] showed similar increases among Class Is and Class IIs in overall (Ar-Gn) and corpus (Go-Gn) lengths between 7 and 10 years of age, but greater increases among Class Is between 10 and 14 years of age. Longitudinal assessments show that the overall mandibular length (Co-Gn) of Class IIs becomes significantly shorter between 10 and 15 years of age [47]. Stahl et al. [45] demonstrated significantly greater increases in overall mandibular length (Co-Gn) and ramus height (Co–Co) during adolescence among Class Is than Class IIs. Bishara [42] found that overall mandibular length (Ar-Pg) was smaller in Class IIs than in Class Is during the mixed and permanent dentition stages, but the differences decreased slightly. Buschang et al. [82] reported small rate differences in the growth of S-Gn between Class Is and Class IIs that accumulated between 6 and 15 years of age.

The differences in overall mandibular length between untreated Class Is and Class IIs are due to differences in condylar growth. The condylion undergoes significantly more overall (14.1 vs. 12.1 mm) growth in Class Is than in Class IIs between 10 and 15 years of age [47]. The yearly difference was small (0.4 mm/yr) and due primarily to more vertical condylar growth in Class Is than in Class IIs. Class I subjects also showed greater modeling change at gonion (7.8 vs. 6.9 mm), again due to greater superior drift of the gonion. The differences between Class Is and Class IIs are primarily due to the reduced growth rates exhibited by hyperdivergent Class IIs; the condylar growth of hypodivergent Class IIs is similar to the growth of hypodivergent Class Is. This helps to explain why hypodivergent Class IIs undergo greater increases in posterior face height between 9 and 18 years of age than hyperdivergent Class IIs, and why hypodivergent Class IIs show greater decreases in facial convexity and more flattening of the MPA than hyperdivergent Class IIs [83].

While Class IIs typically present with greater overjet and slightly greater overbite than Class Is, the changes in overjet and overbite are similar. Stahl et al. [45] showed no Class differences in the adolescent changes of overbite, overjet, or molar relationships. Bishara [42] reported that between the deciduous and mixed dentition, there were only slightly (0.4 mm) greater decreases in overjet among Class II males, and slightly (0.2 mm) greater increases for Class I females. Increases in overbite between the deciduous and permanent dentitions were only slightly smaller (0.2–0.4 mm) in Class IIs than in Class Is.

6.6 Etiology

The norm of reaction reminds us that the same genotype can produce a variety of phenotypes, depending on the environmental circumstances. For example, modern-day Finns exhibit substantially larger gonial and MPAs than Finnish samples from the 15th and 16th centuries [84]. Since the period is insufficient for genetic changes to have occurred, the same genotypes must have been adapting to different environmental factors. The Finnish population also shows marked increases in the prevalence of Class II malocclusion over the past few centuries (Figure 6.12). The skeletal remains of individuals living in the 1600s indicate very low levels of Class II malocclusion, with a prevalence of less than 2% [85]. By 1920, the proportion of Finns with Class II malocclusion had increased to 13.5%, and by 1950 it had increased to almost 24%. The secular trend toward increases in malocclusion over the past few hundred years has been well established [86, 87].

There is little or no evidence that the Bolton tooth-size discrepancy, which is highly heritable [88], is higher or lower than expected among subjects with Class II malocclusion. While there are exceptions, the majority of studies have shown no significant differences in the anterior, posterior, or overall Bolton ratios between Class IIs and Class Is (Table 6.5).

The chondrocranium, another highly heritable component of the craniofacial complex, exhibits growth differences between Class Is and Class IIs. While most of the literature shows no differences in anterior or posterior cranial base lengths, several studies indicate larger cranial base angles among Class IIs (Table 6.6). A larger cranial base angle positions the Class II

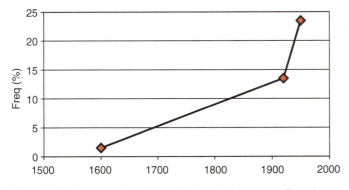

Figure 6.12 Frequencies of Class II malocclusion among Finns born around the year 1600, 1920, and around 1950 (Varrela [85]/with permission of Elsevier).

Table 6.5 Differences (Class II minus Class I) in the anterior, posterior, and overall Bolton ratios.

	Anterior	Posterior	Overall	Ethnicity
Sperry et al. [89]	NS	N/A	NS	US
Crosby and Alexander [90]	NS	N/A	NS	US
Nie and Lin [91]	↓ (−0.7%)	↓ (−1.8%)	↓ (−1.3%)	Chinese
Ta et al. [92]	NS	N/A	NS	Chinese
Alkofide and Hashim [93]	↑ (0.7%) [1]	N/A	NS	Saudi
Araujo and Souki [94]	NS	N/A	NS	Brazil
Uysal and Sari [95]	NS	N/A	NS	Turkey
Al-Khateeb and Al-Khateeb [35]	NS	N/A	NS	Jordan
Fattahi et al. [96]	↓ (−1.7%)	NS	↓ (−1.2%)	Iran
Strujić et al. [97]	NS	NS	↓ (−0.7%)	Croatia
Wedrychowska-Szulc et al. [98]	NS	N/A	NS	Poland
Johe et al. [99]	NS	N/A	NS	US
Summary	NS	(9 to 3)	NS (2 to 1)	NS (9 to 3)

Arrows indicate direction of across the board difference; NS, prob > 0.05; NA, no data available; [1] significant for females only.

Table 6.6 Differences (Class II minus Class I) in cranial base angulation, anterior length, and posterior length.

Article	Cl I/Cl II	Anterior CB	Posterior CB	Angle
Agarwal et al. [100]	52/51	NA	NA	NS
Bacon et al. [101]	41/45	NS	II > I	II > I
Bishara et al. [102]	35/30	NS	NS	NS
Chin et al. [103]	27/30	NS	NS	II > I
Dhoptkar et al. [43]	50/50	II > I	II > I	II > I
Kerr and Hirst [104]	51/34	NA	NA	II > I
Hopkin et al. [105]	96/96	II > I	II > I	II > I
Liu et al. [106]	17/20	I > II	II > I	NS
Menezes [49]	31/37	NS	NS	NS
Ngan et al. [41]	20/20	NS	NS	NS
Polat and Kaya [107]	25/25	NS	NS	NS
Stahl et al. [44]	17/17	NA	NA	II > I
Vandekar et al. [108]	25/25	NA	NA	NS
Wilhelm et al. [109]	22/21	NS	NS	NS
Most common	NS	NS	(6 to 4)	NS

maxilla relatively forward and the mandible relatively back. A larger cranial base angle among Class IIs would also support a genetic predisposition for malocclusion.

To understand the etiology of Class II malocclusion, the hypo- and hyperdivergent subjects must again be considered separately. Skeletally, the Class IIs who are hypodivergent more closely resemble Class Is than their hyperdivergent Class II counterparts. Since the skeletal growth of those who are strictly dental Class IIs is "normal," their molar/canine discrepancies must be due to either 1) deciduous discrepancies too large to self-correct during childhood and adolescence and/or 2) insufficient primate and leeway space allowing for the transition to Class I molar relationships [110–112]. As previously indicated, the Class II dental relationships of subjects with division 2 malocclusion are primarily due to maxillary restriction of mandibular dentoalveolar growth related to incisor inclination. The mandibles of hypodivergent Class IIs typically advance slightly more than their maxillae, resulting in small, cumulative reductions of their AP maxillomandibular relationships. This explains why some Class IIs classified as retrognathic at younger ages, become orthognathic at older ages.

Hypodivergent Class IIs have favorable, more horizontally directed, growth patterns that facilitate treatments. A comparison of favorably growing Class II adolescents and adults treated with the same Tweed edgewise mechanics and four premolar extractions showed that 70% of the molar correction among the adolescents was due to differential mandibular growth; the adult molar corrections were entirely due to tooth movements [113]. Favorable mandibular growth also enhances the outcomes of cervical-pull headgear [114] and functional appliance [54] treatments. Similar enhancements should not be expected for hyperdivergent Class IIs with unfavorable growth patterns.

For most of the hyperdivergent Class IIs, the skeletal manifestations are best explained as development maladaptation to environmental circumstances. Three broad environmental factors have been proposed to explain the development of their malocclusions, including habits, interferences with normal breathing, and decreases in masticatory muscle strength [115].

The development of Class IIs whose AP discrepancies are due primarily to maxillary protrusion may be linked to persistent finger habits. Older (7–16 years) children with persistent thumb-sucking habits show greater tendencies for open-bite malocclusions, a propensity toward Class II molar and canine relationships, proclined upper incisors, and longer maxillae, but their mandibular and palatal plane angles are normal [116]. In other words, Class IIs with persistent finger habits are not necessarily more hyperdivergent. There is also a high prevalence of crossbites among children in the deciduous dentition who habitually suck their fingers [117, 118] or pacifiers [119, 120]. However, most crossbites self-correct if the habit is stopped before the transition to the early mixed dentition, and most children with finger habits after the transitional dentition do not exhibit crossbites after 9 years of age [121, 122].

Airway interferences and decreased masticatory muscle strength provide the most widely recognized explanation for the etiology of hyperdivergent, retrognathic Class IIs. The differential growth of the maxilla and mandible, which best explains the normalization of molar and canine relationships over time, cannot be relied upon in hyperdivergent Class IIs [123]. Due to less than average forward or backward mandibular true rotation, the mandibular teeth of hyperdivergent Class IIs are not displaced sufficiently forward to establish Class I molar and canine relationships.

Airway interferences have been more closely linked than habits with the development of the hyperdivergent retrognathic phenotype [55]. The marked phenotypic similarities reported for subjects with enlarged tonsils, allergic rhinitis, and enlarged adenoids lead to the conclusion that chronic airway interferences produce similar phenotypes. The classic experiment performed by Harvold et al. [124] established a causal link between blocked nasal airways and the development of steeper mandibular planes and larger gonial angles. Multiple studies show that children with enlarged adenoids have increased lower anterior facial heights, larger gonial angles, narrow maxillary arches, smaller SNB angles, retroclined incisors, and larger MPAs than their nose breathing counterparts [125–127]. Following adenoidectomies, spontaneous improvements in the mandibular growth direction, MPAs, arch widths, and incisor inclinations have been reported [126, 128–130].

Chronically enlarged tonsils, sleep apnea, and allergic rhinitis also produce the same hyperdivergent retrognathic phenotype. Behlfelt et al. [131] demonstrated that 10-year-old children with enlarged tonsils were more retrognathic, had longer anterior facial heights, and had larger MPAs than children who do not have enlarged tonsils. Children with obstructive sleep apnea also have steeper MPAs, greater lower anterior face heights, and more retroclined incisors [132], as do children with allergic rhinitis [133–136]. Trask et al. [136] showed that mouth breathers with perennial allergic rhinitis have deeper palates, retroclined lower incisors, smaller SNB and SNPg angles, increased overjet, increased lower face heights, larger gonial angles, and larger MPAs than their siblings. These associations are important because the prevalence of allergic rhinitis ranges between 10% and 20% [137], and it appears to be increasing.

Reduced masticatory muscle force must also be considered as a possible etiologic factor. There is a link between softer diets, reduced muscle function, and hyperdivergence. Experimental studies show that growing animals fed on soft diets exhibit structural differences in their masticatory muscles, lower bite forces, differences in condylar growth, narrower maxillae, and differences in bony modeling [139–137]. Hyperdivergence among humans has also been directly related to reduced muscle size, lower EMG activity, and reduced muscle efficiency [137–143]. Both adults [8, 10] and children [9] with larger MPAs have substantially weaker bite forces. Increased dentoalveolar heights have also been associated with decreased masticatory muscle function [144, 145].

Patients with muscular dystrophy [146, 147] and spinal muscular atrophy [148] most dramatically demonstrate the relationship between muscle function and hyperdivergence. The recessive gene defects that directly weaken the masticatory muscles of these individuals indirectly produce narrow and deep palates, increased anterior facial heights, increased gonial angles, steeper mandibular planes, and malocclusions.

Mandibular posture provides the best and most logical explanation for the same hyperdivergent retrognathic phenotype among subjects with airway blockages and weakened muscles. In addition to the direct experimental support of the relationship between masticatory muscle strength and mandibular posture [145], there is substantial indirect evidence supporting the relationship [149–151]. Mouth breathers reposition their mandibles to breathe, and it is more efficient to lower than protrude or laterotrude the mandible. Experimental obstruction of the upper airway results in lowered resting posture of the mandible, and a 5° increase in the craniocervical extension [152]. If lowered mandibular posture is habitual, and the subject has growth potential, then the dentition, dentoalveolar complex, and mandible will adapt to its changed position (Figure 6.13). Lowering mandibular posture immediately increases the MPA and decreases the posterior-to-anterior face height ratio. Lowered mandibular posture also produces transverse deficiencies over time. As the child grows, a lowered posture further increases anterior face height and the teeth supraerupt to compensate. Whether or not the anterior teeth supraerupt depends, at least in part, on whether the tongue or lips are postured between the teeth, in which case open bites are produced. The mandibular incisors adapt to a

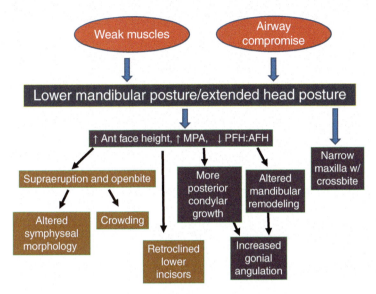

Figure 6.13 Flow chart showing the development of the hyperdivergent retrognathic Class IIs (Buschang et al. [55]/with permission of Elsevier).

lowered mandibular position by retroclining. Retroclination and overeruption cause changes in symphyseal morphology and increase crowding. Lowered mandibular and tongue posture also leads to a narrow maxillary arch with possible crossbites. Finally, a lower posture leads to changes in the mandible's remodeling pattern and a more posteriorly directed condylar growth, which in turn leads to increases in the gonial angle.

References

1 Angle EH. *Treatment of malocclusion of the teeth*. Philadelphia, PA: S.S. White Dental Manufacturing Co, 1907.
2 Ricketts RM. *Orthodontic diagnosis and planning*. Philadelphia, PA: Saunders, 1982.
3 English JD, Buschang PH, Throckmorton GS. Does malocclusion affect masticatory performance? *Angle Orthod* 2002;**72**(1):21–7.
4 Henrikson T, Ekberg EC, Nilner M. Masticatory efficiency and ability in relation to occlusion and mandibular dysfunction in girls. *Int J Prosthodont* 1998;**11**(2):125–32.
5 Owens S, Buschang PH, Throckmorton GS, et al. Masticatory performance and areas of occlusal contact and near contact in subjects with normal occlusion and malocclusion. *Am J Orthod Dentofacial Orthop* 2002;**121**(6):602–9.
6 Lepley CR, Throckmorton GS, Ceen RF, Buschang PH. Relative contribution of occlusion, maximum bite force, and chewing cycle kinematics to masticatory performance. *Am J Orthod Dentofacial Orthop* 2011;**139**(5):606–13.
7 Hisano M, Soma K. Energy-based re-evaluation of Angle's Class I molar relationship. *J Oral Rehabil* 1999; **26**(10):830–5.
8 Proffit WR, Fields HW, Nixon WL. Occlusal forces in normal- and long-face adults. *J Dent Res* 1983;**62**(5):566–70.
9 García-Morales P, Buschang PH, Throckmorton GS, English JD. Maximum bite force, muscle efficiency and mechanical advantage in children with vertical growth patterns. *Eur J Orthod* 2003;**25**(3):265–72.

10 Ingervall B, Minder C. Correlation between maximum bite force and facial morphology in children. *Angle Orthod* 1997;**67**(6):415–22.

11 Czarnecki ST, Nanda RS, Currier GF. Perceptions of a balanced facial profile. *Am J Orthod Dentofacial Orthop* 1993;**104**(2):180–7.

12 Michiels G, Sather AH. Determinants of facial attractiveness in a sample of white women. *Int J Adult Orthodon Orthognath Surg* 1994;**9**(2):95–103.

13 Maple JR, Vig KW, Beck FM, et al. A comparison of providers' and consumers' perceptions of facial-profile attractiveness. *Am J Orthod Dentofacial Orthop* 2005;**128**(6):690–6.

14 Spyropoulos MN, Halazonetis DJ. Significance of the soft tissue profile on facial esthetics. *Am J Orthod Dentofacial Orthop* 2001;**119**(5):464–71.

15 Naini FB, Donaldson AN, McDonald F, Cobourne MT. Influence of chin height on perceived attractiveness in the rethognathic patient, layperson, and clinician. *Angle Orthod* 2012;**82**(1):88–95.

16 Kelly JE, Sanchez M, Van Kirk LE. *An assessment of occlusion of teeth of children*. DHEW publication no 74–1612. Washington, DC: National Center for Health Statistics, 1973.

17 Kelly JE, Harvey C. *An assessment of the teeth of youths 12 to 17 years*. DHEW publication no 77–1644. Washington, DC: National Center for Health Statistics, 1977.

18 Proffit WR, Fields HW Jr, Moray LJ. Prevalence of malocclusion and orthodontic treatment need in the United States: estimates from the NHANES III survey. *Int J Adult Orthodon Orthognath Surg* 1998;**13**(2):97–106.

19 Alhammadi MS, Halboub E, Fayed MS, et al. Global distribution of malocclusion traits: a systematic review. *Dental Press J Orthod* 2018;**23**(6):40 e1–10.

20 Beresford JS. Tooth size and class distinction. *Dent Pract Dent Rec* 1969;**20**(3):113–20.

21 Milacic M, Markovic M. A comparative occlusal and cephalometric study of dental and skeletal anteriorposterior relationships. *Br J Orthod* 1983;**10**(1):53–4.

22 Ast DB, Carlos JP, Cons NC. The prevalence and characteristics of malocclusion among senior high school students in upstate New York. *Am J Orthod* 1965;**51**(6):437–45.

23 Massler M, Frankel JM. Prevalence of malocclusion in children aged 14 to 18 years. *Am J Orthod* 1951;**37**(10):751–68.

24 Mills LF. Epidemiologic studies of occlusion IV. The prevalence of malocclusion in a population of 1,455 school children. *J Dent Res* 1966;**45**(2):332–6.

25 Baldridge J. A study of the relation of the maxillary first permanent molars to the face in Class I and Class II malocclusion. *Angle Orthod* 1941;**11**(2):100–9.

26 Renfroe EW. A study of the facial patterns associated with Class I, Class II, Division 1, and Class II, Division 2 malocclusion. *Angle Orthod* 1948;**18**(1):12–5.

27 Wallis S. Integration of certain variants of the facial skeleton in Cl II, division 2 malocclusion. *Angle Orthod* 1963;**33**(1):60–7.

28 Godiawala RN, Joshi MR. A cephalometric comparison between class II, division 2 malocclusion and normal occlusion. *Angle Orthod* 1974;**44**(3):262–7.

29 Hitchcock HP. The cephalometric distinction of class II, division 2 malocclusion. *Am J Orthod* 1976;**69**(4):447–54.

30 Karlsen AT. Craniofacial characteristics in children with Angle Class II div. 2 malocclusion combined with extreme deep bite. *Angle Orthod* 1994;**64**(2):123–30.

31 Brezniak N, Arad A, Heller M, et al. Pathognomonic cephalometric characteristics of Angle Class II Division 2 malocclusion. *Angle Orthod* 2002;**72**(3):251–7.

32 Fischer-Brandies H, Fischer-Brandies E, Konig A. A cephalometric comparison between Angle Class II division 2 malocclusion and normal occlusion in adults. *Br J Orthod* 1985;**12**(3):158–62.

33 McIntyre GT, Millett DT. Lip shape and position in Class II division 2 maolocclusion. *Angle Orthod* 2006;**76**(5):739–44.

34 Isik F, Nalbantgil D, Sayinsu K, Arun T. A comparative study of cephalometric and arch width characteristics of Class II division 1 and division 2 malocclusions. *Eur J Orthod* 2006;**28**(2):179–83.

35 Al-Khateeb EAA, Al-Khateeb SN. Anteroposterior and vertical components of class II division 1 and division 2 malocclusion. *Angle Orthod* 2009;**79**(5): 859–66.

36 Barbosa LA, Araujo E, Behrents RG, Buschang PH. Longitudinal cephalometric growth of untreated subjects with Class II, division 2, malocclusion. *Am J Orthod Dentofacial Orthop* 2017;**151**(5):914–20.

37 Leighton BC, Adams CP. Incisor inclination in class 2 division 2 malocclusion. *Eur J Orthod* 1986;**8**(2):98–105.

38 Luffingham JK. The lower lip and the maxillary central incisor. *Eur J Orthod* 1982;**4**(4):263–8.

39 Lapatki BG, Mager AS, Shulte-Moenting J, Jonas IE. The importance of the level of the lip line and resting lip pressure in Class II, divisions 2 malocclusion. *J Dent Res* 2002;**81**(5):323–8.

40 McNamara JA Jr. Components of Class II malocclusion in children 8–10 years of age. *Angle Orthod* 1981;**51**(3):177–202.

41 Ngan PW, Byczek W, Scheick J. Longitudinal evaluation of growth changes in Class II division 1 subjects. *Semin Orthod* 1997;**3**(4):222–31.

42 Bishara SE. Mandibular changes in persons with untreated and treated Class II division 1 malocclusion. *Am J Orthod Dentofacial Orthop* 1998;**113**(6):661–73.

43 Dhopatkar A, Bhatia S, Rock P. An investigation into the relationship between the cranial base angle and malocclusion. *Angle Orthod* 2002;**72**(5):456–63.

44 Riesmeijer AM, Prahl-Andersen B, Mascarenhas AK, et al. A comparison of craniofacial Class I and Class II growth patterns. *Am J Orthod Dentofacial Orthop* 2004;**125**(4):463–71.

45 Stahl F, Baccetti T, Franchi L, McNamara JA Jr. Longitudinal growth changes in untreated subjects with Class II division 1 malocclusion. *Am J Orthod Dentofacial Orthop* 2008;**134**(1):125–37.

46 Baccetti T, Stahl F, McNamara JA Jr. Dentofacial growth changes in subjects with untreated Class II malocclusion from late puberty through young adulthood. *Am J Orthod Dentofacial Orthop* 2009;**135**(2):148–54.

47 Jacob HB, Buschang PH. Mandibular growth comparisons of class I and Class II division 1 skeletofacial patterns. *Angle Orthod* 2014;**84**(5):755–61.

48 Yoon SS, Chung CH. Comparison of craniofacial growth of untreated Class I and Class II girls from ages 9 to 18 years: a longitudinal study. *Am J Orthod Dentofacial Orthop* 2015;**147**(2):190–6.

49 Menezes DM. Comparisons of craniofacial features of English children with Angle Class II division 1 and Angle Class I occlusions. *J Dent* 1974;**2**(6):250–4.

50 Vasquez MJ, Baccetti T, Franchi L, McNamara JA Jr. Dentofacial features of class II malocclusion associated with maxillary skeletal protrusion: a longitudinal study at the circumpubertal growth period. *Am J Orthod Dentofacial Orthop* 2009;**135**(5):568.e1–7.

51 Craig EC. The skeletal patterns characteristic of Class I and Class II, division I malocclusions in norma lateralis. *Am J Orthod* 1951;**21**(1):44–56.

52 Nelson WE, Higley LB. The length of mandibular basal bone in normal occlusion and Class I malocclusion compared to Class II, division 1 malocclusion. *Am J Orthod* 1948;**34**(7):610–7.

53 Harris JE, Kowalski CJ, Walker GF. Discrimination between normal and Class II individuals using Steiner's analysis. *Angle Orthod* 1975;**42**(3):212–9.

54. Rogers K, Campbell PM, Tadlock L, et al. Treatment changes of hypo- and hyperdivergent Class II Herbst patients. *Angle Orthod* 2018;**88**(1):3–9.
55. Buschang PH, Jacob HB, Carrillo R. The morphological characteristics, growth, and etiology of the hyperdivergent phenotype. *Semin Orthod* 2013;**19**(4):121–6.
56. Fröhlich FJ. Changes in untreated Class II type malocclusions. *Angle Orthod* 1962;**32**(3):167–79.
57. Bishara SE, Bayati P, Jakobsen JR. Longitudinal comparisons of dental arch changes in normal and untreated Class II, Division 1 subjects and their clinical implications. *Am J Orthod Dentofacial Orthop* 1996;**110**(5):483–9.
58. Baccetti T, Franchi L, McNamara JA Jr, Tollaro I. Early dentofacial features of Class II malocclusion: a longitudinal study from the deciduous through the mixed dentition. *Am J Orthod Dentofacial Orthop* 1997;**111**(5):502–9.
59. Alvaran N, Roldan SI, Buschang PH. Maxillary and mandibular arch widths of Colombians. *Am J Orthod Dentofacial Orthop* 2009;**135**(5):649–56.
60. Beckmann SH, Kuitert RB, Prahl-Andersen B, et al. Alveolar and skeletal dimensions associated with lower face height. *Am J Orthod Dentofacial Orthop* 1998;**113**(5):498–506.
61. Tsunori M, Mashita M, Kasai K. Relationship between facial types and tooth and bone characteristics of the mandible obtained by CT scanning. *Angle Orthod* 1998;**68**(6):557–62.
62. Swasty D, Lee J, Huang JC, et al. Cross-sectional human mandibular morphology as assessed in vivo by cone-beam computed tomography in patients with different vertical facial dimensions. *Am J Orthod Dentofacial Orthop* 2011;**139**(Suppl 4):e377–89.
63. Horner KA, Behrents RG, Kim KB, Buschang PH. Cortical bone and ridge thickness of hyperdivergent and hypodivergent adults. *Am J Orthod Dentofacial Orthop* 2012;**142**(2):170–8.
64. Buschang PH, Martins J. Childhood and adolescent changes of skeletal relationships. *Angle Orthod* 1998;**68**(3):199–208.
65. Nanda SK. Patterns of vertical growth in the face. *Am J Orthod Dentofacial Orthop* 1988;**93**(2):103–16.
66. Buschang PH, Gandini Júnior LG. Mandibular skeletal growth and modelling between 10 and 15 years of age. *Eur J Orthod* 2002;**24**(1):69–79.
67. Bishara SE, Jakobsen JR. Longitudinal changes in three normal facial types. *Am J Orthod* 1985;**88**(6):466–502.
68. Jacob HB, Buschang PH. Vertical craniofacial growth changes in French-Canadian between 10–15 years of age. *Am J Orthod Dentofacial Orthop* 2011;**139**(6):797–805.
69. Rhodes JD. Cephalometric indications of developing skeletal discrepancies in young children. Master's Thesis, Baylor College of Dentistry, Texas A&M Health Science Center, 1990.
70. Björk A, Skieller V. Normal and abnormal growth of the mandible. A synthesis of longitudinal cephalometric implant studies over a period of 25 years. *Eur J Orthod* 1983;**5**(1):1–46.
71. Buschang PH, Jacob HB. Mandibular rotation revisited: what makes it so important? *Semin Orthod* 2014;**20**(4):299–315.
72. Buschang PH, Santos-Pinto A. Condylar growth and glenoid fossa displacement during childhood and adolescence. *Am J Orthod Dentofacial Orthop* 1998;**113**(4):437–42.
73. LaHaye MB, Buschang PH, Alexander RG, Boley JC. Orthodontic treatment changes of chin position in Class II Division 1 patients. *Am J Orthod Dentofacial Orthop* 2006;**130**(6):732–41.
74. Björk A, Skieller V. Facial development and tooth eruption. An implant study at the age of puberty. *Am J Orthod* 1972;**62**:339–83.

75 Lavergne J, Gasson N. A metal implant study of mandibular rotation. *Angle Orthod* 1976;**46**(2):144–50.

76 Ødegaard J. Mandibular rotation studies with the aid of metal implants. *Am J Orthod* 1970;**58**:448–54.

77 Araujo A, Buschang PH, Melo ACM. Adaptive condylar growth and mandibular remodeling changes with bionator therapy – an implant study. *Eur J Orthod* 2004;**26**(5):515–22.

78 Hultgren BW, Isaacson RJ, Erdman AG, Worms FW. Mechanics, growth, and class II corrections. *Am J Orthod* 1978;**74**(4):388–95.

79 Birkebæk L, Melsen B, Terp S. A laminagraphic study of the alterations in the temporo-mandibular joint following activator treatment. *Eur J Orthod* 1984;**6**(4):257–66.

80 Spady M, Buschang PH, Demirjian A, LaPalme L. Mandibular rotation and angular remodeling during childhood and adolescence. *Am J Hum Biol* 1992;**4**:683–9.

81 Wang MK, Buschang PH, Behrents R. Mandibular rotation and remodeling changes during early childhood. *Angle Orthod* 2009;**79**:271–5.

82 Buschang PH, Tanguay R, Demirjian A, et al. Mathematical models of longitudinal mandibular growth for children with normal and untreated Class II, division 1, malocclusion. *Eur J Orthod* 1988;**10**(3):227–34.

83 Chung CH, Wong WW. Craniofacial growth in untreated skeletal Class II subjects: a longitudinal study. *Am J Orthod Dentofacial Orthop* 2002;**122**(6):619–26.

84 Varrela J. Effects of attritive diet on craniofacial morphology: a cephalometric analysis of a Finnish skull sample. *Eur J Orthod* 1990;**12**(2):219–23.

85 Varrela J. Masticatory function and malocclusion: a clinical perspective. *Semin Orthod* 2006;**12**(2):102–9.

86 Welland FJ, Jonke E, Bantleon HP. Secular trend in malocclusion in Austrian men. *Eur J Orthod* 1997;**19**(4):355–9.

87 Corruccini RS. *How anthropology informs the orthodontic diagnosis of malocclusion's causes.* Lewiston, NY: Edwin Mellen Press, 1999.

88 Baydas B, Oktay H, Dağsuyu IM. The effect of heritability on Bolton tooth-size discrepancy. *Eur J Orthod* 2005;**27**(1):98–102.

89 Sperry TP, Worms FW, Isaacson RJ, Speidel TM. Tooth-size discrepancy in mandibular prognathism. *Am J Orthod* 1977;**72**(2):183–90.

90 Crosby DR, Alexander CG. The occurance of tooth size discrepancies among different malocclusion groups. *Am J Orthod Dentofacial Orthop* 1989;**95**(6):457–61.

91 Nie Q, Lin J. Comparison of intermaxillary tooth size discrepancies among different malocclusion groups. *Am J Orthod Dentofacial Orthop* 1999;**116**(5):539–44.

92 Ta TA, Ling JYK, Hägg U. Tooth-size discrepancies among different occlusion groups of southern Chinese children. *Am J Orthod Dentofacial Orthop* 2001;**120**(5):556–8.

93 Alkofide E, Hashim H. Intermaxillary tooth size discrepancies among different malocclusion classes: a comparative study. *J Clin Pediatr Dent* 2002;**26**(4):383–8.

94 Araujo E, Souki M. Bolton anterior tooth size discrepancies among different malocclusion groups. *Angle Orthod* 2003;**73**(3):307–13.

95 Uysal T, Sari Z. Intermaxillary tooth size discrepancy and mesiodistal crown dimensions for a Turkish population. *Am J Orthod Dentofacial Orthop* 2005;**128**(2):226–30.

96 Fattahi HR, Pakshir HR, Hedayati Z. Comparison of tooth size discrepancies among different malocclusion groups. *Eur J Orthod* 2006;**28**(5):491–5.

97 Strujić M, Anić-Milošević S, Meštrović S, Šlaj M. Tooth size discrepancy in orthodontic patients among different malocclusion groups. *Eur J Orthod* 2009;**31**(6):584–9.

98 Wedrychowska-Szulc B, Janiszewska-Olszowska J, Stepien P. Overall and anterior Bolton ratio in Class I, II, and III orthodontic patients. *Eur J Orthod* 2010;**32**(3):313–8.

99 Johe RS, Steinhart T, Sado N, et al. Intermaxillary tooth-size discrepancies in different sexes, malocclusion groups, and ethnicities. *Am J Orthod Dentofacial Orthop* 2010;**138**(5):599–607.

100 Agarwal A, Pandey H, Bajaj K, Pandey L. Changes in cranial base morphology in Class I and Class II division 1 malocclusion. *J Int Oral Health* 2013;**5**(1):39–42.

101 Bacon W, Eiller V, Hildwein M, Dubois G. The cranial base in subjects with dental and skeletal Class II. *Eur J Orthod* 1992;**14**(3):224–8.

102 Bishara SE, Jakobsen JR, Vorhies B, Bayati P. Changes in dentofacial structures in untreated Class II division 1 and normal subjects: a longitudinal study. *Angle Orthod* 1997;**67**(1):55–66.

103 Chin A, Perry S, Liao C, Yang Y. The relationship between the cranial base and jaw base in a Chinese population. *Head Face Med* 2014;**10**(1):1–8.

104 Kerr WJS, Hirst D. Craniofacial characteristics of subjects with normal and postnormal occlusions – A longitudinal study. *Am J Orthod Dentofacial Orthop* 1987;**92**(3):207–12.

105 Hopkins GB, Houston WJB, James GA. The cranial base as an aetiological factor in malocclusion. *Angle Orthod* 1968;**38**(3):250–5.

106 Liu Y, Liu F, Zheng Y, Yu X. Morphological characteristics of the cranial base in sagittal malocclusion. *J Hard Tissue Biol* 2013;**22**(2):249–54.

107 Polat OO, Kaya B. Changes in cranial base morphology in different malocclusions. *Orthod Craniofacial Res* 2007;**10**(4):216–21.

108 Vandekar M, Kulkarni P, Vaid N. Role of cranial base morphology in determining skeletal anteroposterior relationship of the jaws. *J Ind Orthod Soc* 2013;**47**(4):245–8.

109 Wilhelm BM, Beck FM, Lidral AC, Vic KWL. A comparison of cranial base growth in Class I and Class II skeletal patterns. *Am J Orthod Dentofacial Orthop* 2001;**119**(4):401–5.

110 Baume LJ. Physiological tooth migration and its significance for the development of occlusion. II. The biogenesis of accessional dentition. *J Dent Res* 1950;**29**(3):331–7.

111 Baume LJ. Physiological tooth migration and its significance for the development of occlusion. III. The biogenesis of successional dentition. *J Dent Res* 1950;**29**(3):338–48.

112 Moorrees CFA, Grøn AM, Lebret LML, et al. Growth studies of the dentition: a review. *Am J Orthod* 1969;**55**(6):600–16.

113 Harris EF, Dyer GS, Vaden JL. Age effects on orthodontic treatment: skeletodental assessments from the Johnston analysis. *Am J Orthod Dentofacial Orthop* 1991;**100**(6):531–6.

114 Elms TN, Buschang PH, Alexander RG. Long-term stability of Class II, Division 1, nonextraction cervical face-bow therapy: I. Model analysis. *Am J Orthod Dentofacial Orthop* 1996;**109**(3):271–6.

115 Varrela J, Alanen P. Prevention and early treatment in orthodontics: a perspective. *J Dent Res* 1995;**74**(8):1436–8.

116 Subtelny JD. Oral habits. Studies in form, function and therapy. *Angle Orthod* 1973;**43**(4):347–83.

117 Popovich F. The prevalence of sucking habits and its relationship to oral malformations. *Appl Ther* 1966;**8**(8):689–91.

118 Köhler L, Holst K. Malocclusion and sucking habits of four-year-old children. *Acta Paediatr Scand* 1973;**62**(4):373–9.

119 Larsson E. Dummy- and finger-sucking habits in 4-year-olds. *Sven Tandlak Tidskr* 1975;**68**(6):219–24.

120 Svedmyr B. Dummy sucking. A study of its prevalence, duration and malocclusion consequences. *Swed Dent J* 1979;**3**(6):205–10.

121 Larsson E. Dummy- and finger-sucking habits with special attention to their significance for facial growth and occlusion. 7. The effect of earlier dummy- and finger-sucking habit in 16-year-old children compared with children without

earlier sucking habits. *Swed Dent J* 1978;**2**(1):23–33.
122. Larsson E. Prevalence of crossbite among children with prolonged dummy- and finger-sucking habit. *Swed Dent J* 1983;**7**(4):115–9.
123. Tsourakis AK, Johnston LE Jr. Class II malocclusion: the aftermath of a "perfect storm". *Semin Orthod* 2014;**20**(1):59–73.
124. Harvold EP, Tomer BS, Vargevik K, Chierici G. Primate experiments in oral respiration. *Am J Orthod* 1981;**79**(4):359–72.
125. Linder-Aronson S. Adenoids. Their effect on mode of breathing and nasal airflow and their relationship to characteristics of the facial skeleton and the dentition. A biometric, rhino-manometric and cephalometro-radiographic study on children with and without adenoids. *Acta Otolaryngol Suppl* 1970;**265**:1–132.
126. Kerr WJS, McWilliam JS, Linder-Aronson S. Mandibular form and position related to changed mode of breathing – a five-year longitudinal study. *Angle Orthod* 1989;**59**(2):91–6.
127. Arun T, Isik F, Sayinsu K. Vertical growth changes after adenoidectomy. *Angle Orthod* 2003;**73**(2):146–50.
128. Linder-Aronson S. Effects of adenoidectomy on dentition and nasopharynx. *Trans Eur Orthod Soc* 1972:177–86.
129. Linder-Aronson S, Woodside DG, Lundstrom A. Mandibular growth direction following adenoidectomy. *Am J Orthod Dentofacial Orthop* 1986;**89**(4):273–84.
130. Woodside DG, Linder-Aronson S, Lundstrom A, McWilliam J. Mandibular and maxillary growth after changed mode of breathing. *Am J Orthod Dentofacial Orthop* 1991;**100**(1):1–18.
131. Behlfelt K, Linder-Aronson S, McWilliam J, et al. Cranio-facial morphology in children with and without enlarged tonsils. *Eur J Orthod* 1990;**12**(3):233–43.
132. Zettergren-Wijk L, Forsberg CM, Linder-Aronson S. Changes in dentofacial morphology after adeno-/tonsillectomy in young children with obstructive sleep apnea – a 5-year follow-up study. *Eur J Orthod* 2006;**28**(4):319–26.
133. Bresolin D, Shapiro PA, Shapiro GG, et al. Mouth breathing in allergic children: its relationship to dentofacial development. *Am J Orthod* 1983;**83**(4):334–40.
134. Stein E, Flax SJ. Acephalometric study of children with chronic perennial allergic rhinitis. *J Dent Assoc S Afr* 1996;**51**(12):794–801.
135. Harari D, Redlich M, Miri S, et al. The effect of mouth breathing versus nasal breathing on dentofacial and craniofacial development in orthodontic patients. *Laryngoscope* 2010;**120**(10):2089–93.
136. Trask GM, Shapiro GG, Shapiro PA. The effects of perennial allergic rhinitis on dental and skeletal development: a comparison of sibling pairs. *Am J Orthod Dentofacial Orthop* 1987;**92**(4):286–93.
137. Ozdoganoglu T, Songu M. The burden of allergic rhinitis and asthma. *Ther Adv Respir Dis* 2012;**6**(1):11–23.
138. Bouvier M, Hylander WL. The effect of dietary consistency on gross and histologic morphology in the craniofacial region of young rats. *Am J Anat* 1984;**170**:117–26.
139. Yamada K, Kimmel DB. The effect of dietary consistency on bone mass and turnover in the growing rat mandible. *Arch Oral Biol* 1991;**36**(2):129–38.
140. Tuominen M, Kantomaa T, Pirttiniemi P. Effect of food consistency on the shape of the articular eminence and the mandible. An experimental study on the rabbit. *Acta Odontol Scand* 1993;**51**(2):65–72.
141. Ueda HM, Ishizuka Y, Miyamoto K, et al. Relationship between masticatory muscle activity and vertical craniofacial morphology. *Angle Orthod* 1998;**68**(3):233–8.
142. Granger MW, Buschang PH, Throckmorton G, Iannaccone ST. Masticatory muscle function in patients

with spinal muscular atrophy. *Am J Orthod Dentofacial Orthop* 1999;**115**(6):697–702.
143 Throckmorton GS, Ellis E III, Buschang PH. Morphologic and biomechanical correlates with maximum bite forces in orthognathic surgery patients. *J Oral Maxillofac Surg* 2000;**58**(5):515–24.
144 Watt DG, Williams CH. The effects of the physical consistency of food on the growth and development of the mandible and the maxilla of the rat. *Am J Orthod* 1951;**37**(12):895–928.
145 Navarro M, Delgado E, Monje F. Changes in mandibular rotation after muscular resection. Experimental study in rat. *Am J Orthod Dentofacial Orthop* 1995;**108**(4):367–79.
146 Kreiborg S, Jensen BL, Møller E, Björk A. Craniofacial growth in a case of congenital muscular dystrophy. *Am J Orthod* 1978;**74**(2):207–15.
147 Kiliaridis S, Mejersjö C, Thilander B. Muscle function and craniofacial morphology: a clinical study in patients with myotonic dystrophy. *Eur J Orthod* 1989;**11**(3):131–8.
148 Houston K, Buschang PH, Iannaccone ST, Seale NS. Craniofacial morphology of spinal muscular atrophy. *Pediatr Res* 1994;**36**(2):265–9.
149 Kuo AD, Zajac FE. A biomechanical analysis of muscle strength as a limiting factor in standing posture. *J Biomech* 1993;**26**(Suppl 1):137–50.
150 Nallegowda M, Singh U, Handa G, et al. Role of sensory input and muscle strength in maintenance of balance, gait, and posture in Parkinson's disease: A pilot study. *Am J Phys Med Rehabil* 2004;**83**(12):898–908.
151 Yahia A, Jribi S, Ghroubi S, et al. Evaluation of the posture and muscular strength of the trunk and inferior members of patients with chronic lumbar pain. *Joint Bone Spine* 2011;**78**(3):291–7.
152 Linder-Aronson S. Respiratory function in relation to facial morphology and dentition. *Br J Orthod* 1979;**6**(2):59–71.

6.2

Section II: Class II treatment: problems and solutions

Eustáquio A. Araújo, DDS, MDS

Center for Advanced Dental Education, Department of Orthodontics, Saint Louis University, St. Louis, MO, USA

During the Early Treatment Symposium of 2002, Dr. Lysle Johnston clearly summarized the continuing discussion on early treatment with this remark:

> Early or late? Clearly, the timing of many of the treatments to be discussed at this meeting probably would generate little controversy. Indeed, I would argue that the main controversy – and perhaps the reason for the full lecture hall – surrounds the treatment of Class II malocclusion. [1]

The pendulum that regulates the timing of orthodontic treatment has been swinging in different directions for many years. However, at present, it seems to be dramatically swinging toward early interceptive treatment in many situations and for many different reasons. The treatment of Class II malocclusions continues to be the greatest reason for singular debate and singular controversy.

The decision-making on the timing of treatment has, on many occasions, become a passionate issue among academicians as well. Radicalism may negatively reflect on *the excellence goal/effectiveness and efficiency*. No inflexible position will lead a careful clinician to an appropriate decision.

What is the most appropriate time to intervene in Class II malocclusions and how to decide whether to treat or not to treat?

The discussion on treatment timing started in the early 1900s, as presented by Le Roy Johnson in "The diagnosis of malocclusion with reference to early treatment" [2]. In his paper the author discussed interesting concepts of function and form as well as a captivating topic on the bearing of heredity in diagnosis.

More recently, many studies have been presented with the objective of elucidating questions still to be answered. Several randomized clinical trials (RCT) have been documented in the current literature in relation to Class II approaches [3–8].

The conclusions presented lead us to some significant indications:

1) Phase I treatment produces different responses depending on the treatment performed, whether headgear, functional appliance, or no treatment.
2) At the end of phase II, however, this tendency cannot be observed and subjects showed similar results for skeletal and dental corrections.
3) There are no significant differences in the final quality of the results.

Recognizing and Correcting Developing Malocclusions: A Problem-Oriented Approach to Orthodontics, Second Edition. Edited by Eustáquio A. Araújo and Peter H. Buschang.
© 2025 John Wiley & Sons, Inc. Published 2025 by John Wiley & Sons, Inc.

4) Phase I treatment as a means of making the second phase less complicated is questionable.
5) Due to a longer treatment time when phase I and II are considered together, the conclusion is that two-phase treatment does not prove to be more efficient.

Although there is enough evidence that early intervention in Class II malocclusion may not be routinely indicated, many accept the fact that a decision for an early intervention in children with Class II should also be based on other variables, and that each child should be considered separately.

In one of the cited articles, the authors indicate that in the early stages of their treatment protocol, they were so impressed with the positive progress of the treatment that they discussed whether it was ethical to deny treatment to the control group [7].

Nevertheless, in daily practice, it may not be as simple as it might seem. Clinicians are frequently confronted with situations that require decisions, and they must be prepared to answer certain questions:

What should we do for children who present a severe dental/skeletal deviation? What is our responsibility towards those introverted children who constantly suffer bullying and ridicule from peers because of their looks? How do we deal with anxieties of parents who seek an adequate intervention to help their child? Is it appropriate to suggest no treatment for the sake of efficiency (treatment time)?

Orthodontics must be based not only on mastering a system of appliances, but also on a thorough understanding of growth, heredity, and the *physical and psychological development* of the child. It is during this early childhood period that biologic responses are at their peak. With the appropriate diagnosis and careful delivery of forces, much can be accomplished to improve or eliminate an incipient serious problem [9].

It is also during this period that one can strongly impact a child's life and the development of their personality. As mentioned in Chapters 1 and 2, three main instances are important in determining the timing of intervention for developing Class II malocclusions: 1) psychological problems, 2) increased risk of traumatic injury, and 3) developing hyperdivergence. The literature supports these remarks, especially in relation to trauma and psychological problems [10–20]. As for the hyperdivergent facial types in Section I of this chapter, much evidence has been presented. More studies would be welcomed especially in relation to MSIs for intrusion of molars in the mixed dentition. Although some reports refute the idea of early intervention as capable of minimizing the problems, others present optimistic findings [21–28].

Figures 6.14–6.19 illustrate Class II patients with severe malocclusion and unquestionable indication for an earlier intervention, based on the three main reasons to intervene previously described. As orthodontists we are obligated to provide the best for our patients.

Many times, the best treatment does not mean only a better occlusion. We also must consider the development of youngsters with greater self-confidence and who are able to face the world and be winners. There is still a place for early intervention of Class II developing malocclusions when appropriately recommended. As recently presented by Tuncay in *Solving the Puzzle of Class II Malocclusion*,

> "given all the unknowns and all the "knowns," it appears that the best Class II treatment strategy may at best be no different than all other forms of treatment in orthodontics: clinician's judgment within the framework of contributing factors and esthetics." [29]

6.7 Early Class II adjustment

A normal Class I molar occlusion is achieved through different mechanisms. In the early mixed dentition the clinician must be aware of the changes in the dentition as fully described

6.7 Early Class II adjustment | 133

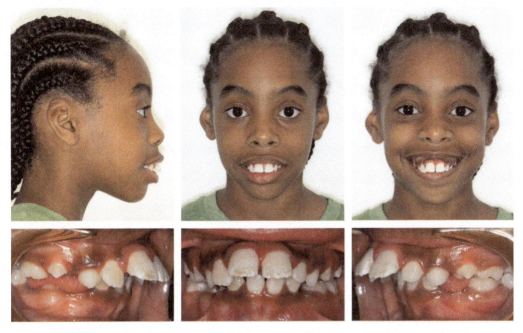

Figure 6.14 Extreme crowding and protrusion. Patient is unable to close her mouth.

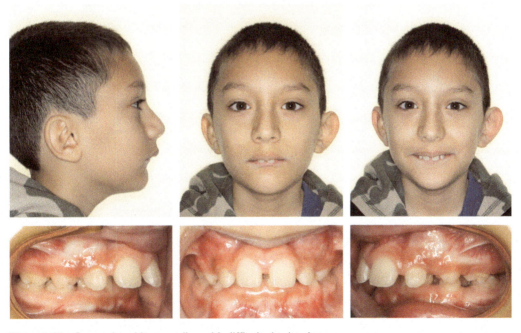

Figure 6.15 Severe deep bite, crowding with difficulty in chewing.

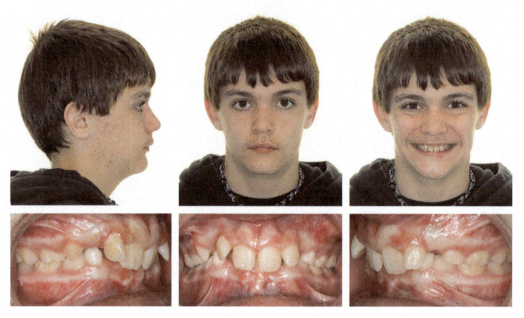

Figure 6.16 Severe Class II division 2 compromising normal growth and development.

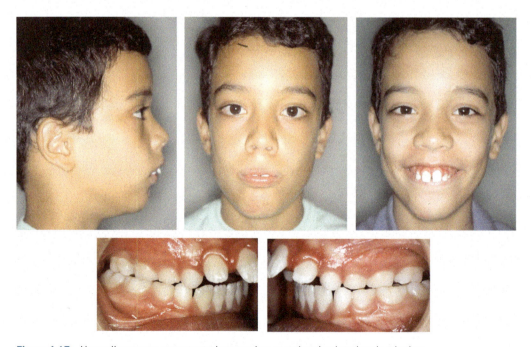

Figure 6.17 Hyperdivergence, accentuated protrusion, emotional-related malocclusion.

6.7 *Early Class II adjustment* | 135

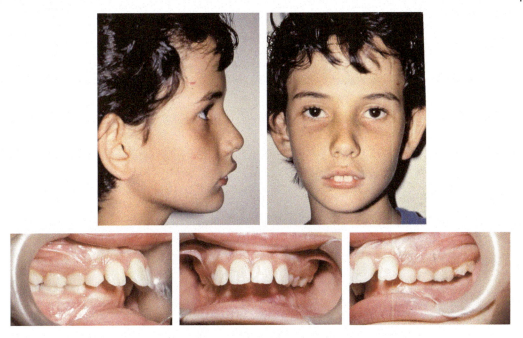

Figure 6.18 Class II deep with Brodie bite, buccal crossbite, on the left segment.

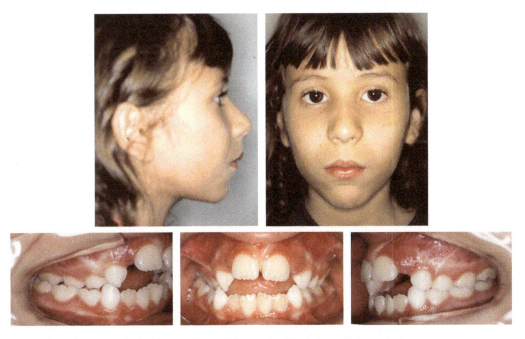

Figure 6.19 Class II, open bite, severe hyperdivergence, unilateral crossbite.

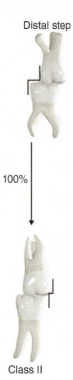

Figure 6.20 Distal step adaptation (Arya et al. [30]/with permission of Elsevier).

in Chapter 2. Studies have indicated that patients presenting with a distal-step relationship of the second deciduous molars in the long run will present a Class II relationship of the permanent molars (Figure 6.20). It has also been confirmed that Class II malocclusions are not "self-correcting" in growing patients [30, 31]. The final molar relationship will depend on the relationship of the terminal planes of the deciduous second molar as well the type of the deciduous dentition–openor closed – in addition to inherited components, and naturally the amount of growth an individual will experience as described and illustrated in Chapter 5.

Growth plays a major role in the correction of the Class II malocclusions. Class II relationships, 70% of the time, may be corrected with growth related interventions [3, 32]. Full-step, less-than-full-step and edge-to-edge Class II malocclusion are normally treated with distinct techniques and protocols.

6.8 Treatment

Certainly, among the most important questions to be answered are those related to the type of Class II treatment to be implemented: *Should the clinician focus the treatment on the maxilla or the mandible? Are treatments of Class II division 1s and Class II division 2s the same? How do we deal with compliance related issues? Are headgears well accepted by the patient? Are functional appliances efficient? Do functional appliances provide a stable and lasting result? Are implant supported appliances indicated for patients in the mixed dentition? How much is too much? How much is not enough?*

As previously mentioned, it has been widely reported that there are few, if any, advantages in the early treatment of Class II patients with either headgears or functional appliances [3–7, 12, 33]. It is important to highlight that even though at the end of a second phase the treatment and control groups showed similar skeletal results, there were initial indications of the treatment being more effective either on the maxilla or mandible, depending on the type of treatment performed. The headgear group showed restriction in the forward movement of the maxilla when compared to control and bionator. The functional (bionator) group showed an increase in mandibular length compared to the control and headgear groups. Although the AP correction for both groups was evident in the first part of the study, this tendency did not continue in the second part of the investigation and treatment.

In conclusion, although phase I produced different responses in relation to growth at the end of phase II, this tendency could not be observed, and the three groups showed similar results for skeletal and dental corrections. The PAR index did not show differences. In relation to phase I, it was reported that no advantages in the final treatment resulted in relation to the outcome itself or to a more simplified second phase. Due to a longer treatment time observed when phase I and II are considered together, the conclusion is that two-phase treatment has not been seen to be more efficient. However, we must ask: Should efficiency surpass necessity?

More recently, other studies have shown that the short-term effects of Class II treatment are significant, but more investigations will add to this longstanding discussion [34–37].

The decisions to treat the maxilla or the mandible must consider the face as the main objective. Indeed, it is imperative to focus on the face. After a complete facial analysis, we need to evaluate the dental imbalance, mainly the proclination of the incisors, the skeletal relationships – SNA and SNB – and the vertical dimensions. It is important to prioritize the face and the major reasons that the patient/family are seeking treatment.

The Class II syndrome, as referred to by Sassouni [38, 39], may be a combination of anteroposterior and vertical deviations. The blend of vertical and anteroposterior variations generates different types of the malocclusion. A publication by Moyers et al. [40] presents several of these combinations (Figure 6.21a–g).

Component analysis of Class II division 1 and Class II division 2, as recently described in the literature, points to the limitations that clinicians must be aware of [41, 42].

Treatment selection will depend on the type of the malocclusion: it ranges from distalization of the maxillary dentition into a Class I, to efforts to manipulate the "lower jaw" orthopaedically until, in severe cases, surgical intervention performed at the right time.

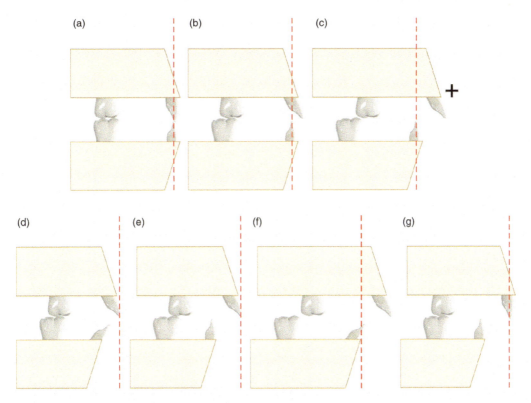

Figure 6.21 Class II combinations. (a) Normal, (b) maxillary dental protraction, (c) midface prognathism, (d) maxillary retrognathism, dental protrusion and mandibular retrognathism, dental procumbency, (e) mandibular retrognathism, maxillary retrognathism and dental protraction, (f) prognathism, dental protraction and dental procumbency, (g) mandibular retrognathism (Moyers et al. [40]/with permission of Elsevier).

The literature presents distinct alternatives for Class II treatment. In the mixed dentition, considering the three conditions previously cited, the clinician may opt for a headgear (cervical or high-pull) alone, a headgear (cervical or high-pull) and four bonded incisors (two-by-four) or any type of mandibular jumping/activator/functional appliance. (See the patients descriptions at the end of this chapter.) Many of these may be compliance related. Patient participation is imperative, as demonstrated in Figure 6.22.

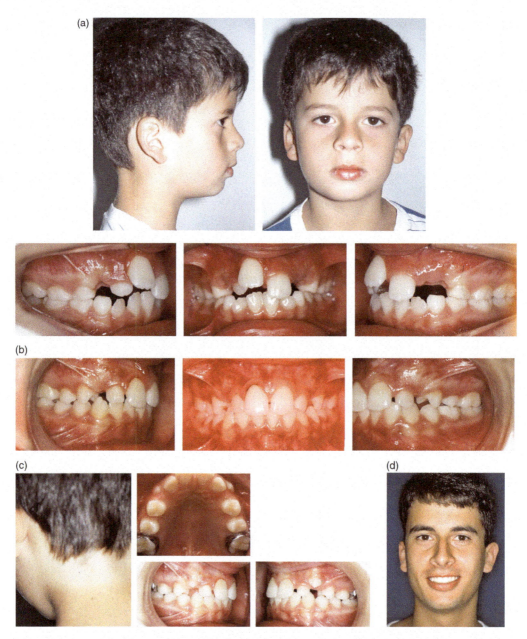

Figure 6.22 Class II division 1 treated with compliance and favorable growth. (a) Initial records, (b) after two-by-four, (c) tan mark and maxillary arch indicating great compliance with cervical pull headgear and buccal segments in Class I, (d) smile at 3 years post treatment.

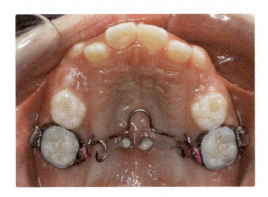

Figure 6.23 Vertical control (intrusion) with MSI and TPA supported device.

As mentioned in Section I, treatment will depend on the patient being hypo- or hyperdivergent. There is no indication of functional appliances for hyperdivergent patients.

Functional or bite-jumping appliances may be indicated for the hypodivergent patients, while an approach to produce an autorotation of the mandible – high-pull headgear, Thurow appliance, and even mini screws for posterior intrusion (Figure 6.23) – are recommended for the hyperdivergent ones. More evidence and clinical trials are needed in relation to intrusion with bone-supported implants or plates. Vertical control is imperative. Patients 2 and 3, at the end of the chapter, illustrate the outcome of treatment without and with planned vertical control.

Clinically speaking, there are two principles that we believe are undisputable. The first is that any Class II functional appliance or bite jumper has an enormous effect on the maxillary dentition. Much of the registered change is dentoalveolar. The second is that any maxillary distalizing appliance anchored on the mandibular dentition establishes "unwanted" proclination of the lower incisors.

Those two principles are clearly evident in Chapter 3, in the discussion of early Class II treatment. The amount of improvement in the Discrepancy Index (DI) observed from the beginning of phase I and the end of phase I was the smallest among the three malocclusion groups, 34.5%. All features of the DI were statistically analyzed, and among the ones that showed a significant reduction in DI score the overjet and the IMPA played an important role in the final result. The IMPA angle, however, demonstrated a statistically significant increase, which indicates that, after treatment, the position of the mandibular incisors was more proclined, contributing to the overjet reduction. Class II correction was partially achieved by growth, and greatly by the dentoalveolar changes described above.

Patient 1
This 8-year-old boy was brought to our clinic to be evaluated. Facially, he presented a convex profile, lack of lip competence due to the protrusion of the maxillary incisors and a retruded mandible. Dentally, a large overjet was present, and with the early loss of deciduous teeth in the lower arch some space was lost. A lip biting habit was also related (Figure 6.24).   The proposed treatment plan included a first phase with a bionator as shown in Figure 6.25. After approximately 1 year with the bionator, and due to the strong commitment of the patient, a much better profile and occlusion could be observed. The cephalometric improvement can also be noticed (Figure 6.26).   With the eruption of the permanent teeth, fixed appliances were placed, managing the spaces and obtaining a good Class I molar and canine relationship (Figure 6.27).

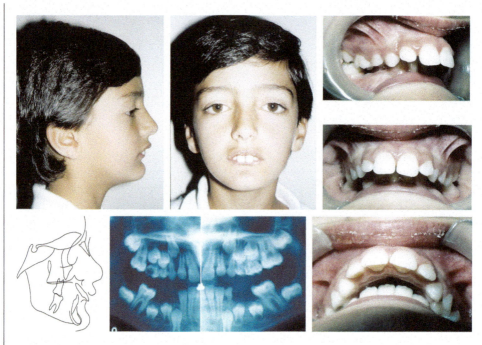

Figure 6.24

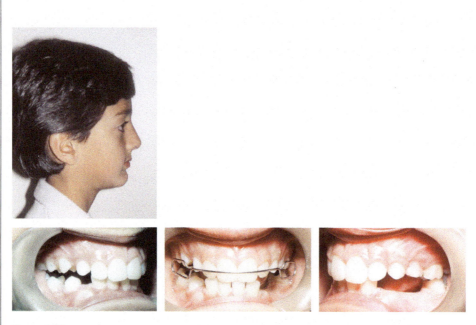

Figure 6.25

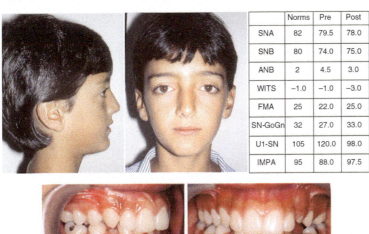

	Norms	Pre	Post
SNA	82	79.5	78.0
SNB	80	74.0	75.0
ANB	2	4.5	3.0
WITS	−1.0	−1.0	−3.0
FMA	25	22.0	25.0
SN-GoGn	32	27.0	33.0
U1-SN	105	120.0	98.0
IMPA	95	88.0	97.5

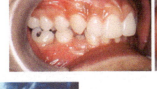
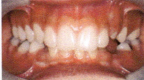
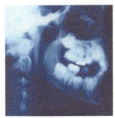

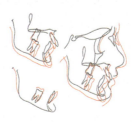

Figure 6.26

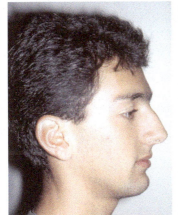
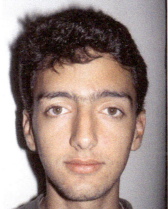
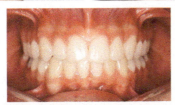
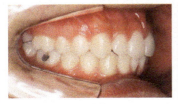
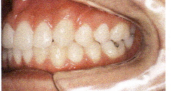

Figure 6.27

Patient 2

This 7y 10m boy was referred to the graduate clinic of PUC Minas in Belo Horizonte, Brazil, with a referral letter from the principal of his school asking for help, and stating that the patient was exposed to ridicule from his peers and was also developing dyslexia, a disorder characterized by impairment to recognize and comprehend written words. According to the referral letter, the disorder could very well be related to his speech problems. Figure 6.28 shows facial and dental features. A convex profile and lack of lip competence can be observed as well as procumbent incisors and gumminess. Dentally a bilateral crossbite could be observed (Figure 6.28d, e) and 15 mm overjet well-demonstrated in Figure 6.28f. The cephalometric film (Figure 6.28g) showed an accentuated hyperdivergence.

Instead of starting his treatment with a maxillary expansion a decision was made to address the overjet initially giving the patient a reason to improve his self-esteem. Along with a two-by-four appliance, a high-pull headgear was given to the patient with the recommendation to wear it for 14 hours/day minimum. The little boy was so involved in improving his malocclusion that he wore for an average of 16 hours/day. Figure 6.29 illustrates the great result obtained in the first 6 months. Note the space mesial to the first molars and the expansion of the maxillary arch as a result of the high-pull biomechanics.

The next step was the removal of the two-by-four and the substitution of the high-pull headgear for a Thurow, a high-pull head gear with total acrylic occlusal coverage. Figure 6.30 illustrates the appliance and the excellent result obtained. The tan mark on the child's face speaks for itself – a great cooperator. Phase I was finished with the patient in Class III molar relationship and no overjet.

At the end of phase II, with fixed appliances, the patient presented an excellent dental relationship and a controlled gingival smile. Retention was done with Hawley's and high-pull head gear, the latter at nighttime only. The face looks considerably better (Figure 6.31).

Figure 6.32 shows the patient 18 years later, and Figure 6.33 illustrates the cephalometric data.

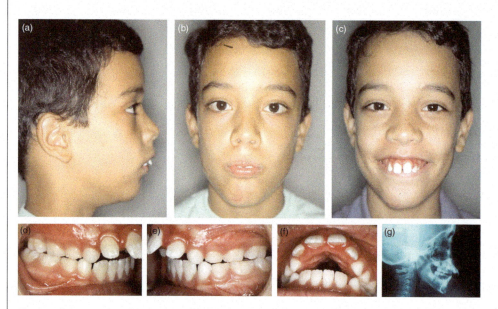

Figure 6.28

6.8 Treatment | 143

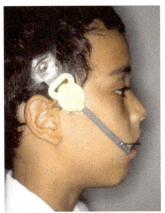
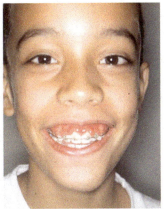
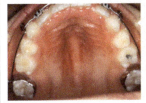
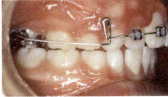
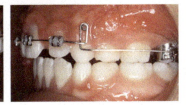

Figure 6.29

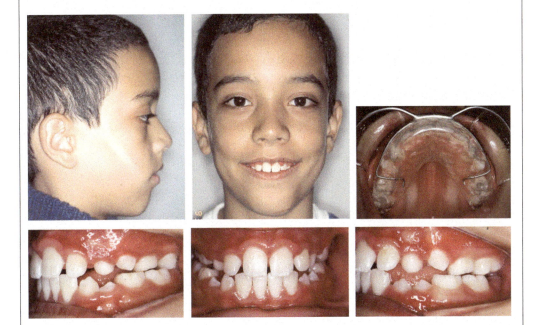

Figure 6.30

6.2 Section II: Class II treatment: problems and solutions

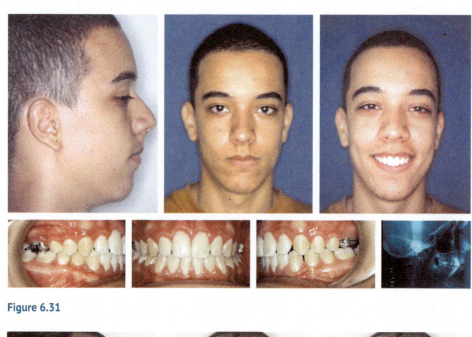

Figure 6.31

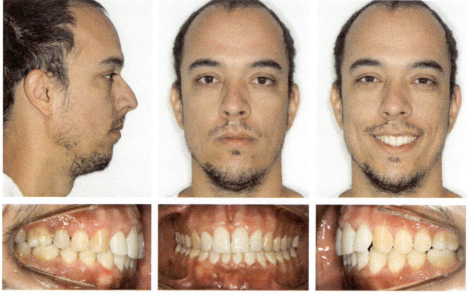

Figure 6.32

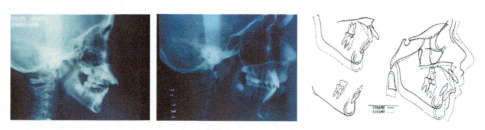

Figure 6.33

Patient 3

This 7-year-old girl was brought to our clinic by her parents, seeking an evaluation. The parents and the family dentist were concerned with the open bite and the "small chin." After all records were studied, a severe hyperdivergence was noted. Facially the patient showed a profile convexity and a small mandible. Dentally, a 7 mm open bite can be noted. Transversally, she presents a constricted maxilla and a unilateral crossbite (Figure 6.34).

During the first phase of treatment a maxillary expansion was completed and retained for 5 months (Figure 6.35). After the expansion was finished, the intervention continued with a high-pull headgear and a LLHA in order to control the vertical and avoid any extrusion of the mandibular molars following the intrusion of the maxillary ones expected to happen with the high-pull force vectors. Figure 6.36 shows the natural correction of the open bite, following the expansion and the headgear therapy associated with the LLHA.

Full orthodontics treatment was initiated later with the presence of the permanent dentition (Figure 6.37). Figure 6.38 presents the facial and dental final results as well as the superimposition. Figure 6.39 shows the occlusion 18 years post-treatment.

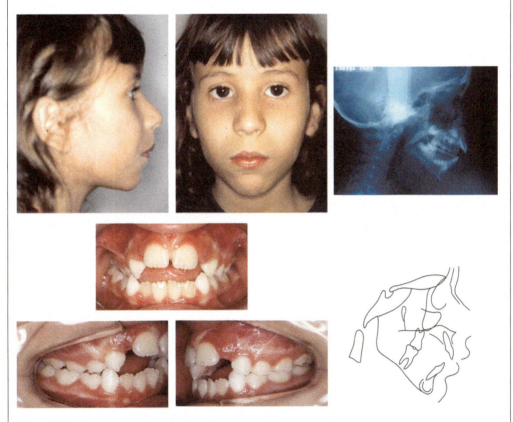

Figure 6.34

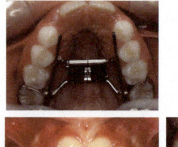
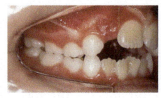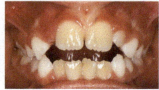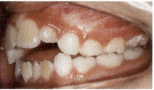

Figure 6.35

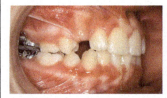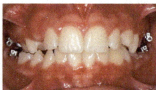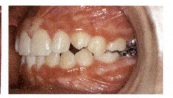

Figure 6.36

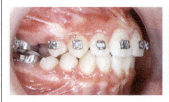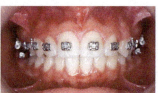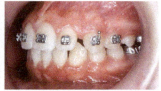

Figure 6.37

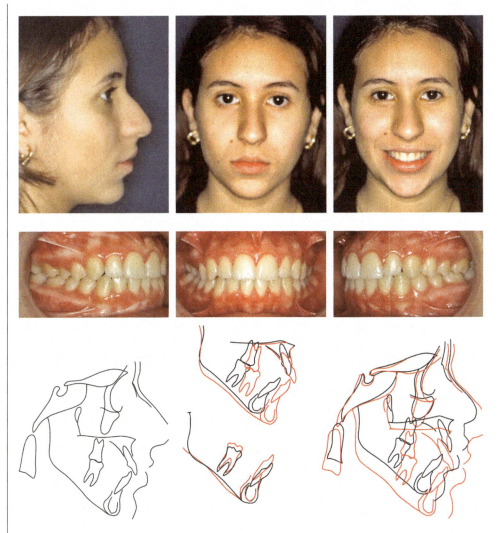

Figure 6.38

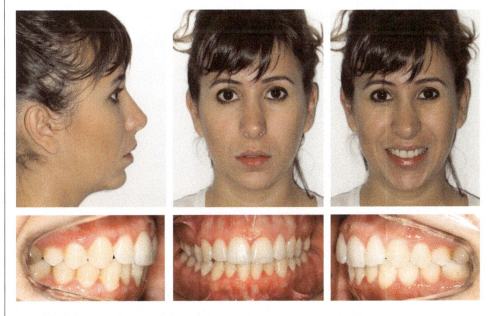

Figure 6.39

Patient 4

This 9-year-old boy was referred to our clinic by his pediatric dentist. The facial analysis shows a Class II facial type, with a retruded mandible and procumbent incisors. Dentally, he presented a severe deep bite, 12 mm overjet and a buccal crossbite on the posterior left segment – a unilateral Brodie bite (Figure 6.40). The first phase of treatment was done with a Frankel 2 appliance. The selection of the Frankel was based on the possibility of expanding the lower left quadrant more than the right quadrant by manipulating the buccal shields distance to the teeth (Figure 6.40h).

After about 1 year of treatment and good cooperation the result was significant, the bite was opened and the patient was in a Class I relationship with the full correction of the Brodie bite. Crossbite elastics were also used to help with the buccolingual relation of the left molars (Figure 6.41).

With the presence of the permanent dentition the patient received full treatment with braces. The final result can be seen in Figure 6.42. The remarkable improving of the face from start to end can be noted in Figure 6.43.

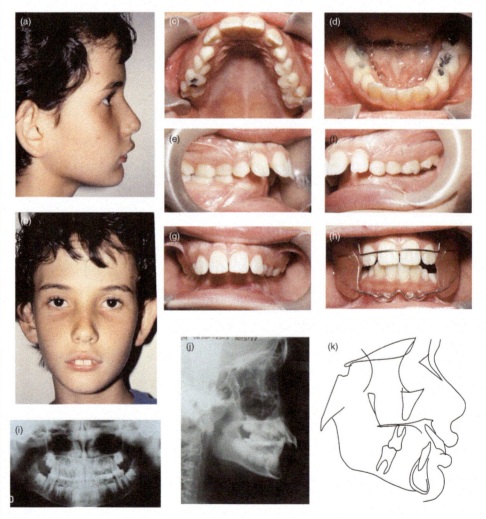

Figure 6.40

6.8 Treatment | 149

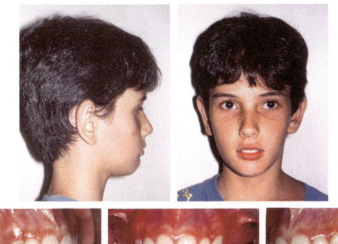

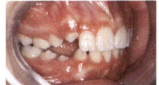 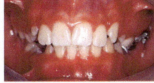 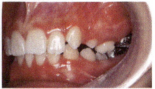

Figure 6.41

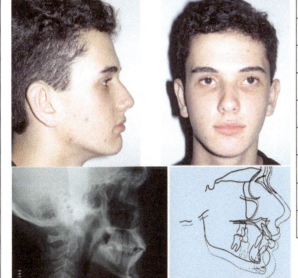

	Norms	Pre	Post
SNA	82	83.5	81.0
SNB	80	77.0	78.0
ANB	2	6.5	3.0
WITS	−1.0	6.0	3.0
FMA	25	24.0	21.0
SN-GoGn	32	30.0	29.0
U1-SN	105	115.0	110.0
IMPA	95	84.0	98.0

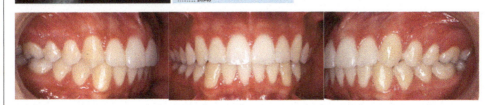

Figure 6.42

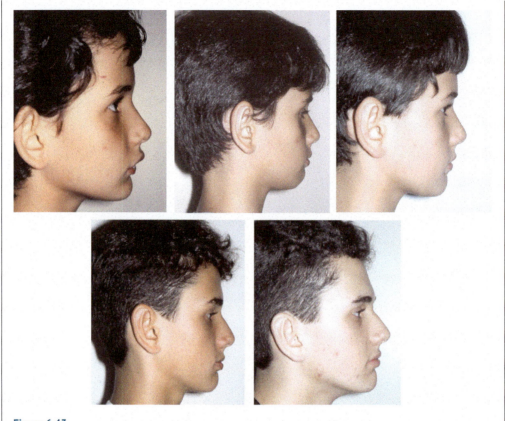

Figure 6.43

Patient 5

Young Class II division 1 patients exposed to the risk of trauma and with low self-esteem may also have their intervention done at an earlier age. This 9y 10m girl presented a convex profile with very pleasant facial appearance. Dentally a severe overjet, proclined maxillary incisors, and spacing as seen in Figure 6.44 can be observed. Initially, the patient was treated with a two-by-four appliance, sliding mechanics and a cervical-pull headgear (Figure 6.45). At the end of phase I the patient received a LLHA and a Nance button and was put in observation for phase II (Figure 6.46). The cephalometric data and the panoramic X-rays are shown in Figure 6.47.

6.8 Treatment | 151

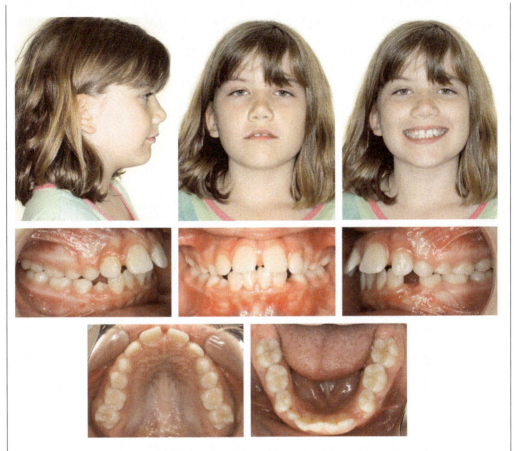

Figure 6.44

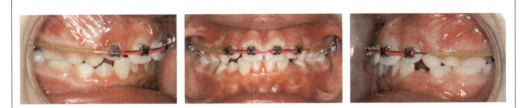

Figure 6.45

6.2 Section II: Class II treatment: problems and solutions

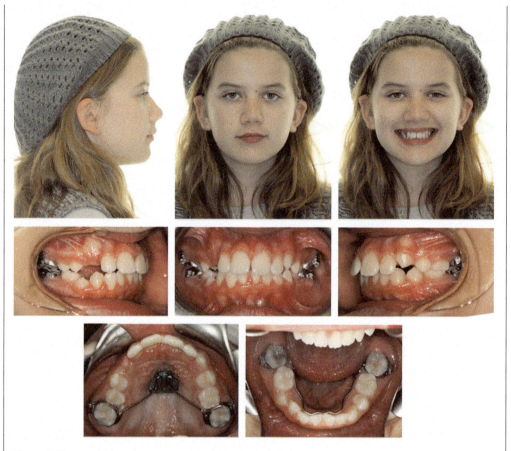

Figure 6.46

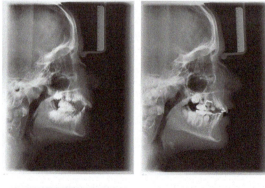

	Norms	Pre	Post
SNA	82	80.0	81.4
SNB	80	77.0	77.3
ANB	2	2.8	4.0
WITS	−1.0	−0.5	0.1
FMA	25	28.2	24.1
SN-GoGn	32	29.7	27.2
U1-SN	105	118.1	107.2
IMPA	95	90.3	98.3

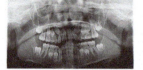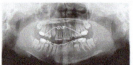

Figure 6.47

6.8 Treatment

Patient 6

This 10-year-old boy presented with a severe Class II division 1 malocclusion. Facially, the patient presented a convex profile and a somewhat retruded chin. Dentally, a severe deep bite was noticed, with procumbent incisors and a deep curve of Spee, as shown in Figure 6.48. After leveling and aligning the incisors a Herbst appliance was inserted. Figure 6.49 illustrates the day of insertion, and Figure 6.50 the occlusion 8 months later. One year from the insertion of the Herbst, the appliance was removed and the patient was placed in active observation (Figure 6.51). The cephalometric changes and the panoramic X-rays can be seen in Figure 6.52.

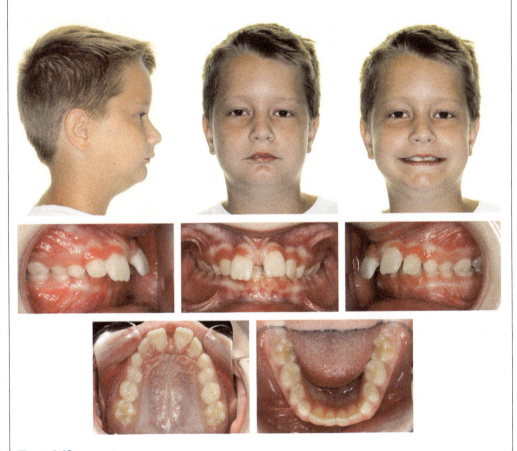

Figure 6.48

6.2 Section II: Class II treatment: problems and solutions

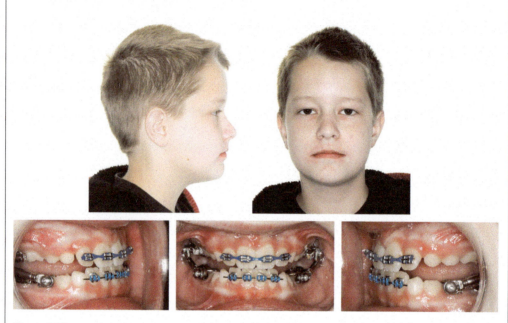

Figure 6.49

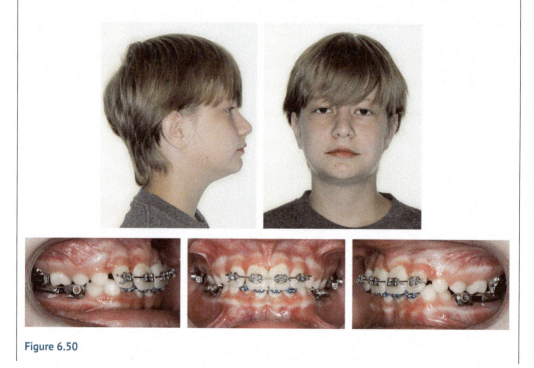

Figure 6.50

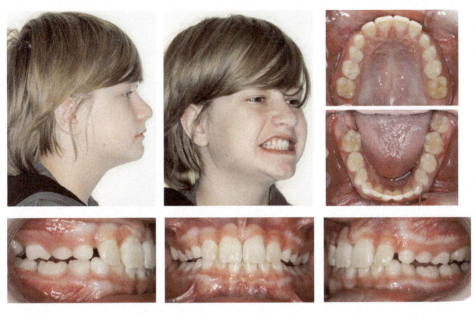

Figure 6.51

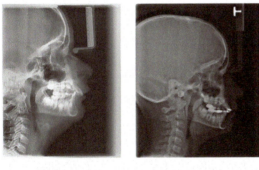

	Norms	Pre	Post
SNA	82	85.6	84.5
SNB	80	79.0	83.3
ANB	2	6.6	1.2
WITS	−1.0	6.3	−2.7
FMA	25	14.8	17.9
SN-GoGn	32	21.6	23.0
U1-SN	105	114.1	108.8
IMPA	95	98.3	99.1

Figure 6.52

Patient 7

Referred by her general dentist, this 7y 9m girl was examined for her "deep bite" and "crooked teeth." Facially she presented a convex profile. Dentally, she had a Class II, division 2 malocclusion with moderate crowding in both arches (Figure 6.53). The treatment plan was composed of a bonded expander and a mandibular lip bumper. At the end of this initial procedure, a two-by-four was placed on both arches

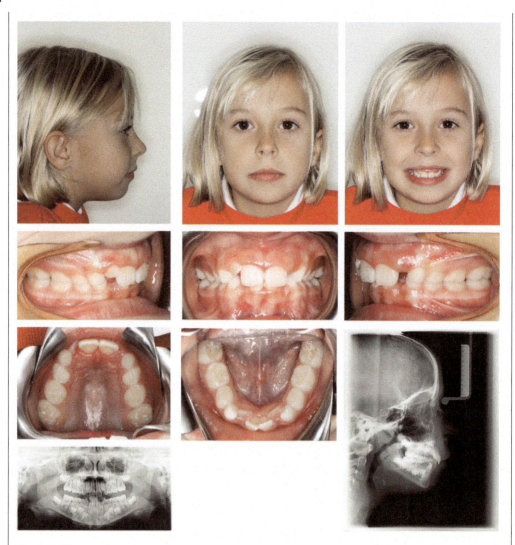

Figure 6.53

(Figure 6.54). The total treatment time was 9 months. The final occlusion pre-phase II, as seen in Figure 6.55, shows a remarkable improvement.

In essence, we can say that Class II children, with good growth potential, may be able to attain an excellent facial and dental result with early treatment. The hyperdivergent ones are normally treated for a longer period of time, with a combination of high-pull headgears, posterior bite blocks, and vertical control including vertical chincups.

Studies on MSI to anchor molar intrusion in the mixed dentition are necessary.

As previously described, the Class II division 2 patients resemble more the Class I patients and are more hypodivergent. Generally, the treatment indicated for them is the alignment of the incisors with a two-by-four appliance with or without a headgear. This depends on the individual case. Any other intervention may have to be re-evaluated until the normal position of the incisors has been established.

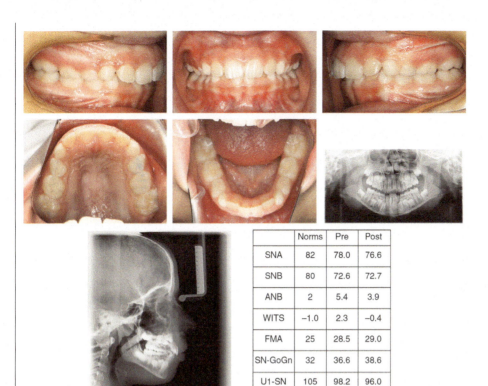

Figure 6.54

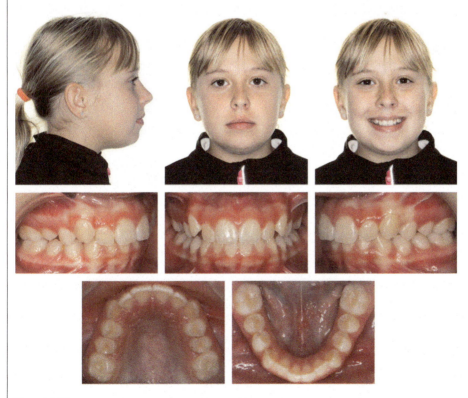

Figure 6.55

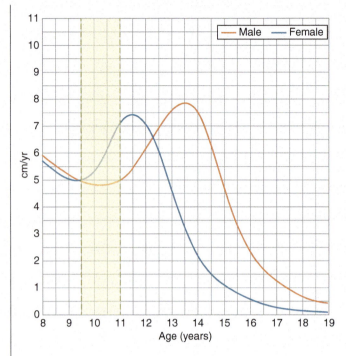

Figure 6.56

It is important to tie our decisions to the growth stage each patient presets. On Figure 6.56 a representation of the growth curves for boys and girls. If growth is critical to achieve a better treatment result, the timings to implement the procedures must respect the dichotomy between boys and girls [43].

The evidence has demonstrated that the most appropriate period to count on *growth as a friend* is during its spurt. Figure 6.56 combines the growth curves with the mean chronologic ages (yellow) for a phase 1 treatment for boys and girls.

The previous sequence of cases illustrated different Class II early treatment approaches. Each case received special attention in an attempt to elucidate possible questionings.

References

1 Johnston LE. Answers in search of questioners. *Am J Orthod Dentofacial Orthop* 2002;**121**(6):552–3.
2 Johnson LR. The diagnosis of malocclusion with reference to early treatment. *J Dent Res* 1921;**3**(1):v–xx.
3 Baccetti T, Franchi L, McNamara JA, Tollaro I. Early dento-facial features of Class II malocclusion: a longitudinal study from the deciduous through the mixed dentition. *Am J Orthod Dentofacial Orthop* 1997 May;**111**(5):502–9.
4 Tulloch JF, Phillips C, Koch G, Proffit WR. The effect of early intervention on skeletal pattern in Class II malocclusion: a randomized clinical trial. *Am J Orthod Dentofacial Orthop* 1997 Apr;**111**(4):391–400.
5 Keeling SD, Wheeler TT, King GJ, et al. Anteroposterior skeletal and dental changes after early Class II treatment with bionators

and headgear. *Am J Orthod Dentofacial Orthop* 1998 Jan;**113**(1):40–50.
6 King GJ, Wheeler TT, McGorray SP, et al. Orthodontists' perceptions of the impact of phase 1 treatment for Class II malocclusion on phase 2 needs. *J Dent Res* 1999 Nov;**78**(11):1745–53.
7 Tulloch JFC, Proffit WR, Phillips C. Outcomes in a 2-phase randomized clinical trial of early Class II treatment. *Am J Orthod Dentofacial Orthop* 2004 Jun;**125**(6):657–67.
8 Harrison JE, O'Brien KD, Worthington HV. Orthodontic treatment for prominent upper front teeth in children. *Cochrane Database Syst Rev* 2007;(3):CD003452.
9 Carlson DS. Biological rationale for early treatment of dentofacial deformities. *Am J Orthod Dentofacial Orthop* 2002 Jun;**121**(6):554–8.
10 Kalha AS. Early orthodontic treatment reduced incisal trauma in children with class II malocclusions. *Evid Based Dent* 2014 Mar;**15**(1):18–20.
11 O'Brien K, Wright JL, Conboy F, et al. The child perception questionnaire is valid for malocclusions in the United Kingdom. *Am J Orthod Dentofacial Orthop* 2006 Apr;**129**(4):536–40.
12 O'Brien K, Macfarlane T, Wright J, et al. Early treatment for Class II malocclusion and perceived improvements in facial profile. *Am J Orthod Dentofacial Orthop* 2009 May;**135**(5):580–5.
13 Tessarollo FR, Feldens CA, Closs LQ. The impact of malocclusion on adolescents' dissatisfaction with dental appearance and oral functions. *Angle Orthod* 2012 May;**82**(3):403–9.
14 de Carvalho Sales Peres SH, Goya S, Cortellazzi KL, et al. Self-perception and malocclusion and their relation to oral appearance and function. *Ciên Saúde Colet* 2011 Oct;**16**(10):4059–66.
15 Ryan FS, Barnard M, Cunningham SJ. Impact of dentofacial deformity and motivation for treatment: a qualitative study. *Am J Orthod Dentofacial Orthop* 2012 Jun;**141**(6):734–42.
16 Seehra J, Fleming PS, Newton T, DiBiase AT. Bullying in orthodontic patients and its relationship to malocclusion, self-esteem and oral health-related quality of life. *J Orthod* 2011 Dec;**38**(4):247–56; quiz 294.
17 Seehra J, Newton JT, Dibiase AT. Interceptive orthodontic treatment in bullied adolescents and its impact on self-esteem and oral-health-related quality of life. *Eur J Orthod* 2013 Oct;**35**(5):615–21.
18 Taghavi Bayat J, Hallberg U, Lindblad F, et al. Daily life impact of malocclusion in Swedish adolescents: a grounded theory study. *Acta Odontol Scand* 2013 Jul;**71**(3–4):792–8.
19 Al-Omari IK, Al-Bitar ZB, Sonbol HN, et al. Impact of bullying due to dentofacial features on oral health-related quality of life. *Am J Orthod Dentofacial Orthop* 2014 Dec;**146**(6):734–9.
20 Petti S. Over two hundred million injuries to anterior teeth attributable to large overjet: a meta-analysis. *Dent Traumatol* 2015 Feb;**31**(1):1–8.
21 Haralabakis NB, Sifakakis IB. The effect of cervical headgear on patients with high or low mandibular plane angles and the "myth" of posterior mandibular rotation. *Am J Orthod Dentofacial Orthop* 2004 Sep;**126**(3):310–7.
22 Kim KR, Muhl ZF. Changes in mandibular growth direction during and after cervical headgear treatment. *Am J Orthod Dentofacial Orthop* 2001 May;**119**(5):522–30.
23 Ulger G, Arun T, Sayinsu K, Isik F. The role of cervical headgear and lower utility arch in the control of the vertical dimension. *Am J Orthod Dentofacial Orthop* 2006 Oct;**130**(4):492–501.
24 Henriques JF, Martins DR, Pinzan A [The cervical headgear action in the mixed dentition on maxilla, mandible and teeth in class II, division 1, malocclusions–a cephalometric study (author's transl.)]. *Ortodontia* 1979 Aug;**12**(2):76–86.

25. Gkantidis N, Halazonetis DJ, Alexandropoulos E, Haralabakis NB. Treatment strategies for patients with hyperdivergent Class II Division 1malocclusion: is vertical dimension affected? *Am J Orthod Dentofacial Orthop* 2011 Sep;**140**(3):346–55.
26. Defraia E, Marinelli A, Baroni G, et al. Early orthodontic treatment of skeletal open-bite malocclusion with the open-bite bionator: a cephalometric study. *Am J Orthod Dentofacial Orthop* 2007 Nov;**132**(5):595–8.
27. Sankey WL, Buschang PH, English J, Owen AH. Early treatment of vertical skeletal dysplasia: the hyperdivergent pheno-type. *Am J Orthod Dentofacial Orthop* 2000 Sep;**118**(3):317–27.
28. Ngan P, Wilson S, Florman M, Wei SH. Treatment of Class II open bite in the mixed dentition with a removable functional appliance and headgear. *Quintessence Int* 1992 May;**23**(5):323–33.
29. Tuncay O. Solving the puzzle of Class II malocclusion. *Semin Orthod* 2014;**20**(4):339–42.
30. Arya BS, Savara BS, Thomas DR. Prediction of first molar occlusion. *Am J Orthod* 1973 Jun;**63**(6):610–21.
31. Bishara SE, Hoppens BJ, Jakobsen JR, Kohout FJ. Changes in the molar relationship between the deciduous and permanent dentitions: a longitudinal study. *Am J Orthod Dentofacial Orthop* 1988 Jan;**93**(1):19–28.
32. McNamara JA. Components of class II malocclusion in children 8–10 years of age. *Angle Orthod* 1981 Jul;**51**(3):177–202.
33. O'Brien K, Wright J, Conboy F, et al. Early treatment for Class II Division 1 malocclusion with the Twin-block appliance: a multi-center, randomized, controlled trial. *Am J Orthod Dentofacial Orthop* 2009 May;**135**(5):573–9.
34. Koretsi V, Zymperdikas VF, Papageorgiou SN, Papadopoulos MA. Treatment effects of removable functional appliances in patients with Class II malocclusion: a systematic review and meta-analysis. *Eur J Orthod* 2015;**37**(4):418–34.
35. Marsico E, Gatto E, Burrascano M, et al. Effectiveness of orthodontic treatment with functional appliances on mandibular growth in the short term. *Am J Orthod Dentofacial Orthop* 2011 Jan;**139**(1):24–36.
36. Antonarakis GS, Kiliaridis S. Short-term anteroposterior treatment effects of functional appliances and extraoral traction on class II malocclusion. A meta-analysis. *Angle Orthod* 2007 Sep;**77**(5):907–14.
37. Vaid N, Doshi V, Vandekar M. Class II treatment with functional appliances: a meta-analysis of short term treatment effects. *Semin Orthod* 2014;**20**(4):324–8.
38. Sassouni V. The Class II syndrome: differential diagnosis and treatment. *Angle Orthod* 1970 Oct;**40**(4):334–41.
39. Sassouni V. A classification of skeletal facial types. *Am J Orthod* 1969 Feb;**55**(2):109–23.
40. Moyers RE, Riolo ML, Guire KE, et al. Differential diagnosis of class II malocclusions. Part 1. Facial types associated with class II malocclusions. *Am J Orthod* 1980 Nov;**78**(5):477–94.
41. Ghafari J, Macari. Component analysis of Class II, Division 1 discloses limitations for transfer to Class I phenotype. *Semin Orthod* 2014;**20**(4):253–71.
42. Ghafari J, Haddad R. Cephalometric and dental analysis of Class II, Division 2 reveals various subtypes of the malocclusion and the primacy of dentoalveolar components. *Semin Orthod* 2014;**20**(4):272–86.
43. Araujo EA, McCray J, Miranda GFPC. Growth: sometimes a friend, sometimes an enemy. *Semin Orthod* 2023 Jun 1;**29**(2):119–36.

7

Recognizing and correcting Class III malocclusions

7.1

Section I: The development, phenotypic characteristics, and etiology of Class III malocclusion

Peter H. Buschang, MA, PhD

Regents Professor Emeritus, Department of Orthodontics, Texas A&M University School of Dentistry, Dallas, TX, USA

7.1 Introduction

Class III malocclusion, also referred to as mesioocclusion, occurs when the mesiobuccal cusps of the maxillary first molars occlude posterior to the mesiobuccal grooves of the mandibular first molars. The entire mandibular dentition occludes mesial to the maxillary dentition and there is an anterior crossbite. Class III permanent molar relationships develop from deciduous flush terminal plane and mesial step relationships (Figure 7.1). While most flush terminal plane relationships in the deciduous dentition develop cusp-to-cusp relations in the mixed dentition, a few will develop normal relations in the early mixed dentition, and of those, a few will develop Class III molar relationships in the permanent dentition. Most subjects with mesial step relations develop normal molar relationships in the mixed dentition, but a few will develop mesial step relations. All of those with mesial step relationships in the mixed dentition will develop Class III molar relationships in the permanent dentition.

Angle [1] originally portrayed Class III malocclusion as having "all the lower teeth occluding mesial to normal the width of one bicuspid, or even more in extreme cases."

He also noted that the lower incisors and canines were inclined lingually and that the skeletal component pertained to lower jaw protrusion. This was a remarkable premonition because the skeletal components of Class III malocclusion are what makes this form of malocclusion among the most difficult to treat.

Class III malocclusion is important and needs to be better understood because it produces detrimental facial esthetics and greater functional deficits than any other form of malocclusion. Its prevalence is not insignificant, especially among certain populations.

Profiles of individuals with Class III malocclusion, especially those with protrusive mandibles, are considered among the least attractive. When 2651 Japanese adults were asked to rank five facial profiles, the mandibular prognathic profile was considered the least attractive, followed by the mandibular retrognathic, bimaxillary protrusive, bimaxillary retrusive, and orthognathic profiles, respectively [2]. Mandibular prognathic profiles were also among the least preferred among the Turkish population [3]. The mandibular prognathic hypodivergent profile is least preferred by laypeople, orthodontists, and surgeons, even more so than the extreme retrognathic

---

Recognizing and Correcting Developing Malocclusions: A Problem-Oriented Approach to Orthodontics,
Second Edition. Edited by Eustáquio A. Araújo and Peter H. Buschang.
© 2025 John Wiley & Sons, Inc. Published 2025 by John Wiley & Sons, Inc.

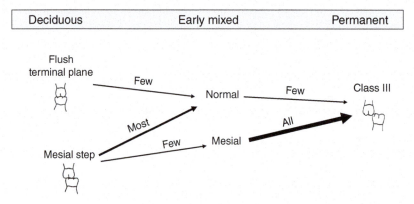

Figure 7.1 Development of Class III molar relationships between the deciduous (mesial steps larger than 0.5–1.0 mm), mixed (mesial relative to normal), and permanent dentitions.

hyperdivergent profile [4]. Appearance is important because it plays a vital role in determining individuals' social status [5–7].

The masticatory function of Class III subjects is also often compromised. Individuals with Class III malocclusion are three times more likely to report difficulties chewing firm foods than individuals with normal occlusion [8]. They are not able to break down food as well as individuals with any other form of occlusion (Figure 7.2). Compared to subjects with untreated normal occlusion, the chewed particle sizes of Class IIIs are approximately 30% larger [8]. Zhou and Fu [9] reported that the masticatory efficiency of Chinese with Class III malocclusion was only 60% of individuals with normal occlusion.

The inability of Class IIIs to efficiently break down foods is due primarily to reduced (by approximately 50%) areas of occlusal contact and near contact [10]. Because the number of occlusal contacts and near contacts is closely associated with muscle and bite forces [11], Class IIIs might be expected to have weaker masticatory muscles. Prognathic surgery patients have been shown to have reduced mechanical advantage of their masticatory muscles [12]. Smaller areas of contact and near contacts are indicative of reduced occlusal support (i.e. force distributed over fewer teeth), which has been linked with reduced masticatory muscle strength and abnormal chewing cycle kinematics [13]. Class IIIs also exhibit abnormal chewing patterns, with a

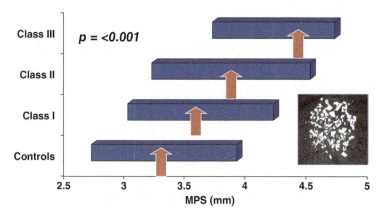

Figure 7.2 Median particle sizes (arrows) and interquartile ranges of subjects of normal occlusion and malocclusion (adapted from English et al. [8]).

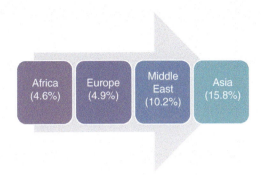

Figure 7.3 Worldwide prevalence estimates of Class III malocclusion based on summary statistics from 24 studies (adapted from Hardy et al. [16]).

high preponderance of chopping, reversed, and contralateral masticatory cycles [14, 15].

The prevalence of Class III malocclusion varies widely between populations, with the highest occurrences reported among Chinese and Malaysians (Figure 7.3). A comprehensive worldwide review found that groups living in southwest Asia exhibit the highest prevalence (15.8%) of Class III malocclusion, followed by Middle Eastern groups (10.2%), Europeans (4.9%), and Africans (4.6%) [16]. A more recent survey shows that the prevalence of Class III malocclusion in Asia (6.3%) to be only slightly higher than in the Americas (6.2%) and Europe (6.2%), all of which are higher than the prevalence in Africa (4.8%) [17]. The best surveys for the USA population were performed by the NCHS in 1973 and 1979. Based on their molar relationships, approximately 4.9% of the white children 6–11 years of age, and 6.0% of the white adolescents 12–17 years of age, exhibited bilateral Class III malocclusion [18, 19]. Approximately 7.0% and 7.7% of black children and adolescents had bilateral Class III malocclusion. Class III malocclusion tended to be slightly more prevalent among males than females; the difference was small (0.2%) but consistent both during childhood and adolescence. Based on overjet, the NHANES III estimated that approximately 4.9% of the white, 8.1% of the black, and 8.3% of the Mexican-American populations have Class III malocclusion [20]. The NHANES estimates indicate that the prevalence of Class III malocclusion increases considerably between 8–11 years and 12–17 years but very little thereafter.

7.2 Characterization of the Class III phenotype

Many earlier studies characterized their Class IIIs samples based on the jaw they thought to be most affected. Sanborn [21], who was among the first to categorize Class IIIs in this manner, reported that the problem was in the mandible 45.5% of the time and in the maxilla 33.3% of the time. Unfortunately, the literature that categorizes Class III subjects in this manner shows no consistent pattern and no dominance of one jaw over the other (Table 7.1). These studies are difficult to compare because they used different methodologies and criteria to categorize their subjects, and only some of them compared the Class III subjects to controls. The best that can be said from these reports is that both jaws appear to be involved.

Whether or not the maxilla is retrusive in Class IIIs remains controversial. Most earlier studies indicate that there are differences between Class IIIs and Class Is, with the average Class III maxilla being more retrusive than the average Class I maxilla (Table 7.2). In contrast, most of the more recent and better-controlled studies have found no Class differences in maxillary position. In combination, the available studies suggest that there probably is a difference (i.e. the Class III maxillae are more retrusive), but that the differences between Class Is and Class IIIs are minor. There are small differences between Class Is and Class IIIs in maxillary size (ANS-PNS), with Class IIIs being smaller. The AP distance of the maxilla from the cranial base indicates no Class differences. The palatal plane angle measured relative to FH may be smaller among Class IIIs, but there are no differences between

Table 7.1 Percentages (most prevalent in bold) of Class IIIs with problems judged to be exclusively in the mandible, exclusively in the maxilla, in both jaws (Combi), or otherwise.

	Md→	Mx←	Combi	Other
Sanborn [21]	**45.2%**	33.3%	9.5%	12%
Dietrich [22]	31%	**37%**	1.5%	31.5%
Jacobson et al. [23]	**49%**	26%	6%	14%
Ellis and McNamara [24]	19.2%	19.5%	**31%**	30.3%
Guyer et al. [25]	20%	22.8%	**34.3%**	22.9%
Bui et al. [26]	35%	**48.8%**	16.2%	N/A
Staudt and Kiliaridis [27]	**47.4%**	19.3%	8.7%	24.6%

Table 7.2 Differences (Class III vs. Class I) in maxillary protrusion, maxillary size, the horizontal distance from the cranial base, and palatal height.

	AP position (SNA)	Size (ANS-PNS)	AP distance from CB	Palatal ht
Sandborn [21]	←	N/A	N/A	N/A
Jacobson [23]	←	↓	N/A	↓
Ellis and McNamara [24]	←	N/A	N/A	N/A
Guyer et al. [25]	←	N/A	↓ (Co-A)	NS
Williams and Andersen [28]	←	↓	N/A	NS
Battagel [29]	NS	N/A	NS	NS
Tollaro et al. [30]	←	N/A	N/A	N/A
Chang et al. [31]	NS	↓	N/A	N/A
Reyes et al. [32]	NS	N/A	NS	NS
Staudt and Kiliaridis [27]	←	N/A	N/A	N/A
Choi et al. [33]	←	NS	N/A	N/A
Wolfe et al. [34]	NS	↓	NS	NS
Most common	←	↓	NS	NS

Class Is and IIIs in the palatal plane angle measured relative to S-N [24, 30]. Most studies evaluating the vertical height of the palatal plane from the cranial base showed no differences between Class Is and Class IIIs.

While the Class III maxilla may be somewhat retrusive and smaller, there is no indication that maxillary retrusion worsens over time. Retrusion, if it exists, appears to be established early. Large cross-sectional evaluations of different age groups indicate that the differences in maxillary position between Class Is and IIIs do not change during childhood and adolescence [25, 29]. Reyes et al. [32], who provide the best cross-sectional comparisons, reported no differences in the SNA angle between Class IIIs and Class Is 6–17 years of age. Based on the longitudinal assessments, Wolfe et al. [34] also found no Class differences in the changes of the SNA angle that occur between 6 and 16 years of age. They showed that the maxilla of Class IIIs was approximately 1.6 mm shorter at 6 years of age, and that this difference was maintained through 16 years of age. Taken as a whole, the available growth data indicate that the maxillae of young Class IIIs are slightly smaller; if there is midfacial retrusion, it is minor, usually established early, and does not worsen over time.

Transversely, it appears that maxillary intercanine widths of Class IIIs and Class Is are similar [35–37]. However, interpremolar and intermolar widths are often smaller in Class IIIs than in individuals with normal occlusion [35–37]. Maxillary skeletal base (interjugal distance) width has also been found to be significantly smaller among Class IIIs. Longitudinal comparisons have shown that posterior maxillary width differences between Class IIIs and Class Is increase between 10 and 14 years of age [38]. Greater posterior arch widths have also been reported among Class IIIs [39] as well as no significant Class differences [40, 41]. The inconsistencies may be due to the vertical makeup of the samples. Chen et al. [42] found that skeletal and dental widths were all significantly smaller among Class IIIs with high mandibular plane angles than among Class IIIs with low angles. In other words, hyperdivergent Class IIIs might be expected to exhibit transverse maxillary deficiencies, while hypodivergent Class IIIs show no differences or excesses.

Class differences in the AP position of the mandible are much greater and more consistent than Class differences in the maxillary AP position. Most studies evaluating the AP position of both the maxilla and mandible have shown that the maxilla is significantly more retrusive among Class IIIs than Class Is (Table 7.3). As indicated, the better cross-sectional studies available show no differences in the SNA angle between Class IIIs and Class Is. For example, Battagel [29], who evaluated 495 untreated Class IIIs, and Reyes et al. [32], who evaluated 949 untreated Class IIIs, showed no differences in maxillary position at any age between 6 and 16 years. In contrast, all of the available studies show that the mandible is significantly more protrusive

Table 7.3 Studies comparing Class IIIs and Class Is for differences in maxillary retrusion and mandibular protrusion.

Retrusion	Maxilla Prob	Protrusion	Mandible Prob	
Sandborn [21]	←3.1°	Sig	→4.2°	Highly sig
Jacobson et al. [23]	←2.6°	Sig	→5.3°	Highly sig
Guyer et al. [25]	←2.2°	Sig	→1.5°	Sig
Williams and Andersen [28]	←2.5 mm	Sig	→3.7 mm	High sig
Battagel [29]	N/A	NS	→3.9°	High sig
Tollaro et al. [30]	←1.1°	Sig	→5–6°	Highly sig
Sugawara and Mitani [43]	N/A	NS	→3.0°	Highly sig
Chang et al. [31]	N/A	NS	→6.5°	Highly sig
Reyes et al. [32]	N/A	NS	→3–4°	Highly sig
Staudt and Kiliaridis [27]	←	Sig	→	Highly sig
Choi et al. [33]	←4.7°	Highly Sig	→1.5°	Sig
Wolfe et al. [34]	N/A	NS	→2.5°	Highly sig

in Class IIIs, with the vast majority showing highly significant differences. The differences in mandibular protrusion between Class IIIs and Class Is are also much greater (often four times or more) than the differences in maxillary retrusion. In summary, the available evidence supports the notion that the AP differences between Class IIIs and Class Is are primarily due to mandibular protrusion, and only secondarily, to maxillary retrusion.

Protrusion is not the only characteristic of the mandible that is consistently different between Class Is and Class IIIs (Table 7.4). All of the studies evaluating overall or total mandibular size (e.g. Co-Gn or Co-Pg) have shown that Class IIIs are significantly larger than Class Is. While most studies indicate that the corpus is longer in Class IIIs than Class Is, the literature remains unclear whether there are differences in ramus height. Class differences in vertical relationships are more clear-cut. Class IIIs have larger mandibular plane and gonial angles than Class Is. Class IIIs are clearly mandibular prognathic and hyperdivergent.

The available studies suggest that the increased overall mandibular length found among Class IIIs worsens over time (Figure 7.4). Importantly, the differences in overall length between Class IIIs and Class Is do not appear to be due to excessive condylar growth. In this regard, it is important to remember that the condyle is a growth site (i.e. not a growth center), responsive to biomechanical and environmental stresses [44, 45]. Studies evaluating the growth of ramus height have reported both significant and nonsignificant differences between Class IIIs and Class Is (Table 7.4). Wolfe et al. [34], who followed well-matched groups longitudinally, showed that ramus height was approximately 1.4 mm greater in 6- to 8-year-old Class IIIs than Class Is and that the differences maintained through 14–16 years of age. If excessive condylar growth were the primary causative factor, ramus height should show larger and more consistent Class differences. More importantly, the differences should be increasing over time, as the differences in overall mandibular length do (Figure 7.4). The data provided by Björk and Skieller [46],

Table 7.4 Differences (Class III minus Class I) in mandibular protrusion, total size, ramus height, corpus length, mandibular plane angle, and gonial angle.

	Protrusion	Total size	Ramus Ht	Corpus Lt	MPA	Gonial angle
Sandborn [21]	→	N/A	NS	NS	N/A	↑
Jacobson et al. [23]	→	↑	NS	NS	↑	↑
Ellis and McNamara [24]	→	N/A	N/A	N/A	↑	N/A
Guyer et al. [25]	→	↑	↑	↑	↑	↑
Williams and Andersen [28]	→	↑	NS	NS	N/A	N/A
Battagel [29]	→	↑	N/A	N/A	↑	↑
Tollaro et al. [30]	→	↑	↑	↑	N/A	NS
Chang et al. [31]	→	↑	NS	↑	↑	↑
Reyes et al. [32]	→	↑	N/A	N/A	NS	N/A
Staudt and Kiliaridis [27]	→	N/A	N/A	N/A	↑	↑
Choi et al. [33]	→	↑	↑	N/A	NS	NS
Wolfe et al. [34]	→	↑	↑	↑	↑	↑
Most common	→	↑	—	↑	↑	↑

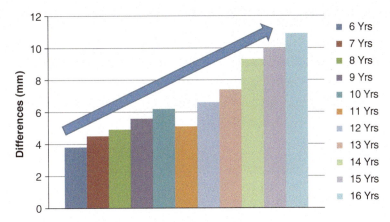

Figure 7.4 Differences (Class III minus Class I) in overall mandibular length between 6 and 16 years of age (adapted from Reyes et al. [32]).

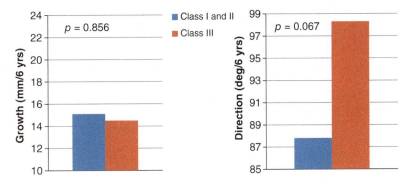

Figure 7.5 Total condylar growth and condylar growth direction based on mandibular superimpositions on metallic implants, adjusted for sex differences (Björk and Skieller [46]/with permission of Elsevier).

who superimposed the subjects' mandibles on metallic implants, shows more posterior condylar growth in Class IIIs than Class Is or Class IIs, but no differences in growth rates (Figure 7.5).

Class IIIs have excessively large overall mandibular lengths because their condyles grow in a more posterior direction. The more posterior the direction of condylar growth, the greater the increase in overall mandibular length. For example, 10 mm of condylar growth can increase overall length by up to 10 mm if it is directed more posteriorly along the original vector, but it increases overall length by only 0.5 mm if directed more anteriorly (Figure 7.6). As previously noted, the occlusion of Class IIIs is less stable, which causes them to posture their mandibles in a more anterior/inferior position. McNamara and Carlson [47] were the first to show that when the mandible is clinically protruded, the condylar cartilage adapts by assuming a more posterior direction of growth. Functional appliances, which also posture the mandible forward and down, alter condylar growth in a more posterior direction [48].

Finally, there are consistent differences in incisor relationships between Class IIIs and Class Is. The upper incisors of Class IIIs are usually proclined and the lower incisors are retroclined (Table 7.5). Since the interincisor angles are usually greater among Class IIIs, the differences in lower incisor retroclination between Class IIIs and Class Is must be greater than the differences in upper incisor proclination.

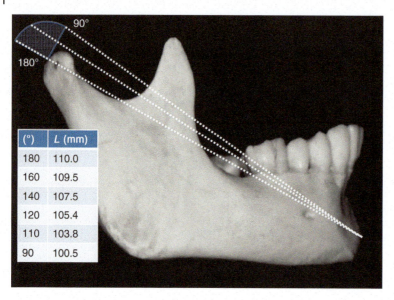

Figure 7.6 Changes in overall mandibular length (L) depending on 10 mm of condylar growth in various directions.

Table 7.5 Differences (Class III minus Class I) in upper incisor angulation, lower incisor angulation, and interincisal angulation.

	U1 Inc	IMPA	U1/L1
Sandborn [21]	↑	↓	↑
Jacobson et al. [23]	↑	↓	N/A
Ellis and McNamara [24]	↑	↓	N/A
Guyer et al. [25]	↑	↓	NS
Battagel [29]	↑	↓	N/A
Mouakeh [49]	↑	↓	↑
Chang et al. [31]	↑	↓	N/A
Staudt and Kiliaridis [27]	↑	↓	N/A
Choi et al. [33]	↑	↓	↑
Most common	↑	↑	↑

7.3 Class III development

Class III malocclusion often develops during the primary dentition. Angle [50] wrote that it occurs with the emergence of the first permanent molars or even earlier. There is substantial literature supporting the existence of Class III malocclusion in the primary dentition. Three-dimensional analyses show that differences between Class III and non-Class IIIs are evident by 5–6 years of age [51]. Guyer et al. [25] noted that the maxillary retrusion and mandibular protrusion that characterize 13- to 15-year-old Class IIIs are already evident in 5- to 7-year-olds. Interestingly, Sugawara and Mitani [43] reported greater differences (i.e. mandibular protrusion, mandibular length) between 7-year-old Class Is and Class IIIs than their 10-year-old counterparts. Japanese samples show that the AP discrepancies are already established when the second deciduous molars erupt [52].

Class III molar relationships worsen over time, and the changes appear to be growth-related (Figure 7.7). As previously shown, the large-scale epidemiological studies conducted in the 1970s evaluating molar relationships showed that the prevalence of Class III malocclusion was higher in youths 12–17 years of age than children at 6–11 years old. More recently, the NHANES III showed that the prevalence of Class III malocclusion increases between

7.3 Class III development

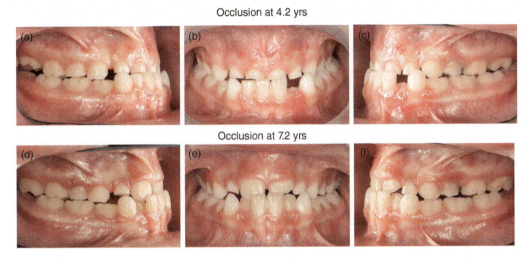

Figure 7.7 Lateral (a, c, d, and f) and frontal (b and e) intraoral views showing worsening of Class III malocclusion in an untreated male patient followed between 4y 2m and 7y 2m (courtesy of Dr. Samuel Roldan).

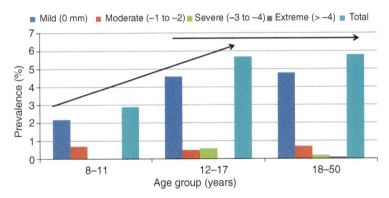

Figure 7.8 NHANES III estimates of Class III malocclusion among US children, adolescents, and adults (Proffit et al. [20]/Quintessence Publishing Company, Inc.).

childhood (8–11 years) and adolescence (12–17 years) but not thereafter (Figure 7.8) [20]. Longitudinal evaluations of 22 untreated Class IIIs show that the molar relationships worsened by 3.3 mm between 8.5 and 15.2 years of age [53].

Most, but not all, Class III skeletal relationships also worsen over time. Baccetti et al. [53] showed worsening for the Wits appraisal (−2 mm) and ANB angle (−1.9°) of Class IIIs evaluated at 8.5 and 15.2 years of age. In contrast, Wolfe et al. [34], who longitudinally evaluated 42 untreated Class IIIs, showed that the ANB angle decreased by approximately 0.25 deg/yr between 6 and 16 years of age (Figure 7.9). Importantly, the decreases in the ANB angle that occurred over time were the same in Class IIIs as in Class Is. In other words, the differences between Class IIIs and Class Is were already established by 6–8 years of age and were maintained through 17 years of age. The large cross-sectional sample evaluated by Reyes et al. [32] also shows that the differences in the ANB angle that exist between Class IIIs and Class Is do not increase over time.

In contrast, Class differences in the Wits appraisal and maxillo-mandibular differential

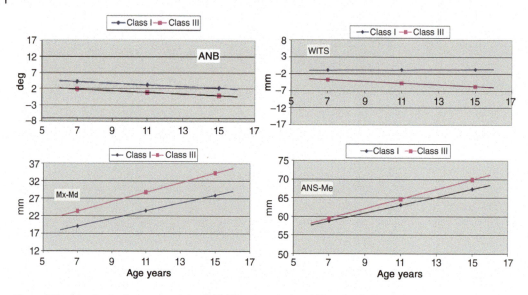

Figure 7.9 Longitudinal changes of the ANB, Wits appraisal, maxillomandibular differential, and lower face height of untreated Class IIIs and matched Class Is (Wolfe et al. [34]/EH Angle Orthodontists Research & Education Foundation, Inc.).

increase over time. The maxillo-mandibular differential increases in both Class IIIs and Class Is, but the increase is significantly greater among Class IIIs (Figure 7.9). The Wits appraisal shows little or no change among Class Is and decreases among Class IIIs. Larger cross-sectional Class III Japanese samples [52], evaluated at various times between the eruption of the first permanent incisors and the completed eruption of the third molars, show the same changes in the ANB angle (1.9°) as Class Is but greater than expected changes of the Wits (5.5 mm) appraisal.

The Wits appraisal and the maxillomandibular differential of Class IIIs worsen over time, while the ANB angle does not, due to the associated vertical growth changes that are occurring. As indicated earlier, most studies evaluating the vertical aspects of Class III malocclusion have found larger mandibular plane and gonial angles among Class IIIs (Table 7.4). The longitudinal evaluations by Wolfe et al. [34] showed greater-than-expected increases in lower facial height among Class IIIs. This indicates that Class IIIs not only are more hyperdivergent than Class Is but also that they continue to become more hyperdivergent over time. In other words, their mandibles do not undergo as much forward true rotation or their mandibles might even be rotating backwards. True forward rotation is the primary determinant of anterior chin displacement; during childhood, the chin is displaced forward 1.2 mm for every degree of forward rotation that occurs [54]. The ANB angle does not change as much as the Wits or maxillomandibular differential, because vertical growth masks the development discrepancies in overall length.

7.4 Etiology

Nongenetic growth disturbances and genetic factors determine the etiology of Class III malocclusion (Figure 7.10). Regarding nongenetic disturbances, anything that prevents the midface from being displaced anteriorly can produce Class III skeletal and dental relationships. For example, it has been well established that cleft lip/palate surgery produces Class III malocclusion due to midfacial retrusion.

Non-genetic growth disturbances

- Prevention of midfacial anterior displacement
- Habitual postural positioning

Genetic factors

- Congenital maxillary synostoses
- Primary cartilage growth
- Tooth sizes

Figure 7.10 Nongenetic disturbances and genetic factors that explain the etiology of Class III malocclusion.

Doğan et al. [55] showed that children who had unilateral cleft lip and palate closures at 3 and 12 months, respectively, had shorter and more posteriorly positioned maxillae than untreated controls. The midfacial deficiencies are related to the scar tissues produced by the palatal and lip surgery, which inhibits or restricts the normal anterior displacement of the maxilla that occurs during growth. Scar tissues in the posterior pharyngeal region could also serve as a tether, restricting the normal anterior and inferior displacement of the posterior maxilla that occurs. The midfacial retrusion that characterizes cleft patients is iatrogenic. Individuals with unoperated clefts have relatively normal facial growth potential [56]. Trauma that causes premature synostosis of midfacial sutures can also prevent midfacial displacements. For example, Ousterhout and Vargervik [57] reported maxillary hypoplasia secondary to midfacial trauma among children who had normal facial proportions before their accidents.

Habitual anterior posturing of the mandible is probably the primary cause of Class III malocclusion. Patients who present with anterior crossbite and Class III malocclusion often posture their mandibles forward when occluding. If this is identified early, the mandible can often be manipulated back into a centric relation (Figure 7.11). There are various factors that could cause patients to habitually posture their mandibles forward. Occlusal relations, especially the anterior, need to be considered etiological factors. As previously indicated, the limited posterior contacts and near contact make Class III occlusions less stable and forward posturing of the mandible more likely. Airway issues also need to be considered. Angle [50], for example, considered lower airway disturbances to be the major etiological factors explaining Class III malocclusion. He thought that enlarged tonsils cause children to protrude the tongue and, in turn, the mandible. It has been well established that enlarged tonsils cause patients to posture the tongue

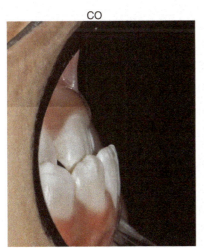
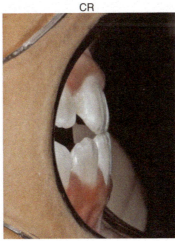

Figure 7.11 Pretreatment records of a patient who habitually postures her mandible forward (2 mm CO/CR discrepancy) into centric occlusion.

forward to maintain their airways. Any airway disturbance could cause individuals to posture their mandible forward. When Harvold et al. eliminated the possibility of nasal breathing, primates postured their mandibles in various ways, with some posturing anteriorly [58]. There may also be other environmental factors that could cause subjects to posture their mandible in a more anterior position. Cone-beam computed tomography has shown children with Class III malocclusion have significantly larger oropharyngeal airways than Class Is [59].

Unlike Class I and Class II malocclusions, for which no genetic basis has been established, Class III malocclusion "runs in families." Population studies show that approximately 11–13% of Class III relatives were affected [60, 61]. Studies of Class III monozygotic twin pairs demonstrate a lack of concordance [62] and variable expressivity [63] of the malocclusion. Importantly, genetics does not directly determine the excessive amounts of mandibular growth that characterize Class III subjects. Their genes predispose them to Class III malocclusion.

Genetically, there are three ways that individuals may be predisposed to developing Class III malocclusion. Subjects with maxillary retrusion could have a genetic predisposition for synostosis of the sutures. Mutations of the fibroblast growth factor signaling molecules have been found in patients diagnosed with Crouzon, Pfeiffer, and Jackson–Weiss craniosynostosis syndromes [64]. These same individuals could also have synostoses of the circumaxillary and intermaxillary sutures. Premature synostosis of the premaxillary-maxillary, nasal-frontal, and maxillary-palatine sutures has been reported in mouse models of Pfeiffer and Apert syndromes [65].

Genetic factors also play a dominant role in the development of the chondrocranium. Growth of the synchondroses, like other primary cartilages, is largely under genetic control. Most of the available literature indicates that the cranial base angle of Class IIIs is significantly smaller than the cranial base angle of Class Is (Figure 7.12; Table 7.6). The largest available cross-sectional study of untreated subjects 6–16 years of age showed that the cranial base angle of Class IIIs was approximately 7° smaller than the cranial base angle of Class Is [32]. A smaller cranial base angle effectively repositions the maxilla and mandible more posteriorly and anteriorly, respectively (Figure 7.13). Although more limited, there is also some evidence that cranial base lengths of Class IIIs may be shorter, which would also predispose subjects to skeletal discrepancies.

The nasal septum is also a growth center that plays an important role in midfacial growth

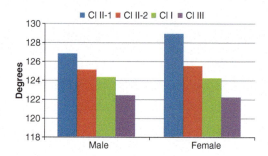

Figure 7.12 Cranial base angle (N-S-Ba) of subjects with Class I, Class II, and Class III malocclusion (Hopkins et al. [66]/with permission of Elsevier).

Table 7.6 Differences (Class III minus Class I) in cranial base angulation, anterior length, and posterior length.

	Angle	Anterior	Posterior
Sandborn [21]	N/A	↓	N/A
Hopkins et al. [66]	↓	↓	↓
Guyer et al. [25]	NS	NS	↑
Williams and Andersen [28]	↓	NS	↓
Battagel [29]	↓	NS	N/A
Tollaro et al. [30]	NS	NS	N/A
Mouakeh [49]	NS	↓	↓
Chang et al. [31]	↓	NS	↓
Reyes et al. [32]	↓	↓	N/A
Staudt and Kiliaridis [27]	↓	N/A	N/A
Wolfe et al. [34]	NS	NS	N/A

displacements. In their classic work, Wexler and Sarnat [67] showed that removal of the nasal septum limited midfacial growth of rabbits. Some individuals may have a genetic predisposition for maxillary deficiencies that result in Class III malocclusion.

Along with endochondral bone (i.e. bone formed from primary cartilage), tooth size is also highly heritable. Townsend and Brown [68] have estimated that approximately 64% of the variability in permanent tooth size can be attributed to genetic factors. More recently, Baydas et al. [69] showed that both the overall and anterior Bolton ratios were highly heritable. A review of the available literature shows that most studies evaluating the Bolton ratios of Class IIIs and Class Is report significant differences (Table 7.7). The anterior, posterior, and overall ratios tend to be higher among Class IIIs, and the differences apply worldwide. Importantly, the differences are due to relatively larger mandibular than maxillary tooth size [78].

The key to understanding the development of Class III malocclusion may be the cusp–fossa relationships of teeth (Figure 7.14). Whether the skeletal discrepancies are due to mandibular protrusion, maxillary retrusion, or a combination of both, the occlusion of

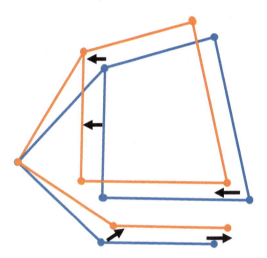

Figure 7.13 Relative effects of a smaller cranial base angle, bringing the maxillary back and the mandible forward.

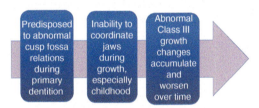

Figure 7.14 Importance of cusp–fossa relationships to the development of Class III dental and skeletal malocclusion.

Table 7.7 Differences (Class III minus Class I) in the anterior, posterior, and overall Bolton ratios.

	Anterior	Posterior	Overall	Ethnicity
Sperry et al. [70]	NS	N/A	↑	US
Nie and Lin [71]	↑	↑	↑	Chinese
Ta et al. [72]	↑	N/A	↑	Chinese
Araujo and Souki [73]	↑	N/A	↑	Brazil
Uysal and Sari [36]	NS	N/A	NS	Turkey
Al-Khateeb and Alhaija [41]	NS	N/A	NS	Jordan
Fattahi et al. [74]	↑	↑	↑	Iran
Strujić et al. [75]	↑	↑	↑	Croatia
Wedrychowska-Szulc et al. [76]	↑	N/A	↑	Poland
Johe et al. [77]	NS	N/A	NS	US

↑, across the board difference; ↑, limited differences; NS, not statistically significant.

Class IIIs will be compromised. It has been experimentally shown that a more prognathic mandible is produced and a more mesial occlusion develops when interdigitation is eliminated by grinding the cusps of the posterior teeth and canines of primates [79]. In other words, the lack of proper interdigitation of the posterior teeth plays a prominent role in the development of Class III malocclusion. Both the foregoing nongenetic disturbances and genetic factors make it difficult for the teeth of Class IIIs to fit together.

How the teeth fit together influences the maxillomandibular skeletal relationships? Tooth cusps do not improve the ability to chew and break down foods. Anthropologists have shown that attritional occlusion with flat occlusal surfaces was the norm among both prehistoric and nonindustrialized groups [80]. Occlusal wear was the norm for most of the human history. Based on their extensive work with Australian Aboriginals, Begg and Kesling [81] were among the first orthodontists to claim that cusps diminish rather than enhance masticatory efficiency. They found that the role of high cusps was to help guide the teeth into their occlusal relationships. From an evolutionary perspective, the cusps fitting together serve primarily to stabilize the relationship of the upper and lower jaws during growth [80]. By the time the second molar erupts, the enamel on the occlusal surface of the first molar had often worn off in prehistoric groups, and the cusps of the second molar were often worn off when the third molar erupted. Since the crown pattern of the first molar has been among the most stable over the past 20 million years [82], the cusp–fossa relationships of the first molars appear to be the most important. This indicates that treatments that establish stable Class I molar relationships and simultaneously address the etiology of the problem hold great potential for longer-term stability (Figure 7.15).

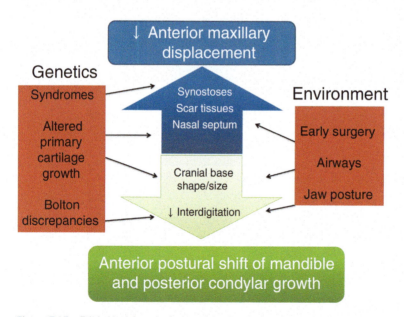

Figure 7.15 Etiological factors that explain the development of Class III malocclusion.

References

1. Angle EH. Classification of malocclusion. *Dental Cosmos* 1899;**41**:248–64.
2. Mantzikos T. Esthetic soft tissue profile preferences among the Japanese population. *Am J Orthod Dentofacial Orthop* 1998;**114**(1):1–7.
3. Türkkahraman H, Gökalp H. Facial profile preferences among various layers of Turkish population. *Angle Orthod* 2004;**74**(6):640–7.
4. Maple JR, Vig KWL, Beck M, et al. A comparison of providers' and consumers' perceptions of facial-profile attractiveness. *Am J Orthod Dentofacial Orthop* 2005;**128**(6):690–6.
5. Dion K, Berscheid E, Walster E. What is beautiful is good. *J Pers Soc Psychol* 1972;**24**(3):285–90.
6. Albino JE, Alley TR, Tedesco LA, et al. Esthetic issues in behavioral dentistry. *Ann Behav Med* 1990;**12**:148–55.
7. Shaw WC. The influence of children's dentofacial appearance on their social attractiveness as judged by peers and lay adults. *Am J Orthod* 1981;**79**(4):399–415.
8. English JD, Buschang PH, Throckmorton GS. Does malocclusion affect masticatory performance? *Angle Orthod* 2002;**72**(1):21–7.
9. Zhou Y, Fu M. Masticatory efficiency in skeletal class III malocclusion. *Zhonghua Kou Qiang Yi Xue Za Zhi* 1995;**30**(2):72–4.
10. Owens S, Buschang PH, Throckmorton GS, et al. Masticatory performance and areas of occlusal contact and near contact in subjects with normal occlusion and malocclusion. *Am J Orthod Dentofacial Orthop* 2002;**121**(6):602–9.
11. Bakke M, Holm B, Jensen BL, et al. Unilateral, isometric bite force in 8–69-year-old women and men related to occlusal factors. *Scand J Dent Res* 1990;**98**(2):149–58.
12. Ellis E, Throckmorten GS, Sinn DP. Bite forces before and after surgical correction of mandibular prognathism. *J Oral Maxillofac Surg* 1996;**54**(2):176–81.
13. Lepley CR, Throckmorton GS, Ceen RF, Buschang PH. Relative contribution of occlusion, maximum bite force, and chewing cycle kinematics to masticatory performance. *Am J Orthod Dentofacial Orthop* 2011;**139**:606–13.
14. Proeschel PA. Chewing patterns in subjects with normal occlusion and with malocclusion. *Semin Orthod* 2006;**12**(2):138–49.
15. Ahlgren J. Pattern of chewing and malocclusion of teeth. A clinical study. *Acta Odontol Scand* 1967;**25**(1):3–13.
16. Hardy DK, Cubas YP, Orellana MF. Prevalence of angle class III malocclusion: a systematic review and meta analysis. *Open J Epidem* 2012;**2**:75–82.
17. Alhammadi MS, Halboub E, Fayed MS, et al. Global distribution of malocclusion traits: A systematic review. *Dental Press J Orthod* 2018;**23**(6):40 e1–10.
18. Kelly JE, Sanchez M, VanKirk LE. National Center for Health Statistics: an assessment of the occlusion of the teeth of children 6–11 years, United States. In: *Vital and health. Statistics*. Series 11-No. 130. DHEW Pub. No. (HRA) 74–1612. Washington, DC: Health Resources Administration, 1973.
19. Kelly JE. An assessment of the occlusion of the teeth of youths 12–17 years, United States. In: *Vital and health. Statistics*. Series 11-No. 162. DHEW Pub. No. (HRA) 74–1644. Washington, DC: Health Resources Administration, 1973.
20. Proffit WR, Fields HW Jr, Moray LJ. Prevalence of malocclusion and orthodontic treatment need in the United States: estimates from the NHANES III survey. *Int J Adult Orthodon Orthognath Surg* 1998;**13**(2):97–106.

21. Sanborn RT. Differences between the facial skeletal patterns of Class III malocclusion and normal occlusion. *Angle Orthod* 1955;**25**(4):208–21.
22. Dietrich UC. Morphological variability of skeletal Class III relationships as revealed by cephalometric analysis. *Trans Eur Orthod Soc* 1970;**46**:131–43.
23. Jacobson A, Evans WG, Preston CB, Sadowsky PL. Mandibular prognathism. *Am J Orthod* 1974;**66**(2):140–71.
24. Ellis E, McNamara JA Jr. Components of adult Class III malocclusion. *J Oral Maxillofac Surg* 1984;**42**:295–305.
25. Guyer EC, Ellis ED III, McNamara JA Jr, Behrents RG. Components of Class II malocclusion in juveniles and adolescents. *Angle Orthod* 1986;**56**(1):7–30.
26. Bui C, King T, Proffit W, Frazier-Bowers S. Phenotypic characterization of Class III patients. *Angle Orthod* 2006;**76**(4):564–9.
27. Staudt CB, Kiliaridis S. Different skeletal types underlying Class III malocclusion in a random population. *Am J Orthod Dentofacial Orthop* 2009;**136**(5):715–21.
28. Williams S, Andersen CE. The morphology of the potential skeletal pattern in the growing child. *Am J Orthod* 1986;**89**(4):302–11.
29. Battagel J. The aetiological factors in Class III malocclusion. *Eur J Orthod* 1993;**15**(5):347–70.
30. Tollaro I, Baccetti T, Bassarelli V, Franchi L. Class III malocclusion in the deciduous dentition, a morphological and correlation study. *Eur J Orthod* 1994;**16**(5):401–8.
31. Chang HP, Liu PH, Yang YH, et al. Craniofacial morphometric analysis of mandibular prognathism. *J Oral Rehabil* 2006;**33**(3):183–93.
32. Reyes BC, Baccetti T, McNamara JA. An estimate of cranio-facial growth in Class III malocclusion. *Angle Orthod* 2006;**76**(4):577–84.
33. Choi HJ, Kim JY, Yoo SE, et al. Cephalometric characteristics of Korean children with Class III malocclusion in the deciduous dentition. *Angle Orthod* 2010;**80**(1):86–90.
34. Wolfe SM, Araujo E, Behrents RG, Buschang PH. Cranio-facial growth of Class II subjects six to sixteen years of age. *Angle Orthod* 2011;**81**(2):211–6.
35. Kuntz TR, Staley RN, Bigelow HF, et al. Arch widths in adults with Class I crowded and Class III malocclusions compared with normal occlusion. *Angle Orthod* 2008;**78**(4):597–603.
36. Uysal T, Sari Z. Intermaxillary tooth size discrepancy and mesiodistal crown dimensions for a Turkish population. *Am J Orthod Dentofacial Orthop* 2005;**128**(2):226–30.
37. Herren P, Jordi-Guilloud T. Quantitative determination of dental arch by polygon measurements in the ideal and anomalous arch. *SSO Schweiz Monatsschr Zahnheilkd* 1973;**83**(6):682–709.
38. Chen F, Terada K, Yang L, Saito I. Dental arch widths and mandibular-maxillary base widths in class III malocclusion from ages 10–14. *Am J Orthod Dentofacial Orthop* 2008;**133**(1):65–9.
39. Braun S, Hnat WP, Fender DE, Legan HL. The form of the human dental arch. *Angle Orthod* 1998;**68**(1):29–36.
40. Basaran G, Hamamci N, Hamamci O. Comparison of dental arch widths in different types of malocclusion. *World J Orthod* 2008;**9**(1):e20–8.
41. Al-Khateeb SN, Alhija ESJA. Tooth size discrepancies and arch parameters among different malocclusions in a Jordanian sample. *Angle Orthod* 2006;**76**(3):459–65.
42. Chen F, Terada K, Wu L, Saito I. Dental arch widths and mandibular-maxillary base width in Class III malocclusions with low, average and high MP-SN angles. *Angle Orthod* 2007;**77**(1):36–41.
43. Sugawara J, Mitani H. Facial growth of skeletal Class II malocclusion and the effects, limitations, and long-term dentofacial adaptations to chincap therapy. *Semin Orthod* 1997;**3**(4):244–54.
44. Copray JCVM, Jansen HWB, Duterloo HS. Growth and growth pressure of

mandibular condylar and some primary cartilages of the rat in vitro. *Am J Orthod Dentofacial Orthop* 1986;**90**(1):19–28.
45. Peltomäki T, Kylämarkula S, Vinkka-Puhakka H, et al. Tissue-separating capacity of growth cartilages. *Eur J Orthod* 1997;**19**(5):473–81.
46. Björk A, Skieller V. Facial development and tooth eruption – An implant study at the age of puberty. *Am J Orthod* 1972;**62**(4):339–83.
47. McNamara JA Jr, Carlson DS. Quantitative analysis of temporomandibular joint adaptation to protrusive function. *Am J Orthod* 1979;**76**(6):593–611.
48. Araujo A, Buschang PH, Melo ACM. Adaptive condylar growth and mandibular remodeling changes with bionator therapy – an implant study. *Eur J Orthod* 2004;**26**(5):515–22.
49. Mouakeh M. Cephalometric evaluation of craniofacial pattern of Syrian children with Class III malocclusion. *Am J Orthod Dentofacial Orthop* 2001;**119**(6):640–9.
50. Angle EH. *Treatment of malocclusion of the teeth*. Philadelphia, PA: S.S. White Dental Manufacturing Co, 1907.
51. Krenta B, Primožič J, Zhurov A, et al. Three-dimensional evaluation of facial morphology in children age 5–6 yeas with a Class III malocclusion. *Eur J Orthod* 2014;**36**(2):133–9.
52. Miyajima K, McNamara JA Jr, Sana M, Murata S. An estimation of craniofacial growth in the untreated Class III female with anterior crossbite. *Am J Orthod Dentofacial Orthop* 1997;**112**(4):425–34.
53. Baccetti T, Franchi L, McNamara JA Jr. Growth in the untreated Class III subject. *Semin Orthod* 2007;**13**(3):130–42.
54. Buschang PH, Jacob HB. Mandibular rotation revisited: what makes it so important? *Semin Orthod* 2014;**20**(4):299–315.
55. Doğan S, Oncağ G, Akin Y. Craniofacial development in children with unilateral cleft lip and palate. *Br J Oral Maxillofac Surg* 2006;**44**(1):28–33.
56. Shetye PR. Facial growth of adults with unoperated clefts. *Clin Plast Surg* 2004;**31**(2):361–71.
57. Ousterhout DK, Vargervik K. Maxillary hypoplasia secondary to midfacial trauma in childhood. *Plast Reconstr Surg* 1987;**80**(4):491–7.
58. Harvold EP, Tomer BS, Vargevik K, Chierici G. Primate experiments in oral respiration. *Am J Orthod* 1981;**79**(4):359–72.
59. Iwasaki T, Hayasaki H, Takemoto Y, et al. Oropharyngeal airway in children with Class III malocclusion evaluated by cone-beam computed tomography. *Am J Orthod Dentofacial Orthop* 2009;**136**:318.e1–9.
60. Watanabe M, Suda N, Ohyama K. Mandibular prognathism in Japanese families ascertained through orthognathically treated patients. *Am J Orthod Dentofacial Orthop* 2005;**128**:466–70.
61. Cruz RM, Krieger H, Ferreira R, et al. Major gene and multifactorial inheritance of mandibular prognathism. *Am J Med Genet A* 2008;**146A**:71–7.
62. Korkhaus G. Anthropologic and odontologic studies of twins. *Int J Orthod Oral Surg Radiogr*. 1930;**16**:640–7.
63. Jena AK, Duggal R, Mathur VP, Parkash H. Class III malocclusion: genetics or environment? A twin study. *J Indican Soc Pedod Prev Dent* 2005;**23**:27–30.
64. Eswarakumar VP, Lax I, Schlessinger J. Cellular signaling by fibroblast growth factor receptors. *Cytokine Growth Factor Rev* 2005;**16**(2):139–49.
65. Purushothaman R, Cox TC, Maga AM, Cunningham ML. Facial suture synostosis of newborn Fgfr1(P250R/+) and Fgfr2(S252W/+) mouse models of Pfeiffer and Apert syndromes. *Birth Defects Res A Clin Mol Teratol* 2011;**91**(7):603–9.
66. Hopkins GB, Houston WJB, James GA. The cranial base as an aetiological factor in malocclusion. *Angle Orthod* 1968;**38**(3):250–5.
67. Wexler MR, Sarnat BG. Rabbit snout growth. Effect of injury to septovomeral region. *Arch Otolaryngol* 1961;**74**:305–13.

68 Townsend GC, Brown T. Heritability of permanent tooth size. *Am J Phys Anthropol* 1978;**49**(4):497–504.
69 Baydas B, Oktay H, Dağsuyu IM. The effect of heritability on Bolton tooth-size discrepancy. *Eur J Orthod* 2005;**27**(1):98–102.
70 Sperry TP, Worms FW, Isaacson RJ, Speidel TM. Tooth-size discrepancy in mandibular prognathism. *Am J Orthod* 1977;**72**(2):183–90.
71 Nie Q, Lin J. Comparison of intermaxillary tooth size discrepancies among different malocclusion groups. *Am J Orthod Dentofacial Orthop* 1999;**116**(5):539–44.
72 Ta TA, Ling JYK, Hägg U. Tooth-size discrepancies among different occlusion groups of southern Chinese children. *Am J Orthod Dentofacial Orthop* 2001;**120**(5):556–8.
73 Araujo E, Souki M. Bolton anterior tooth size discrepancies among different malocclusion groups. *Angle Orthod* 2003;**73**(3):307–13.
74 Fattahi HR, Pakshir HR, Hedayati Z. Comparison of tooth size discrepancies among different malocclusion groups. *Eur J Orthod* 2006;**28**(5):491–5.
75 Strujić M, Anić-Milošević S, Meštrović S, Šlaj M. Tooth size discrepancy in orthodontic patients among different malocclusion groups. *Eur J Orthod* 2009;**31**(6):584–9.
76 Wedrychowska-Szulc B, Janiszewska-Olszowska J, Stepien P. Overall and anterior Bolton ratio in Class I, II, and III orthodontic patients. *Eur J Orthod* 2010;**32**(3):313–8.
77 Johe RS, Steinhart T, Sado N, et al. Intermaxillary tooth-size discrepancies in different sexes, malocclusion groups, and ethnicies. *Am J Orthod Dentofacial Orthop* 2010;**138**(5):599–607.
78 Lavelle CLB. Maxillary and mandibular tooth size in different racial groups and in different occlusal categories. *Am J Orthod* 1972;**61**(1):29–37.
79 Ostyn JM, Maltha JC, van't Hof MA, van der Linden FPGM. The role of interdigitation in sagittal growth of the maxillomandibular complex in *Macaca fascicularis*. *Am J Orthod Dentofacial Orthop* 1996;**109**(1):71–8.
80 Brace CL. Occlusion to the anthropological eye. In: McNamara JA Jr (ed), *The biology of occlusal development*. Ann Arbor, MI: Center Human Growth and Development, University of Michigan, 1977. p. 179–209.
81 Begg PR, Kesling PC. *Begg's orthodontic theory and technique*. 2nd edn. Philadelphia, PA: WB Saunders, 1971.
82 Gregory WK, Hellman M. The dentition of Dryopithecus and the origin of man. *Anthropol. Pap. Am. Mus. Nat. Hist.* 1926;**28**:1–23.

7.2

Section II: Class III treatment: problems and solutions
Eustáquio A. Araújo, DDS, MDS

Center for Advanced Dental Education, Department of Orthodontics, Saint Louis University, St. Louis, MO, USA

The skeletal pattern of "children with protruding chins" has been reported since 1757 when Bourdet [1] described the characteristics of the malocclusion. Later, in the early 1900s, Angle [2] defined Class III malocclusion as "the relation of the jaws with all the lower teeth occluding mesial to normally the width of one premolar or even more in extreme cases."

In the first section of this chapter, the prevalence of this malocclusion has been fully described as reported in the literature [3–9].

Class III deviations are frequently classified among the most challenging mechanical problems in orthodontics. In addition, it seems to predispose more patients to low indices of self-esteem (Figure 7.16) [10, 11].

Nonsurgical approaches for developing Class IIIs require a meticulous diagnosis protocol and thoughtful decision-making in relation to treatment modalities and timing. There is no consensus among different authors in relation to the problem, even though the literature on this matter is extensive. An untreated Class III usually worsens over time as demonstrated in Figures 7.17 and 7.18. It can be observed that a malocclusion that was initially believed to be mild to moderate at age 9 became much more severe at age 16 and was expected to be treated with surgery. Although it is impossible to predict if an early orthodontic/orthopedic intervention would be able to alter the course of the establishment of the malocclusion, it is the clinician's responsibility to study each patient carefully. Among the studies that analyze Class III growth and compare it with Class I growth, those by Baccetti et al. [12] and Wolfe et al. [13] unequivocally demonstrate that Class III malocclusions tend to become more severe with time as growth continues.

The development of the Class III malocclusion has been extensively described in the preamble to this chapter by Buschang.

Are there reasons for early intervention even with the risk of unfavorable growth in the future?

Till now, nonsurgical Class III treatments are essentially a camouflaging of the discrepancy, with the objective of obtaining a better dental relationship and a more harmonious face. These treatments are initiated during the early mixed dentition to provide ample time and flexibility for maxillary expansion and protraction as well as redirection of the mandibular growth in a more clockwise direction (Figure 7.19).

Patients with normal or hypodivergent vertical profiles are the ones who benefit the most from early interventions. Those with hyperdivergent faces and patterns of growth may experience a decrease in the severity of their problem, but they may still have to undergo some type of orthognathic surgery.

Recognizing and Correcting Developing Malocclusions: A Problem-Oriented Approach to Orthodontics, Second Edition. Edited by Eustáquio A. Araújo and Peter H. Buschang.
© 2025 John Wiley & Sons, Inc. Published 2025 by John Wiley & Sons, Inc.

7.2 Section II: Class III treatment: problems and solutions

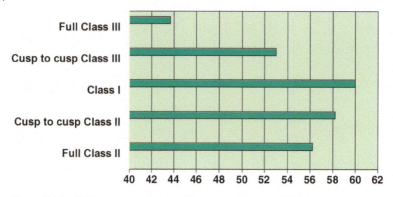

Figure 7.16 Self-esteem evaluation (Graber and Lucker [10]/with permission of Elsevier).

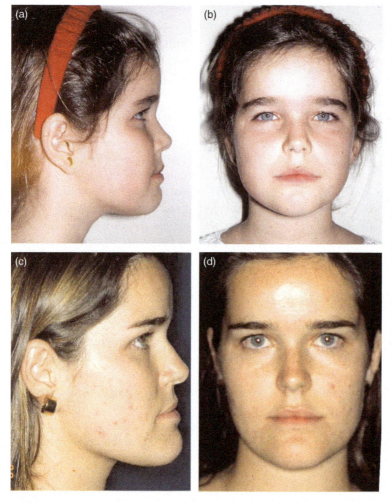

Figure 7.17 Untreated Class III, (a, b) prepubertal and (c, d) postpubertal.

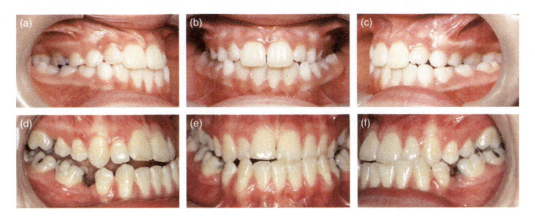

Figure 7.18 Intraoral composite of untreated Class III: (a–c) prepubertal and (d–f) postpubertal.

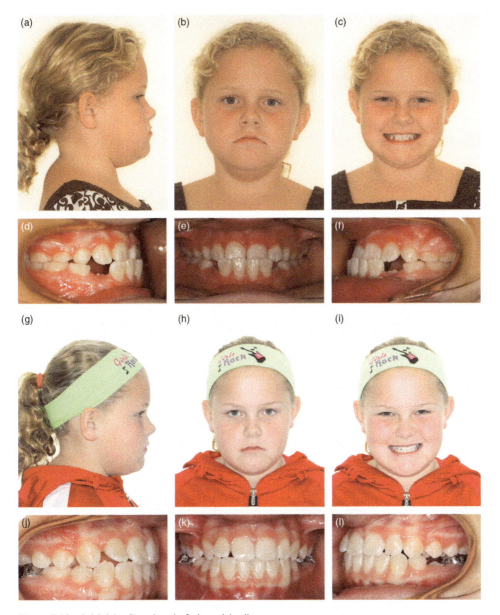

Figure 7.19 Initial (a–f) and end of phase I (g–l).

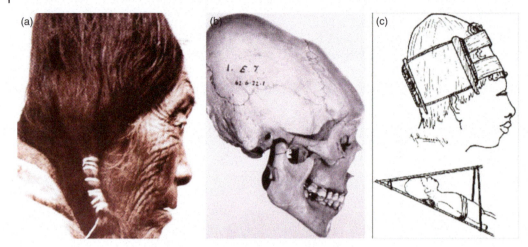

Figure 7.20 Induced cranium deformation (from [15]).

With all the unpredictability and important variables included in the Class III development, how can we decide whether to treat or not at an early age?

Answers to this question are strongly related to psychological issues. Intervention can lead to increased self-esteem, that would normally be followed by a higher degree of social acceptance. Bullying has become recognized as a major social disorder, and those affected by a "different" facial appearance may be targeted more than others. Dion showed that children favor "prettier" girls and "cuter" boys [14]. They tend to pick attractive children for friends and express dislike for the unattractive ones, based on the appearance alone. Albino also stresses that "Emotional well-being is directly related to facial and dental esthetics" [11].

Another reason to defend a primary intervention is the reestablishment of correct function as early as possible. Untreated premature contacts with either lateral or forward functional deviations must be addressed early, preferably as soon as detected, in order to avoid asymmetrical growth and an unwanted direction of growth. Growth can be unpredictable and, when not controlled, may be the cause of much frustration.

The controversy on this matter is basically centered on the likelihood of changing or restraining growth in Class III. An interesting review of cultural and ancient ways of changing growth direction has been presented by Sassouni [15]. Orthopedic resources have been used in order to alter the shape of parts of the human body [15, 16] (Figures 7.20 and 7.21).

Reports like these are thought-provoking, and they increase the number of questions to be pursued. How much of the growth change we

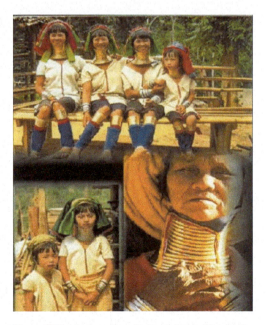

Figure 7.21 Induced neck elongation with metal rings? A Thailand ancient tradition.

see is genetically related and how much is environmental? As clinicians, we may interfere in the environmental or external factors, but we are still incapable of manipulating hereditary traits.

Our protocol for treating Class III developing malocclusions consists of ten points that, for many years, we have affectionately named *The Ten Commandments of the Class III*: 1) diagnosis; 2) communication; 3) early intervention; 4) orthopedic maxillary expansion; 5) face mask and/or chincup orthopedics; 6) leeway space control; 7) orthodontic mechanics; 8) finishing; 9) retention, and 10) growth reevaluation.

7.5 Diagnosis

Records must be kept with extreme diligence in order to minimize errors that could possibly influence diagnosis. It is imperative that impeccable attention be paid to detail.

Facial, cephalometric, and dental diagnostics are routine in our daily practice. In Class III individuals, however, it becomes indispensable to add to this routine a thorough and detailed functional diagnosis and a meaningful heredity study. A functional diagnosis with an accurate assessment of the centric occlusion (CO) or maximum intercuspation (MIP), and centric relation (CR) is crucial in determining the severity of the deviation as well as providing information for planning the correct treatment. A family study is vital in assessing previous history of Class III as well as treatments and surgeries and their results. It is important to examine the parents and older siblings, if possible. A cephalometric study of these family members when available may provide valuable information as to the likely growth pattern of the patient, which can be useful in deciding on the treatment plan. Let us introduce each phase of the diagnosis in a more didactic format.

7.5.1 Facial diagnosis

Facial evaluation is normally capable of providing the first indications of the origin of the discrepancy—maxillary retrusion, mandibular protrusion, or a combination of both [16]. A natural head position is warranted with the visual or optic plane [15] as parallel as possible to the floor.

In the Class III individuals, the photographic study must be duplicated, once in CR and then in CO (Figure 7.22).

7.5.2 Cephalometric diagnosis

It really does not matter which analysis is used, since they all include traditional measurements that quantify skeletal discrepancy. Some specificities, however, can be taken from various analyses [17, 18] (Figure 7.23).

It is highly recommended to have two cephalometric registrations – one in CR and one in CO. Because Class III treatments attempt to camouflage the skeletal deviations, the evaluations of the cephalograms in CR and CO are an important tool in identifying the limits of the procedures to be implemented, as shown in Figure 7.22.

Class III camouflage orthodontic treatment consists of a clockwise rotation of the mandible, proclination of the maxillary incisors, and retroclination of the mandibular ones. The amount of the clockwise rotation and of the inclination of the incisors is limited because lip competence must be maintained. The loss of lip seal indicates excessive rotation.

7.5.3 Dental diagnosis

A complete dental diagnosis includes photographs, radiographs, models, either physical or digital. Good records are imperative for diagnosis and communication.

The dental casts are evaluated intra- and interarch. On the panoramic radiograph, the number of teeth, anomalies, and congenitally missing and supernumerary teeth are assessed. These registrations are important for a good Bolton analysis and setups when necessary [19–22].

The interarch assessment considers the maxilla-to-mandible relationships – transverse,

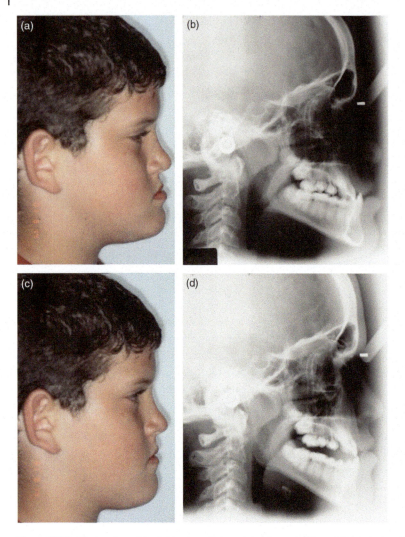

Figure 7.22 Pretreatment facial and cephalometric views: (a, b) centric occlusion (CO), (c, d) centric relation (CR).

anteroposterior, and vertical – and determines the severity of the deviations in all planes (Figure 7.24a,b).

7.5.4 Functional diagnosis

In Class III individuals, it becomes indispensable to add to the evaluation a thorough and detailed functional diagnosis. Premature contacts are typically identified in both the deciduous and the transitional dentition. The persistence of these deviations may very well be the long-term cause of asymmetries. Prematurities can displace the mandible not only sideways but also in a more anterior position. Any crossbite with functional shift of the mandible should be corrected early.

A pseudo-Class III malocclusion is characterized by the presence of an anterior crossbite due to a premature contact and a forward displacement of the mandible. It should be detected early and corrected immediately. Normally, the correction takes a short to moderate amount of time (Figure 7.25a,b).

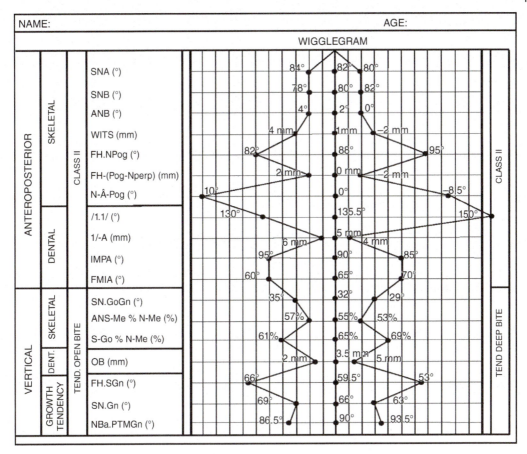

Figure 7.23 Cephalometric wigglegram with measurements derived from several analyses (Amaral [17]/SciELO).

A more severe anterior slide, when combined with other parameters, indicates forward mandibular displacement. It can be compared to a Class II functional appliance stimulating an undesired direction of mandibular growth and strongly affecting the development of the (mal) occlusion. The dynamics is comparable to the idea of "a permanent activator," which may very well stimulate unwanted growth patterns and the onset of a skeletal Class III malocclusion (Figure 7.26a,b).

In the deciduous dentition, occlusal equilibration to eliminate any premature contact may be very helpful. Correct function must be reestablished at the earliest age possible. A comprehensive dynamic functional evaluation is mandatory. Videos may also facilitate the communication process with the families.

7.5.5 Hereditary diagnosis

Class III malocclusions are the most predisposed deviations in dentistry [23]. In severe dental-skeletal deviations, heredity studies can be of great relevance [24–26]. Important studies by Krogman [26] led to a better understanding of the role of heredity in growth and development. It has been noted that "An option to increase the reliability of the data obtained from the patient – our number one source of information – is a detailed examination of the data obtained from his/her family." [27]. Broadie [28] also indicated

7.2 Section II: Class III treatment: problems and solutions

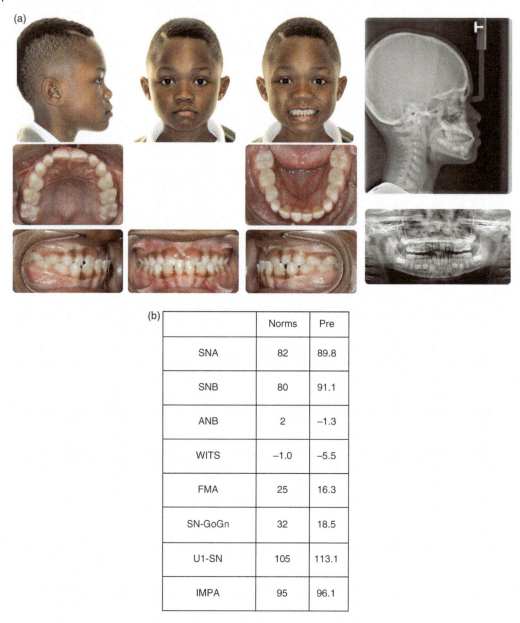

	Norms	Pre
SNA	82	89.8
SNB	80	91.1
ANB	2	−1.3
WITS	−1.0	−5.5
FMA	25	16.3
SN-GoGn	32	18.5
U1-SN	105	113.1
IMPA	95	96.1

Figure 7.24 (a, b) Composite of pretreatment records.

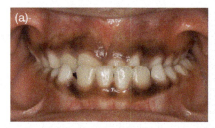 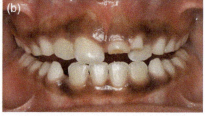

Figure 7.25 Examples of bite registrations in (a) CO and (b) CR. Note the midline deviation discrepancy between CO and CR.

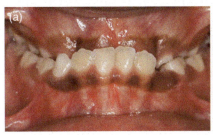 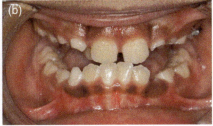

Figure 7.26 Unfavorable development of an anterior shift as demonstrated on the functional evaluations in CO (a) and CR (b).

	Measurement	Parent	Child
Angular	Gonial Angle		
	Facial Angle		
	Y-axis		
	SNA		
	SNB		
	ANB		
Linear	Corpus length		
	Ramus height		
	Total facial height		
	Upper facial height		
	Lower facial height		
	Maxillary length		
	Mandibular length		
	Overbite		
	Overjet		

Figure 7.27 Hereditary analysis: cephalometric comparison of parents and child.

that "within a family it is possible to distinguish individuals with more favorable or less favorable growth when examining other members of the family."

Based on the foregoing observations and the study by Mossey [29], a comparative analysis can be performed as demonstrated in Figure 7.27.

Craniofacial inheritance is influenced by both genetics and environment, but it is difficult to determine the exact contribution of each factor. As professionals whose therapies intervene directly with individuals, orthodontists become actors of the environment. Early interventions are an attempt to minimize the severity of the problems. The family treatment history is also a good reference for diagnosis. The images shown in Figure 7.28 are a good representation of a resemblance between child and father.

7.6 Communication

During the consultation, the family is shown the results of the examinations and the alternatives for treatment. It is important to build a strong relationship of mutual trust between all parties and all must be aware of the steps of treatment. The dialogue must be frank, honest, and centered on evidence and probabilities. The referring dentist must also be contacted and updated on the treatment. The communication process should include three points: 1) the necessity of the intervention and establishment of goals for the treatment; 2) a full explanation that it is impossible to have a secure prognosis owing to variables such as growth and compliance; and 3) the real possibility of relapse or rebound after the intervention owing to uncontrolled genetic growth factors. The protocol and informed consent should also indicate that a second intervention when growth has completed is likely. The nature of this intervention will depend on the amount of growth and deviation. It can be a fast and simpler low complexity treatment or, in the case of a severe rebound, it may require a surgical intervention.

The informed consent must include references to different phases of treatment, duration of treatment, and continuous observation.

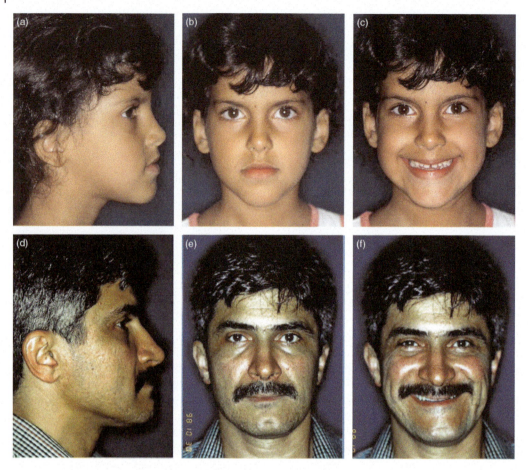

Figure 7.28 Facial resemblance between father and daughter.

Furthermore, the importance of the retention protocol with periodic cephalograms and visits to the orthodontist must be emphasized.

7.7 Early intervention

The timing of the intervention in a developing Class III is unquestionably important and influences the treatment outcome. "Early" must not be understood as "premature." Actually, it is probably the most adequate time to intervene in a developing malocclusion.

In Class III malocclusions, the transverse dimension should be addressed first since discrepancy between the maxillary and the mandibular arches is usually present. It is important to intervene to establish compatible arches. Many morphologic changes occur during the transitional dentition, and interceptive procedures can be successful. Figure 7.29a–l illustrates an early intervention.

7.8 Orthopedic maxillary expansion

The maxilla plays such a large role in the appearance and harmony of the face that it is vital to understand its role in facial development as well as the possibility of applying orthopedic forces during its development [30]. Its growth process allows easier and more effective interventions at earlier ages. Maxillary

7.8 Orthopedic maxillary expansion | 189

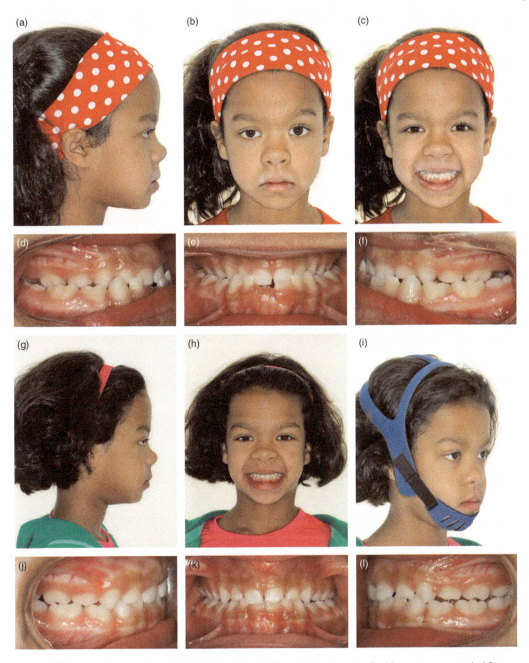

Figure 7.29 Early intervention: (a–f) Initial and (g–l) End of phase I and soft chincup recommended for the retention phase.

constriction can stem from genetic, developmental, environmental, or even iatrogenic factors [31].

Rapid maxillary expansion (RME) is one the most common treatment modalities used in orthodontic practice today. Angell was the first to describe an orthopedic effect resulting in gaining arch length space in 1860 [32], but its use in the United States had been largely abandoned by the early 1900s.

It was not until the 1950s that the use of RME reemerged in the USA for orthodontic practitioners [33]. RME has proven to be an effective and reliable method of skeletally increasing the transverse dimension in patients with narrow maxilla. Maxillary expansion becomes crucial for the harmony of the occlusion, especially in Class III malocclusions.

Since the advent of RME, appliances have been designed, remodeled, and revamped with the intent of minimizing unwanted tooth movements, and maximizing those that are beneficial. Presently, the distinction between different types of fixed rapid expanders resides on their attachment: tooth-borne, purely bone supported, or hybrid. The most commonly used appliances are still the tooth-borne banded or bonded ones. A banded expander can be cemented to two or four supporting teeth and may be a purely metal one – Hyrax – or have acrylic pads on the palate – Haas-type expander.

If a patient is in the mixed dentition and the option is a banded appliance, two molar bands are used and an occlusal rest is placed on the anterior part of the expander to be bonded to the first deciduous molars if present. The anterior rest increases the stability of the appliance. Four bands are more frequently used in older patients, utilizing molars and premolars, or when the first deciduous molars have an anatomy capable of bearing bands. As for the novel hybrid device, two bands and two mini screws serve as anchorage for the expansion [34–36].

Different types of expanders can be seen in Figure 7.30a–d.

Bonded expanders are well accepted and widely used in many practices. The jackscrew is typically the same in either the banded or bonded expanders. The selection criteria depend on professional preference, patient acceptance, and stability of the appliance.

The expansion benefits the patient not only in the dentition and basal bone but also in possible improvements of the respiratory function due to the expansion of the nasal cavity [34]. Maxillary expansion has the effect of moving the maxilla forward as it expands, which can slightly improve the Class III relationship. The maxillary expansion is recommended not only when the maxilla is in crossbite but also to help in its orthopedic traction.

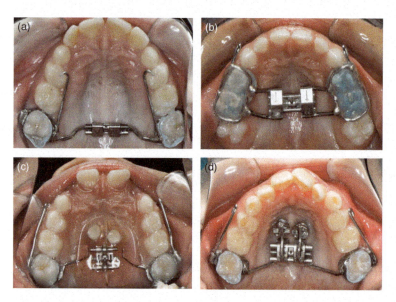

Figure 7.30 Palatal expanders: top row (a), miniexpander and (b) bonded expander. On the bottom (c, d), two types of hybrid (MSI and bands) expanders.

7.9 Face mask and/or chincup orthopedics

Face mask therapy is often performed with the assistance of a palatal suture expander, and it attempts to protract the deficient maxilla and to enhance its forward displacement.

When the mandible is excessive and the maxilla is normal in size and position, the use of a chincup, although controversial, may be considered. This therapy attempts to retard or redirect the growth of the oversized mandible backward and/or downward.

When confronted with a combination of mandibular excess and maxillary deficiency, the orthodontist may use both the chincup and face mask. In these cases, it is recommended to work with the face mask initially or, if preferred, to utilize the Hickham chincup and protraction device [35]. This therapy attempts to apply the effects of chincup and face mask to the respective jaw simultaneously.

7.9.1 The face mask

The orthopedic protraction of the maxilla associated with the maxillary expansion has been widely accepted in our daily practices. It normally results in a beneficial contribution to the treatment of Class IIIs in mixed dentition. Although it is widely accepted, there is a lack of consensus on the effectiveness of this protocol. The question of protraction with or without an associated RME protocol is still debated [36–40]. Presently, a hybrid appliance, bands, and MSIs, have been reported [37], but further studies are necessary.

If a child is still very young, up to 7–8 years of age – the most recommended age for better results – our protocol is a slower expansion that may start with one turn a day or one turn every other day. It all depends on the patient's attitude toward the treatment and the desire of the professional not to establish an aggressive protocol.

As for the decision on banded vs. bonded RPE, a recent publication comparing the two found that they are equally effective in increasing maxillary width [41]. However, depending on the desired effect on the mandible dimensions, one appliance may be more effective than the other. Although the maxillary expansion is similar, they produce different responses on the untreated mandibular arch. The banded Haas-type expander demonstrated significant mandibular arch width gain in the molar region. The bonded type showed the mandibular arch width remaining stable or even achieving a slight decrease at the intermolar level. The bonded RME also demonstrated significant loss in arch perimeter and arch depth in the transitional dentition. The results indicate that with a protraction face mask, a bonded maxillary appliance may produce better results, with the elimination of occlusal interdigitation. If the face mask therapy is used with a Hyrax, Haas, or Hybrid, the use of an acrylic coverage or Essix type of appliance on the mandibular arch may eliminate detrimental occlusal interference.

The most common types of the face mask are the Petite, the Delaire, or the Hickham chincup with protraction hooks. The soft chincup is also a helpful device (Figure 7.31a–d).

The Petite and Delaire can be easily purchased from numerous vendors. The Hickham is generally a custom-made appliance and takes more chair time to fabricate and adjust.

The protraction protocol has been extensively described in the literature [38, 39, 42]. We recommend an average wear time of 14–16 hours/day with a force in the order of 250 g initially and, after 2 weeks, 400 g per side. Figure 7.32 shows the recommended direction and the point of force application. The angle of applied force ranges from 30° to 45° to the occlusal plane. Considering that the dento-maxillary center of resistance is normally located in the region above the second premolar and first molar, it is desirable that the resultant of the force runs through the same area, to avoid unwanted rotations of the maxillary complex.

Buccal hooks on the maxillary expander serve as anchorage for the elastics to connect

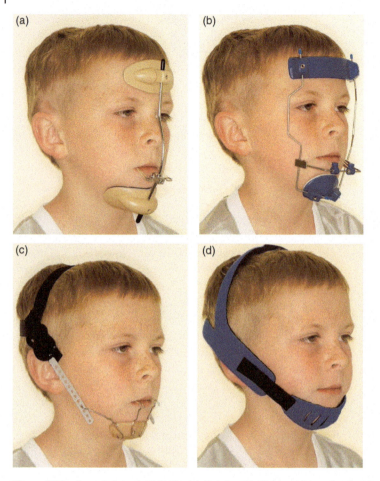

Figure 7.31 From left to right Petite (a), Delaire (b), Hickham (c), and soft chincup (d).

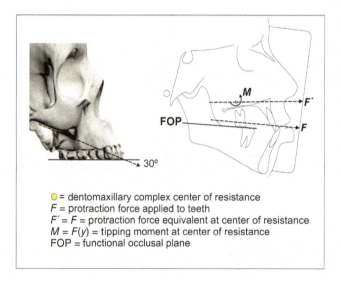

Figure 7.32 Direction of force for the protraction face mask.

○ = dentomaxillary complex center of resistance
F = protraction force applied to teeth
$F' = F$ = protraction force equivalent at center of resistance
$M = F(y)$ = tipping moment at center of resistance
FOP = functional occlusal plane

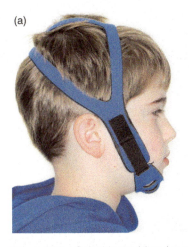
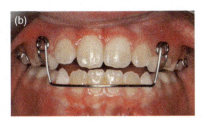

Figure 7.33 Soft chincup (a) and modified Class III Hawley (b).

the maxilla to the face mask to achieve the protraction. The position of these hooks must be at the level of the maxillary canines.

Skeletal and dental effects of face-mask therapy include protraction of the dento-maxillary complex (2–4 mm), rotation of maxilla, proclination of the maxillary incisors, a retroclination of the mandibular incisors, and a clockwise autorotation of the mandible. This clockwise autorotation of the mandible is possibly the most desired mandibular response for an effective camouflaging in nonsurgical Class III protocols.

The duration of the maxillary protraction should be about 10–12 months. After this active period, a soft chincup (Figure 7.33) is recommended for nighttime wear (12 hours/day) during the phase I retention period until the patient is ready for a phase II treatment. A mandibular plastic full-coverage Essix type retainer should be worn to eliminate occlusal interference and assist in the positive effects of the chincup. Along with the chincup, a modified Hawley appliance is recommended for the daytime (Figure 7.33). If the malocclusion is not severe, a normal Hawley may be prescribed.

7.9.2 The chincup

The controversy concerning chincup therapy, although still present, seems to have dissipated somewhat [43, 44]. Among the controversies, the most likely to cause discussion is the possible harm to the temporomandibular joint (TMJ) [45]. It must be understood that the chincup force is not physiologic, so it is reasonable to consider that some disorders may occur. Mitani [46] has indicated that noise, clicking, or some pain at the TMJ may be observed during the first 6 months of treatment in about 35% of chincup patients. Also, if the chincup force is too high and is delivered for a long period of time, the chance of joint problems increases. For these reasons, the suggested protocol is a nighttime wear only, and if any signs of TMJ problems are detected the magnitude of the force should be reduced [44, 46–49].

Another report describes that 18% of 160 chincup patients were found to present with some type of TMJ disorder during retention. The same study indicates that the incidence of TMJ disorders in a general untreated population of children is 10–25% [49]. So the chincup group is within the range of normality and may not be more likely to develop TMJ problems.

Studies finding problems with the chincup therapy as well as others that find no negative effects of the appliance use are part of the orthodontic literature [44, 46, 50–55].

The soft chincup, as shown in Figure 7.33, is more gentle and it has been one of our selected retention appliances after phase I and even after phase II, if growth is still present.

The effects of the chincup vary considerably with the individual's facial type. Hyperdivergent

Class III skeletal types are among those that may be contraindicated as the long vertical pattern may be accentuated.

One of the effects of the chincup is a possible decrease in the gonial angle, so the chincup may make the short face even shorter in severely hypodivergent patients.

The chincup therapy can be seen as a procedure that may minimize the severity of the Class III malocclusion, but alone will not be able to correct the malocclusion. Effects of the chincup appear to be more significant at younger ages. The chincup is also used as a postural regulator to keep the patient from protruding the mandible and potentially causing more unfavorable growth.

Some characteristics have been described to identify individuals with a "bad" Class III, who would most likely not benefit from an interceptive Class III intervention: 1) chin protruded with a sharp chin angle; 2) long and shallow mandible; 3) gonial angle widely opened and steep mandibular plane; 4) inclined ramal plane; 5) long and thin condylar neck; 6) narrow ramus; 7) corpus with triangular shape in the lateral view; 8) lower incisors with very severe lingual inclination; and 9) cranial base angle extremely acute and closed spheno-occipital synchondrosis [36, 44].

7.10 Leeway space control

There is a consensus on the importance of the second deciduous molars or "E's" in the development of the occlusion [56]. Gianelly has also shown that the proper and timely use of the E-space allows an increase in the number of cases that can be treated by nonextraction [57]. The benefits generated from the correct and wise manipulation of this space are great. It does not matter if the orthodontic treatment is done in one or two phases. Even those who oppose two-phase treatments agree about taking advantage of nature's "generosity." In Class III corrections or interceptions, any extra space in the mandibular arch is welcome.

The concluding four "commandments" of the protocol are more related to the second phase of treatment in the permanent dentition.

For the sake of completion, a brief description of each will be given here. In chapter 5, section II, new interesting findings on the E space have benn reported.

7.11 Orthodontic mechanics

After all these steps and recommendations, it is the time to consider mechanical alternatives. The orthodontist faces important options and must design a treatment plan with a sequence of events that are intended to decrease the severity of the malocclusion, intercepting it, and later correcting it, if possible, in a nonsurgical way.

On many occasions, the patient and family must be aware that in order to camouflage the deviation and to achieve a stable and functional result, extraction of permanent teeth in the future may be necessary. However, in some patients, it is possible to obtain a good result with a nonextraction approach with or without the use of interproximal reduction (IPR) to gain space.

7.12 Finishing

A good finish with a well-interdigitated occlusion not only adds quality to the treatment but also minimizes retention problems. According to Haas [33], the occlusal force vectors and the inclined planes of the posterior teeth cause interferences capable of generating more stability after orthodontic treatment. Also, overcorrection of the overjet, if possible, will help guard against relapse. An ideal distribution of spaces of the maxillary incisors is important if there is a mandibular excess Bolton relationship, which is common with the Class III malocclusion as shown in Figure 7.34 [19].

7.13 Retention

The retention protocol between the first and second phases has been previously presented. The use of a soft chincup with a mandibular plastic occlusal coverage at night and a normal or a modified Hawley (Figure 7.33) is recommended for the daytime.

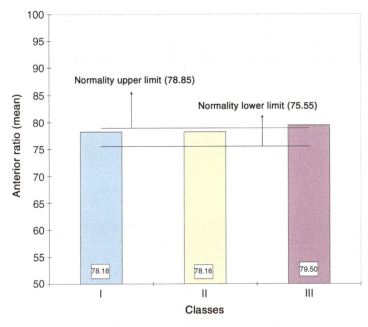

Figure 7.34 Bolton relationship for different occlusion types.

After the second phase of comprehensive orthodontic treatment, a maxillary wraparound Hawley retainer is effective in preserving the occlusal contacts, and a mandibular fixed retainer is a simple method for retention in the mandibular arch. The best retention, however, may be a natural and stable well-interdigitated occlusion.

7.14 Growth reevaluation

The final "commandment" is tied to the initial informed consent. It is important to reevaluate growth and/or any changes that may have occurred due to growth and development on an ongoing basis. The evaluation must be done by the superimposition of sequential cephalograms. The compound superimposition of the maxilla and mandible as one unit may also provide a reliable way of studying the displacement of the mandible in relation to the maxilla [58].

This reevaluation will determine if the occlusion is being maintained, and there is no need for further intervention, or if a retreatment with or without extractions is needed, or if there is an indication for orthognathic surgery in cases of extreme severity and patient desire.

Patient 1

This first case report illustrates the importance of an early intervention. A 7-year-old boy was brought to our clinic by his parents, referred by the pediatric dentist, to evaluate his occlusion and determine the correct time to start an interceptive treatment. All records were taken. The facial profile was somewhat concave. The cephalometric measurements showed a developing Class III and in the dental evaluation we could detect the anterior crossbite, a unilateral posterior crossbite, and the presence of a clear CR/CO discrepancy (Figure 7.35).

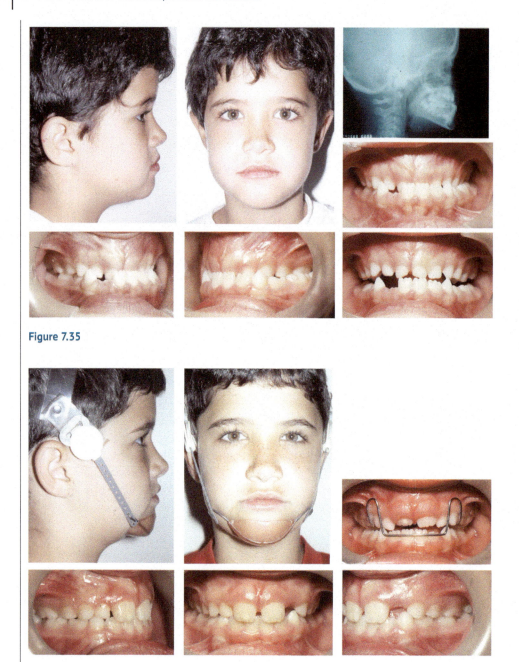

Figure 7.35

Figure 7.36

The recommendation was to start treatment immediately, using a removable expander with an inverted labial bow. In 6 months, the crossbite was corrected and a chincup for nighttime wear was recommended. From that point on the patient was put in observation without retainers but with the required use of the chincup for bed time (Figure 7.36). With the development of the occlusion, a LLHA was placed with the objective of holding the possible mesial drifting of the mandibular molars upon the loss of the second deciduous molars. Figure 7.37 illustrates the sequential development of the occlusion from the moment the LLHA was placed until final treatment.

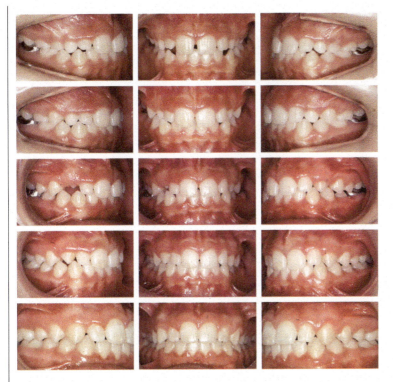

Figure 7.37

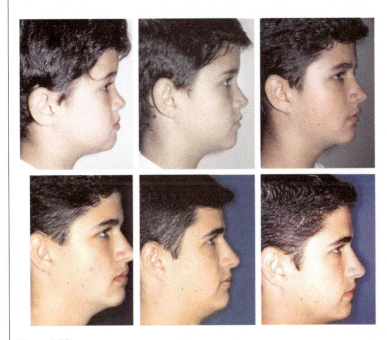

Figure 7.38

When the permanent occlusion was complete, the patient went through about 14 months of orthodontic treatment. The final evaluation shows a balanced profile, a solid Class I occlusion and very good stability, as demonstrated in the 4- and 6-year retention illustrations. Figure 7.38 shows the facial profile from start to finish, and Figure 7.39 illustrates 4 and 6 years of retention, respectively. The initial and intermediate cephalograms and the analysis are shown in Figure 7.40.

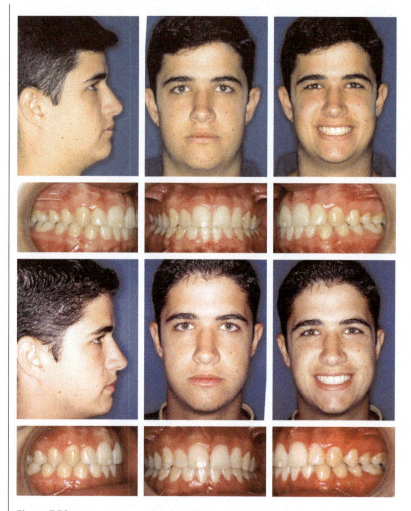

Figure 7.39

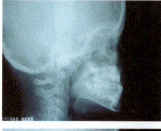

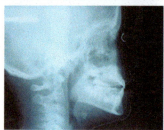

	Norms	Pre	Post
SNA	82	79.7	81.2
SNB	80	82.5	81.4
ANB	2	−2.8	−0.8
WITS	−1.0	−5.0	−4.3
FMA	25	23.5	23.6
SN-GoGn	32	27.3	30.7
U1-SN	105	104.4	105.6
IMPA	95	84.7	85.4

Figure 7.40

7.14 Growth reevaluation

Patient 2

This 12y 1m girl and her parents presented to our clinic referred by "the previous orthodontist for a possible nonsurgical procedure." She had a straight profile and a complete crossbite with the presence of a few deciduous teeth. A skeletal Class III was diagnosed, as demonstrated in the cephalometry. Initial records are shown in Figure 7.41.

After a thorough communication with the family, where we stressed the uncertainty of the prognosis and the possibility of a future surgical intervention, a treatment plan was presented. In the first stage, a palatal expansion and a protraction Hickham chincup were indicated. In 4 months, the maxilla was

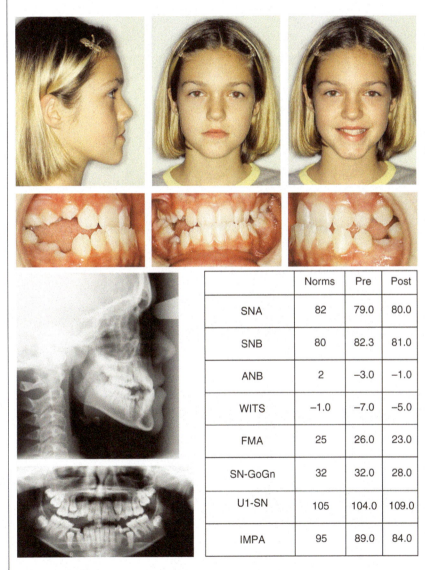

	Norms	Pre	Post
SNA	82	79.0	80.0
SNB	80	82.3	81.0
ANB	2	−3.0	−1.0
WITS	−1.0	−7.0	−5.0
FMA	25	26.0	23.0
SN-GoGn	32	32.0	28.0
U1-SN	105	104.0	109.0
IMPA	95	89.0	84.0

Figure 7.41

expanded and positive overjet was obtained (Figure 7.42).

After the extractions of the remaining deciduous teeth, a new evaluation was done, and treatment proceeded with the extraction of the mandibular first molars. The rationale behind this extraction pattern was the uncertainty about her growth. Since the patient ruled out any surgical option, the decision to preserve the mandibular premolars was taken. The presence of good third molars was essential. Figure 7.43 shows the images after

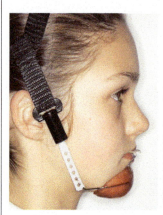
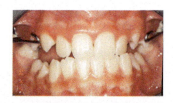
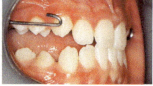
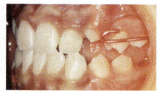

Figure 7.42

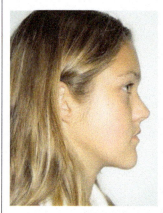
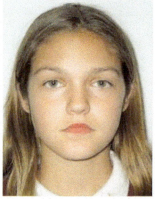
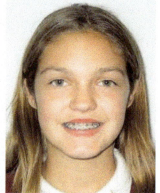
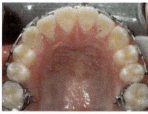
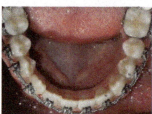
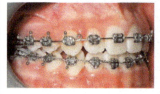
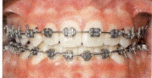
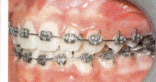

Figure 7.43

20 months of treatment, with all the spaces closed. Figure 7.44 illustrates the case at the end of treatment and Figure 7.45 illustrates the case at the 10 years posttreatment.

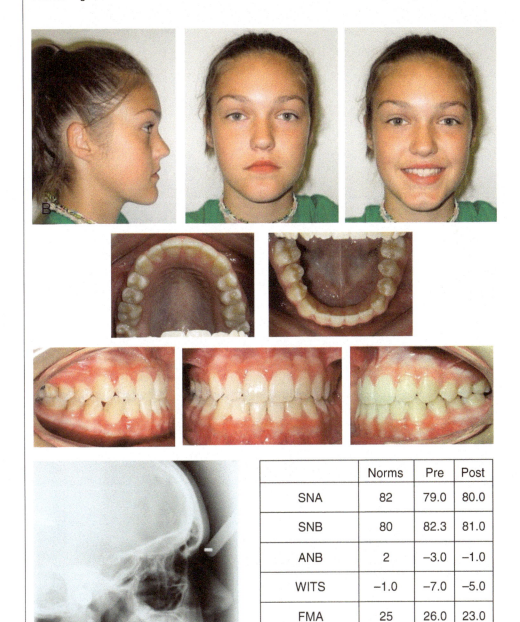

	Norms	Pre	Post
SNA	82	79.0	80.0
SNB	80	82.3	81.0
ANB	2	−3.0	−1.0
WITS	−1.0	−7.0	−5.0
FMA	25	26.0	23.0
SN-GoGn	32	32.0	28.0
U1-SN	105	104.0	109.0
IMPA	95	89.0	84.0

Figure 7.44

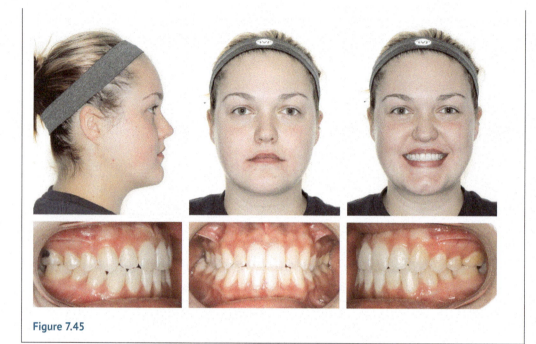

Figure 7.45

Patient 3

This 6-year-old girl was referred by the pediatric dentist to be evaluated. A complete series of records was requested. The functional diagnosis showed a minimum premature contact, and the family analysis showed a high resemblance between the patient and her father, as demonstrated in Figure 7.28 of this Section II. The patient was in the early mixed dentition and presented a Class III with total crossbite (Figure 7.46).

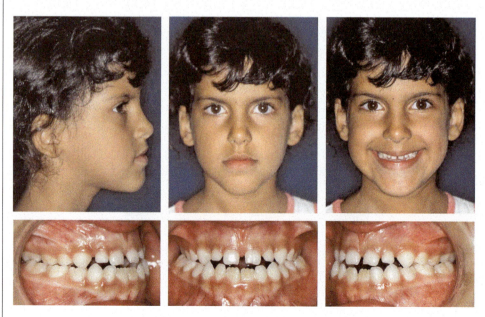

Figure 7.46

Initially, RME was indicated (Figure 7.47) and it was decided to supervise her growth with chincup only, as illustrated in the sequence shown in Figure 7.48. This was the only treatment until the time she was about to lose the Es. Figure 7.49 shows the cephalometric numbers and the superimposition comparing the beginning and end of phase I. A full fixed appliance was used and removed after 20 months (Figure 7.50). Figure 7.51 shows the patient 18 years later.

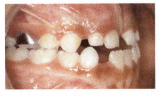
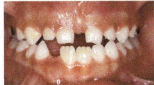
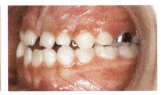

Figure 7.47

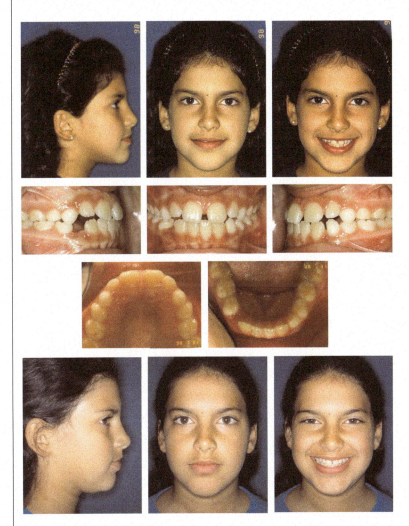

Figure 7.48

7.2 Section II: Class III treatment: problems and solutions

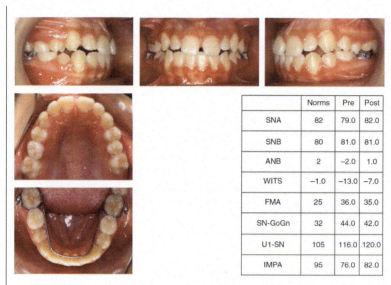

	Norms	Pre	Post
SNA	82	79.0	82.0
SNB	80	81.0	81.0
ANB	2	−2.0	1.0
WITS	−1.0	−13.0	−7.0
FMA	25	36.0	35.0
SN-GoGn	32	44.0	42.0
U1-SN	105	116.0	120.0
IMPA	95	76.0	82.0

Figure 7.48 (Continued)

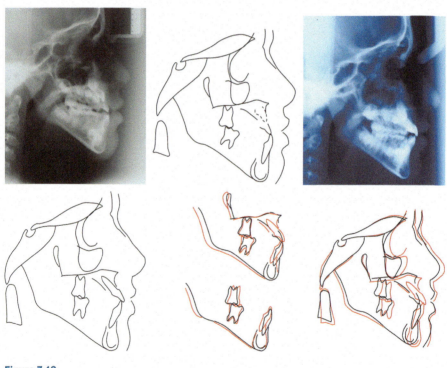

Figure 7.49

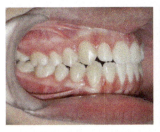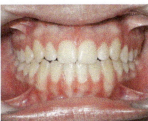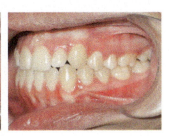

Figure 7.50

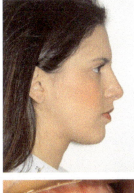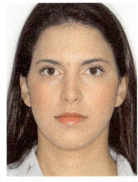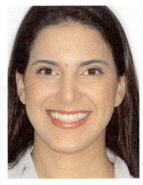
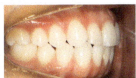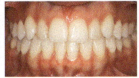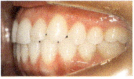

Figure 7.51

Patient 4

As mentioned earlier, early intervention in Class IIIs is one of the factors that may be able to help the clinician to succeed. This 5y 9m youngster happened to be in our clinic with his sister, when a severe malocclusion was noticed. The family was updated on the severity of his malocclusion and opted to have records taken. Figure 7.52 shows the initial facial and dental records. A concave profile can be noticed. The patient was in his late deciduous dentition. In the AP dental evaluation, a severe mesial step is clear. Transversely, there is a complete crossbite and vertically a developing open bite.

The cephalometric analysis shows a skeletal Class III, a large negative Wits, and a negative ANB. A tendency to hyperdivergence is also present (Figure 7.53). There was no functional shift detected and the family had little, if any, indication of Class III familial pattern.

The proposed treatment plan included a bonded RME and face mask for maxillary traction for 14 hours/day. Six months later, positive results could be observed (Figure 7.54).

7.2 Section II: Class III treatment: problems and solutions

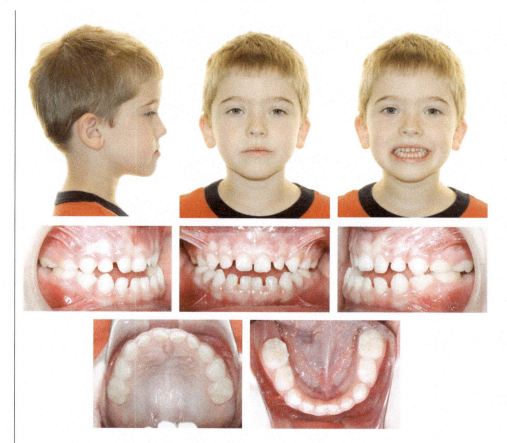

Figure 7.52

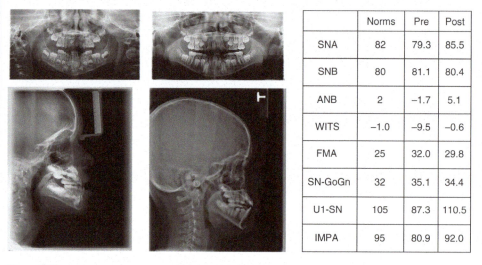

	Norms	Pre	Post
SNA	82	79.3	85.5
SNB	80	81.1	80.4
ANB	2	−1.7	5.1
WITS	−1.0	−9.5	−0.6
FMA	25	32.0	29.8
SN-GoGn	32	35.1	34.4
U1-SN	105	87.3	110.5
IMPA	95	80.9	92.0

Figure 7.53

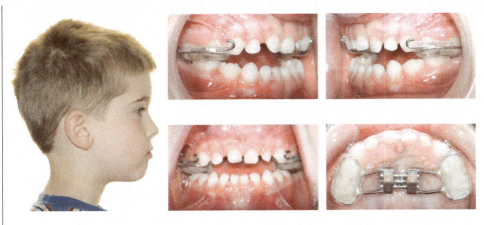

Figure 7.54

With 11 months of treatment, the patient showed a remarkable improvement, the expander was removed and the protraction was stopped. The patient was given a soft chincup for retention with the instructions to wear it 12 hours (nighttime) and to report any discomfort (Figure 7.55). Figure 7.53 shows the cephalometric comparison between the two time points.

With the eruption of the incisors, an irregularity was detected and a two-by-four was placed in order to align them (Figure 7.56). A modified Hawley as shown in Figure 7.33 was prescribed and delivered for daytime wear.

Figure 7.57 shows a progress stage close to initiation of phase II. Note the LLHA to preserve the E-space.

Figure 7.58 shows the initial records for Phase II. It can be noted an improvement of the open bite, an appropriate overjet, Angle Class I molar relation on the right side, a slightly Class II molar relation on the left side. This scenario would probably have had a much higher complexity if Phase I had not taken place at the appropriate time.

Another treatment phase was implemented with fixed appliances and Class III mechanics. The treatment was performed in 16 months achieving the main goals; an adequate overbite and overjet, Class I molar and canines and a pleasant facial balance (Figure 7.59). Considering that growth can sometimes be a friend and sometimes an enemy, the patient was closely monitored in retention.

Eight years after the end of Phase II, a severe relapse took place, mostly due to his late growth associated with the Class III pattern. As mentioned on page 187 (Section 7.6), the patient and family were aware of that possibility. A retreatment would occur closer to the time/age when a surgical procedure could be successfully done.

Figure 7.60 shows the preretreatment records, where a concave profile, full step Class III molars and canines, anterior crossbite, and an open bite are present and also an asymmetric growth was noted.

As the golden standard for growth assessment, a hand and wrist radiograph were taken (Figure 7.61), demonstrating that there was no growth left, what led to the final preparation for a mandibular setback surgery. Figure 7.62 shows the presurgery records and Figure 7.63 shows the 1-month postsurgery evaluation. Final records were taken 6 months after surgery time when the debonding took place (Figure 7.64).

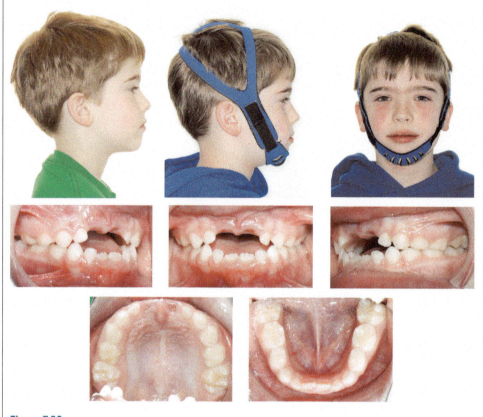

Figure 7.55

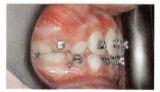 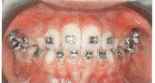 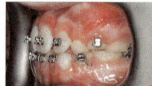

Figure 7.56

A straight profile, molar and canines' Class I, adequate overbite and overjet are now present, and stability should no longer be an issue.

This case illustrates that orthodontics does not change growth, but it can partially control it by minimizing its effects and redirecting its direction when necessary.

The relapse occurred at a time that the patient was more mature and aware of its possibility. During the patient's early teens, he showed a pleasant profile creating a protective measure for bullying and helping to build up confidence and a positive psychological attitude.

7.14 Growth reevaluation | 209

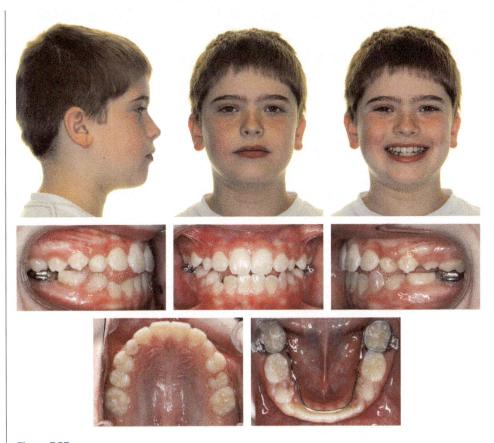

Figure 7.57

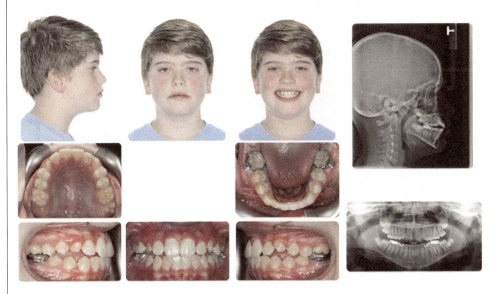

Figure 7.58

7.2 Section II: Class III treatment: problems and solutions

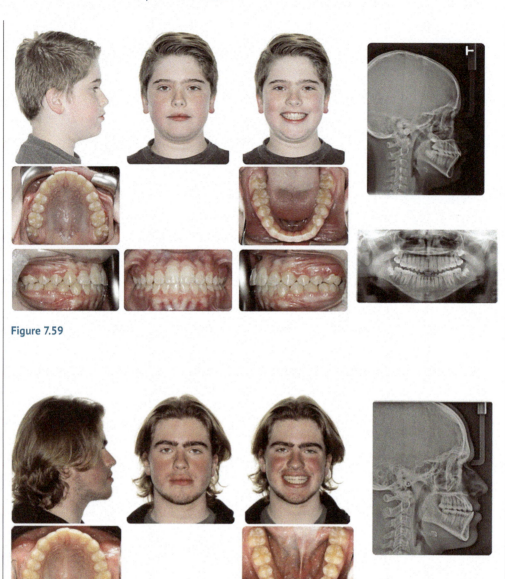

Figure 7.59

Figure 7.60

7.14 Growth reevaluation | 211

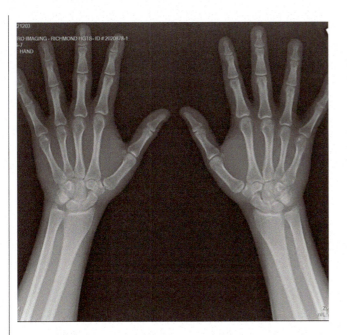

Figure 7.61

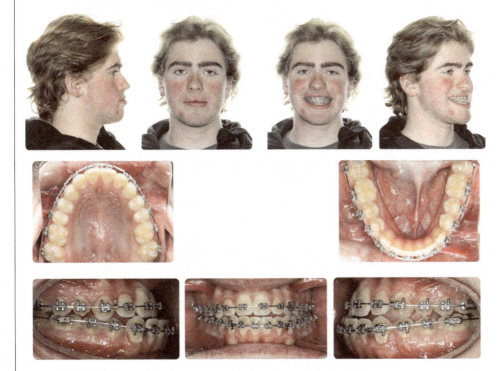

Figure 7.62

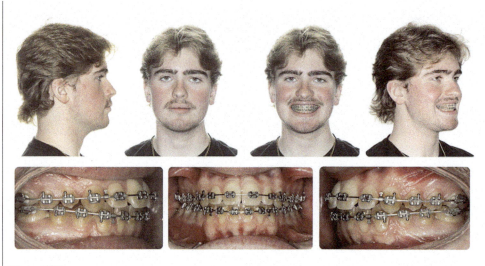

Figure 7.63

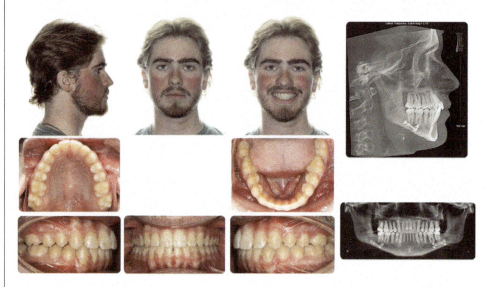

Figure 7.64

Patient 5

A novel approach for early intervention in Class IIIs is introduced in the treatment of this 5-year-old girl who presented a good profile but a severe dental crossbite. The images are courtesy of Dr. Tarcisio Junqueira from Brazil (Figure 7.65).

Figure 7.66 shows the appliances used at this early age: a maxillary expander protraction device with posterior and anterior hooks fixed on the Es and, on the mandibular arch, a sturdy plastic coverage with hooks at the canine level. During the day, the Class III

7.14 Growth reevaluation

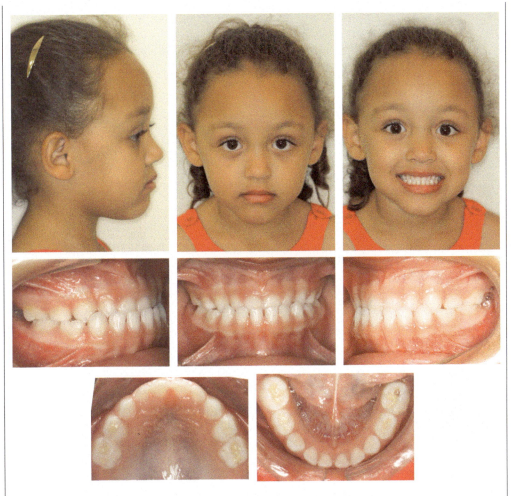

Figure 7.65

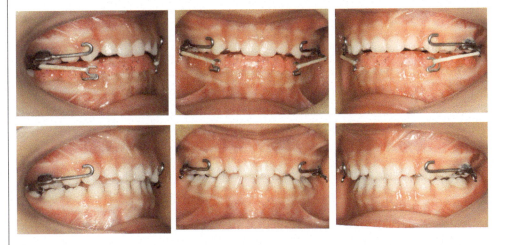

Figure 7.66

elastics are placed on the upper and lower hooks, and at nighttime, a facemask therapy is implemented.

After 10 months, the correction was achieved and the patient was recommended to wear a chincup and a Frankel III for 12 hours (nighttime) (Figure 7.67). Five years later, as shown in Figure 7.68, the occlusion is stable and the patient is waiting for the best time to initiate the phase II treatment.

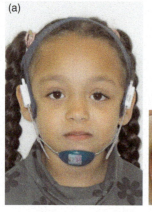
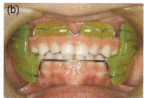

Figure 7.67

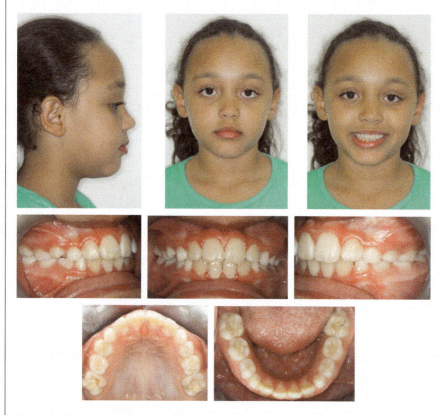

Figure 7.68

Patient 6

The treatment for this 8-year-old patient was simply a palatal expansion and a two-by-four as the patient did not cooperate with the facemask. Initial records show the Class III molar relationship and an anterior crossbite characterizing a pseudo Class III (Figure 7.69). At the removal of the appliances, a positive overbite and overjet were obtained (Figure 7.70). Figure 7.71a–f shows the patient's 3 years postretention and Figure 7.71g–l shows the patient's 5 years postretention. No other treatment has been rendered up to this point.

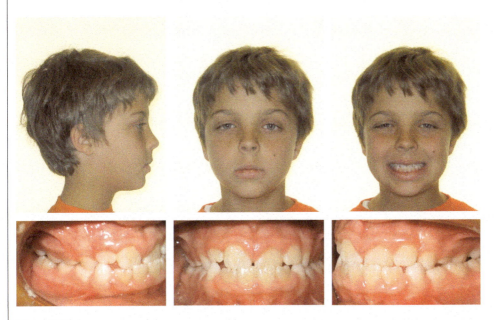

Figure 7.69

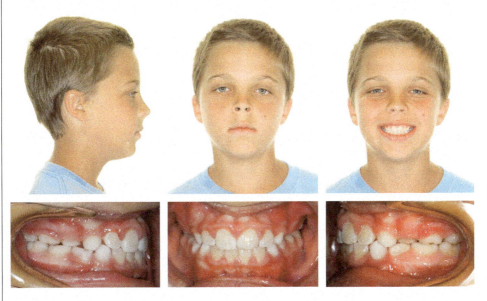

Figure 7.70

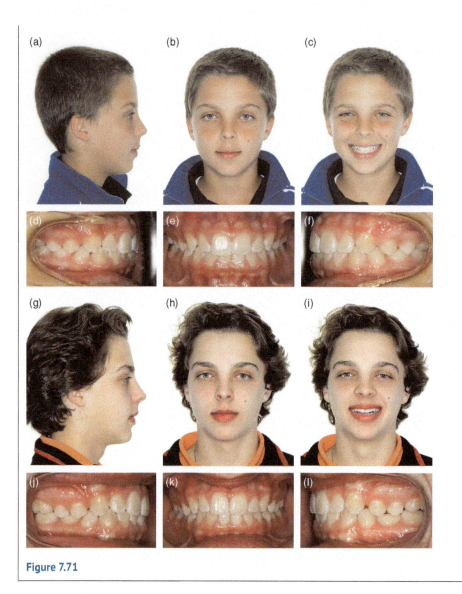

Figure 7.71

Patient 7

This 8y 10m boy came to our clinic to be evaluated for his "underbite." Although the dental malocclusion was severe enough to warrant immediate intervention, the face was well balanced with minimum midface retrusion. The dental evaluation showed a severe mesial step, maxillary crowding with the absence of space for the permanent laterals, and complete crossbite except for the left posterior segment (Figure 7.72).

The initial and final of phase I cephalometric and dental panoramic evaluation are shown in Figure 7.73.

The recommended treatment consisted of maxillary expansion and protraction using a bonded RME. After the expansion had ceased and consolidated, a two-by-four appliance was placed to align the maxillary teeth as shown in Figure 7.74.

Figure 7.75 illustrates the patient 15 months from the start of treatment, with an excellent and stable result.

7.14 Growth reevaluation | 217

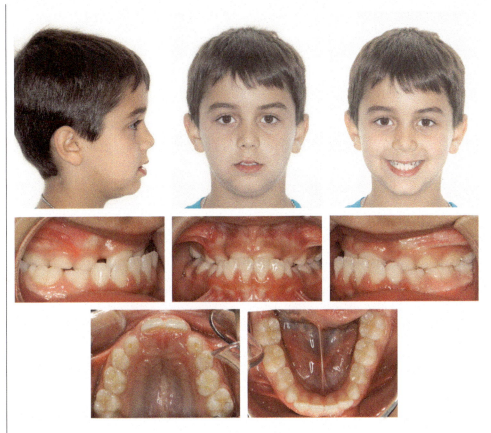

Figure 7.72

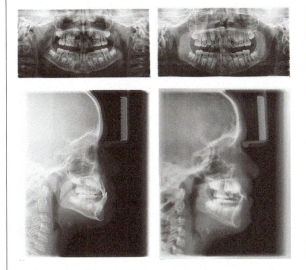

	Norms	Pre	Post
SNA	82	73.9	77.0
SNB	80	75.3	74.3
ANB	2	−1.4	2.7
WITS	−1.0	−3.2	2.6
FMA	25	28.9	32.8
SN-GoGn	32	34.2	40.4
U1-SN	105	80.2	107.6
IMPA	95	90.0	79.8

Figure 7.73

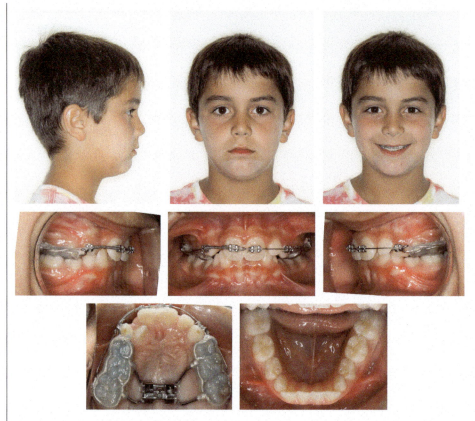

Figure 7.74

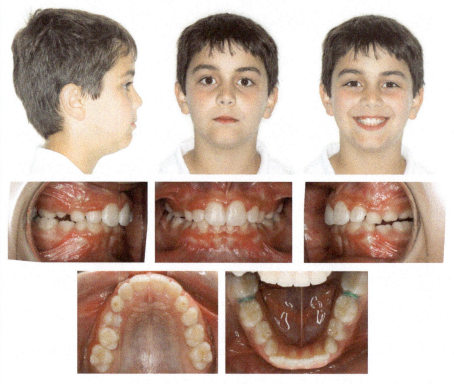

Figure 7.75

Patient 8

The initial evaluation of this 5y 10m girl showed a balanced facial appearance but a dental Class III open bite with premature contact on the deciduous canines (Figure 7.76). An initial expansion with a maxillary Schwarz was initiated. Progress records show improvement (Figure 7.77a–c) and 12 months later the crossbite was under control (Figure 7.77d–f). At this point, a chin-cup was recommended. Figure 7.78a–g show the facial and dental progress at two distinct times. Figure 7.79 shows the patient in the permanent dentition. No fixed appliances were used up to that time.

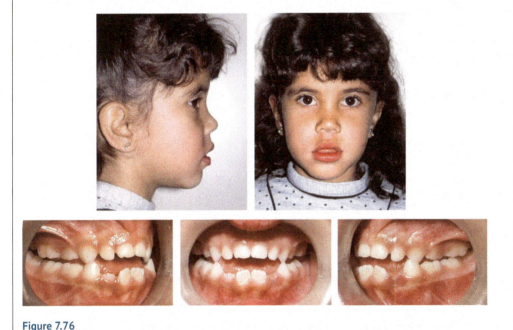

Figure 7.76

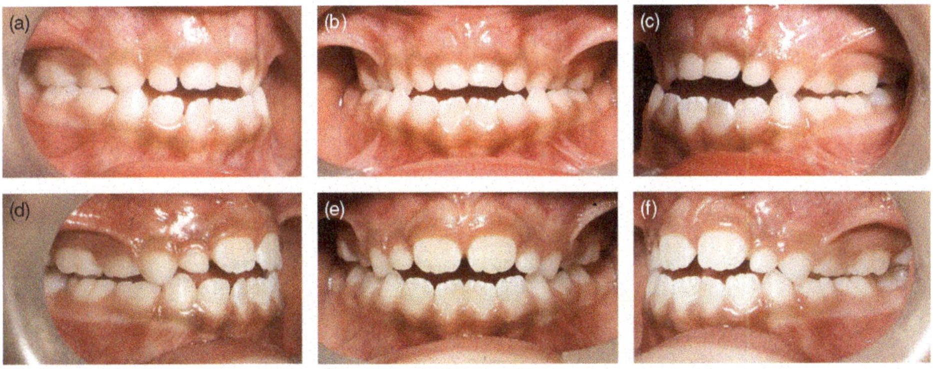

Figure 7.77

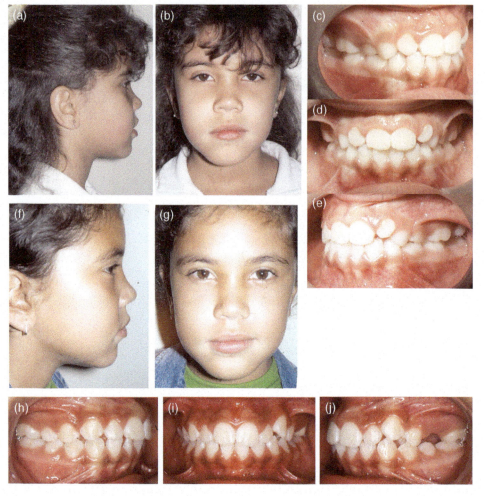

Figure 7.78

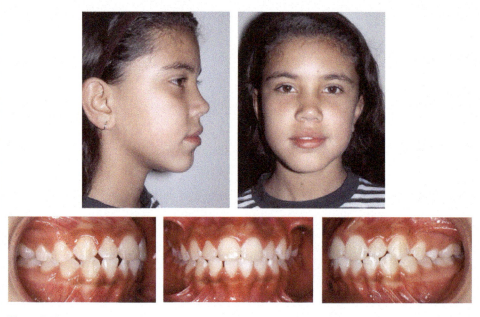

Figure 7.79

References

1. Bourdet B. *Research observation of all areas of the art of the dentist*. Paris: Chez Jean-Thomas Herissant, 1757. p. 358pp.
2. Angle EH. Classification of malocclusion. *Dent Cosmos* 1899;**41**:248.
3. Huber RE, Reynolds JW. A dentofacial study of male students at the University of Michigan in the physical hardening program. *Am J Orthod Oral Surg* 1946 Jan;**32**:1–21.
4. Hardy D, Cubas Y, Orellana M. Prevalence of Angle Class III malocclusion: a systematic review and meta-analysis. *Open J Epidemiol* 2012;**2**:75–82.
5. Watkinson S, Harrison JE, Furness S, Worthington HV. Orthodontic treatment for prominent lower front teeth (Class III malocclusion) in children. *Cochrane Database Syst Rev* 2013;**9**:CD003451.
6. Kelly J, Sanchez M, Van Kirk L. *An assessment of the occlusion of teeth of children 6–11 years*. DHEW Publication No. (HRA) 74-1617. Washington, DC: National Center for Health Statistics, 1973.
7. Kelly J, Harvey C. An assessment of the occlusion of the teeth in youths 12–17 years, United States. *US Dep Health Educ Welf Ed* 1977.
8. Proffit WR, Fields HW Jr, Moray LJ. Prevalence of malocclusion and orthodontic treatment need in the United States: estimates from the NHANES III survey. *Int J Adult Orthodon Orthognath Surg* 1998;**13**(2):97–106.
9. Mills LF. Epidemiologic studies of occlusion. IV. The prevalence of malocclusion in a population of 1,455 school children. *J Dent Res* 1966 Apr;**45**(2):332–6.
10. Graber LW, Lucker GW. Dental esthetic self-evaluation and satisfaction. *Am J Orthod* 1980 Feb;**77**(2):163–73.
11. Albino JE. Psychosocial factors in orthodontic treatment. *N Y State Dent J* 1984 Oct;**50**(8):486–7, 489.
12. Baccetti T, Franchi L, McNamara JA Jr. Growth in the untreated Class III subject. *Semin Orthod* 2007;**13**:130–42.
13. Wolfe SM, Araújo E, Behrents RG, Buschang PH. Craniofacial growth of Class III subjects six to sixteen years of age. *Angle Orthod* 2011 Mar;**81**(2):211–6.
14. Dion KK. Young children's stereotyping of facial attractiveness. *Dev Psychol* 1973;**9**:183–8.
15. Sassouni V. *Dentofacial orthopedics*. Pittsburgh, PA: C.O.T Publications, 1971.
16. Janzen EK, Bluher JA. The cephalometric, anatomic, and histologic changes in *Macaca mulatta* after application of a continuous-acting retraction force on the mandible. *Am J Orthod* 1965 Nov;**51**(11):823–55.
17. Amaral RL. *Avaliação cefalométrica através de um Wigglegram: uma nova proposta [Literature]*. Belo Horizonte: Pontifícia Universidade Católica de Minas Gerais, 1998.
18. Sassouni V. *Orthopedics in dental practice*. St. Louis, MO: C.V. Mosby, 1971.
19. Araújo E, Souki M. Bolton anterior tooth size discrepancies among different malocclusion groups. *Angle Orthod* 2003 Jun;**73**(3):307–13.
20. Bolton WA. The clinical application of a tooth size analysis. *Am J Orthod* 1962 Jul;**48**(7):504–29.
21. Nie Q, Lin J. Comparison of intermaxillary tooth size discrepancies among different malocclusion groups. *Am J Orthod Dentofacial Orthop* 1999 Nov;**116**(5):539–44.
22. Sperry TP, Worms FW, Isaacson RJ, Speidel TM. Tooth-size discrepancy in mandibular prognathism. *Am J Orthod* 1977 Aug;**72**(2):183–90.
23. Salzmann JA. Genetic consideration in clinical orthodontics. *Am J Orthod* 1978 Oct;**4**(74):467–8.
24. Araújo EA. Hereditariedade em Ortodontia. In: Sakai E et al. (eds), *Nova visão em Ortodontia e Ortopedia Facial*. Soc Paulista de Ortodontia: São Paulo, 2000.
25. Harris JE, Kowalski CJ, Walker SJ. Intrafamilial dentofacial associations for Class II, Division 1 probands. *Am J Orthod* 1975 May;**67**(5):563–70.

26. Krogman WM. *Child growth*. Ann Arbor, MI: University of Michigan Press, 1972.
27. Harris JE, Kowalski CJ. All in the family: use of familial information in orthodontic diagnosis, case assessment, and treatment planning. *Am J Orthod* 1976 May;**69**(5):493–510.
28. Broadie AG. On the growth pattern of the human head: from the third month to the eight year of life. *Am J Anat* 1941 Mar;**68**(2):209–62.
29. Mossey PA. The heritability of malocclusion: part 2. The influence of genetics in malocclusion. *Br J Orthod* 1999 Sep;**26**(3):195–203.
30. Proffit WR, Fields HW, Sarver DM. *Contemporary orthodontics*. 4th edn. St. Louis, MO: Mosby, Inc, 2007.
31. Betts NJ, Vanarsdall RL, Barber HD, et al. Diagnosis and treatment of transverse maxillary deficiency. *Int J Adult Orthodon Orthognath Surg* 1995;**10**(2):75–96.
32. Timms DJ, Emerson C. Angell (1822–1903), founding father of rapid maxillary expansion. *Dent Hist* 1997 May;**32**:3–12.
33. Haas AJ. The treatment of maxillary deficiency by opening the mid-palatal suture. *Angle Orthod* 1965 Jul;**35**:200–17.
34. Krebs A. Midpalatal suture expansion studies by the implant method over a seven-year period. *Rep Congr Eur Orthod Soc* 1964;**40**:131–42.
35. Hickham JH. Maxillary protraction therapy: diagnosis and treatment. *J Clin Orthod* 1991 Feb;**25**(2):102–13.
36. Ngan P. Biomechanics of maxillary expansion and protraction in Class III patients. *Am J Orthod Dentofacial Orthop* 2002 Jun;**121**(6):582–3.
37. Wilmes B, Nienkemper M, Ludwig B, et al. Early Class III treatment with a hybrid hyrax-mentoplate combination. *J Clin Orthod* 2011 Jan;**45**(1):15–21; quiz 39.
38. Turley PK. Orthopedic correction of Class III malocclusion with palatal expansion and custom protraction headgear. *J Clin Orthod* 1988 May;**22**(5):314–25.
39. Gautam P, Valiathan A, Adhikari R. Craniofacial displacement in response to varying headgear forces evaluated biomechanically with finite element analysis. *Am J Orthod Dentofacial Orthop* 2009 Apr;**135**(4):507–15.
40. Vaughn GA, Mason B, Moon H-B, Turley PK. The effects of maxillary protraction therapy with or without rapid palatal expansion: a prospective, randomized clinical trial. *Am J Orthod Dentofacial Orthop* 2005 Sep;**128**(3):299–309.
41. Miller CL, Araújo EA, Behrents RG, et al. Mandibular arch dimensions following bonded and banded rapid maxillary expansion. *J World Fed Orthod* 2014;**3**:119–23.
42. Anne Mandall N, Cousley R, DiBiase A, et al. Is early Class III protraction facemask treatment effective? A multicentre, randomized, controlled trial: 3-year follow-up. *J Orthod* 2012 Sep;**39**(3):176–85.
43. Liu ZP, Li CJ, Hu HK, et al. Efficacy of short-term chincup therapy for mandibular growth retardation in Class III malocclusion. *Angle Orthod* 2011 Jan;**81**(1):162–8.
44. Mitani H. Early application of chincap therapy to skeletal Class III malocclusion. *Am J Orthod Dentofacial Orthop* 2002 Jun;**121**(6):584–5.
45. Tanne K, Lu YC, Tanaka E, Sakuda M. Biomechanical changes of the mandible from orthopaedic chincup force studied in a three-dimensional finite element model. *Eur J Orthod* 1993 Dec;**15**(6):527–33.
46. Araújo EA. Interview with Hideo Mitani. *Rev Dent Press Orthodon Orthop Facial* 2002 May;**5**(3):1–6.
47. Fukazawa H, Mukaiyama T, Kurita T, et al. [Evaluation on facial pattern of early childhood patients with T. M. J. dysfunction occurred after anterior crossbite correction]. *Nihon Ago Kansetsu Gakkai Zasshi* 1989;**1**(1):66–78.
48. Mitani H, Fukazawa H. Effects of chincap force on the timing and amount of mandibular growth associated with anterior reversed occlusion (Class III malocclusion)

during puberty. *Am J Orthod Dentofacial Orthop* 1986 Dec;**90**(6):454–63.

49 Mukaiyama T, Fukazawa H, Mizoguchi I, Mitani H [Prevalence of temporomandibular joint dysfunction for 6–10-year old Japanese children with chincap orthodontic treatment]. *Nihon Kyōsei Shika Gakkai Zasshi J Jpn Orthod Soc* 1988 Jun;**47**(2):425–32.

50 Mimura H, Deguchi T. Morphologic adaptation of temporomandibular joint after chincup therapy. *Am J Orthod Dentofacial Orthop* 1996 Nov;**110**(5):541–6.

51 Arat ZM, Akçam MO, Gökalp H. Long-term effects of chin cap therapy on the temporomandibular joints. *Eur J Orthod* 2003 Oct;**25**(5):471–5.

52 Deguchi T, Uematsu S, Kawahara Y, Mimura H. Clinical evaluation of temporomandibular joint disorders (TMD) in patients treated with chincup. *Angle Orthod* 1998 Feb;**68**(1):91–4.

53 Deguchi T, McNamara JA. Craniofacial adaptations induced by chincup therapy in Class III patients. *Am J Orthod Dentofacial Orthop* 1999 Feb;**115**(2):175–82.

54 Deguchi T, Kuroda T, Hunt NP, Graber TM. Long-term application of chincup force alters the morphology of the dolichofacial Class III mandible. *Am J Orthod Dentofacial Orthop* 1999 Dec;**116**(6):610–5.

55 Reynders RM. Orthodontics and temporomandibular disorders: a review of the literature (1966–1988). *Am J Orthod Dentofacial Orthop* 1990 Jun;**97**(6):463–71.

56 Moreira RC, Araújo EA. Freqüência das exodontias em tratamentos ortodônticos realizados na clínica do Curso de Especialização em Ortodontia do Centro de Odontologia e Pesquisa da Pontifícia Universidade Católica de Minas Gerais. *Rev Bras Orthod Orthop Dentofacial* 2000;**3**(2):49–53.

57 Gianelly AA. Treatment of crowding in the mixed dentition. *Am J Orthod Dentofacial Orthop* 2002 Jun;**121**(6):569–71.

58 Araújo EA, Kim BJ, Wolf G. Two superimposition methods to assess Class III treatment. *Semin Orthod* 2007 Sep;**13**(3):200–8.

8

Special topics

8.1

Section I: Habit control: the role of function in open-bite treatment

Ildeu Andrade, Jr., DDS, MS, PhD[1] and Eustáquio A. Araújo, DDS, MDS[2]

[1] Department of Orthodontics, School of Dental Medicine, University of Pittsburgh, Pittsburgh, PA, USA
[2] Center for Advanced Dental Education, Saint Louis University, St. Louis, MO, USA

In psychology, a habit is an automatic pattern of behavior in reaction to a specific situation. It may be inherited or acquired through frequent repetition, and it may occur consciously at first, then unconsciously [1]. According to the American Academy of Pediatric Dentistry, oral habit behaviors include digit-sucking, pacifier, lip-sucking and biting, nail-biting, bruxism, self-injurious habits, mouth breathing, and tongue thrusting.

Oral habits have long been recognized to be associated with dentoalveolar and/or skeletal deformation in some patients. The amount of dentoalveolar-skeletal deformation is related to the frequency, duration, direction, and intensity of certain habits [2]. According to Brodie [3], patterns of facial growth are established early in development. However, there is still controversy about whether oral habits can cause skeletal malocclusions. Cephalometric studies show that most anterior open bite subjects present characteristics of both dentoalveolar and skeletal increased vertical dimensions [4, 5]. A previous study has suggested that, in the presence of a prolonged sucking habit, a facial hyperdivergence might modulate the appearance and severity of a developing malocclusion [6].

Conversely, skeletal open bite subjects do not necessarily have a negative overbite [7].

8.1 Nutritive vs. nonnutritive sucking habits

The habit of sucking is the first coordinated muscular activity of the infant. There are essentially two forms of sucking: the nutritive form, which provides essential nutrients, and non-nutritive sucking (e.g. finger or pacifier sucking), which is considered normal in infants and young children and is usually associated with their need to satisfy the urge for contact and security.

Relationships between nonnutritive sucking habits and dentoalveolar abnormalities have been extensively studied [8–13]. Changes that can occur to the dentoalveolar structures may include an anterior or posterior open bite, interference of normal tooth position and eruption, increased overjet, greater maxillary arch depth, narrowed maxillary arch widths, shallower palatal depths, increased mandibular arch width, Class II malocclusion, and crossbites.

Recognizing and Correcting Developing Malocclusions: A Problem-Oriented Approach to Orthodontics,
Second Edition. Edited by Eustáquio A. Araújo and Peter H. Buschang.
© 2025 John Wiley & Sons, Inc. Published 2025 by John Wiley & Sons, Inc.

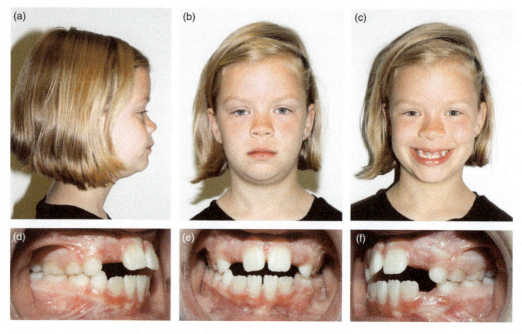

Figure 8.1 (a–f) 9y 2m girl with history of thumb sucking.

Nonnutritive sucking habits until 3 years of age are normal, but persistence of these habits beyond age 3 significantly increases the probability of developing undesirable dentoalveolar characteristics at the end of the deciduous dentition stage [14]. Since they create a mechanical obstacle for the eruption of anterior teeth, associated with a forward resting posture of the tongue, prolonged nonnutritive sucking habits often result in an anterior open bite [10, 15, 16].

Figure 8.1 presents a typical case of a child with prolonged digital habits. This child continued a thumb-sucking habit beyond 3 years of age and presents with an anterior open bite, a Class II canine relationship, and an increased overjet.

In digital sucking, depending on the direction that the force is applied and how the hand rests on the dental arches, the thumb or finger pushes the lower incisors lingually and the upper incisors labially. Moreover, the mandible is positioned downward, allowing a greater eruption of posterior teeth. While the tongue is lowered vertically away from the posterior maxillary teeth, an increased cheek pressure may be observed (the buccinator muscle contracts during sucking), and the equilibrium that controls the dental arch width dimensions is altered [15].

8.2 Tongue physiology

The tongue plays an important role in physiological functions such as breathing, mastication, deglutition, and speech. In normal deglutition, the tip of the tongue rests on the lingual part of the maxillary anterior dentoalveolar area and the center portion of the tongue sequentially elevates from front to back [17]; during swallowing, the teeth briefly touch with minimal contraction of the perioral muscles, and there is neither a tongue thrust nor a continuous forward posture.

However, in most anterior open bite patients, the tongue tip protrudes without contacting the alveolar ridge during deglutition in order to seal off the front of the mouth during swallowing, which prevents food or liquids from escaping. In addition, the posterior aspect of the tongue exhibits a decelerated movement after the bolus passes through the esophagus opening. During deglutition, the tongue's movements primarily involve up-and-down motions in each region, facilitating bolus propulsion [18, 19].

8.3 Tongue thrusting and forward resting posture of the tongue

Tongue thrusting is a predominant swallowing pattern in infants [20]. It is a normal transitional stage in swallowing, and the mature or adult swallow pattern appears in some normal children as early as age 3 but is not present in the majority until about age 6.

The tongue thrusting habit is a condition in which the tongue makes contact with anterior teeth during swallowing [21]. Tongue thrusting is commonly indicated by a forward tongue position, a swallow characterized by tongue thrust, the contraction of perioral muscles (such as hyperactive mentalis and orbicularis oris), excessive buccinator hyperactivity, and swallowing without the usual momentary tooth contact [22].

However, the brief duration of tongue-thrust swallowing is insufficient to influence the position of the teeth. Tongue pressure against the teeth during swallowing lasts around 1 s. A typical individual swallows 1000 times per day, which totals only a few minutes of pressure over the teeth, not nearly enough to affect the equilibrium. Meanwhile, in cases where there is a forward resting posture of the tongue, this pressure lasts much longer and may affect tooth position either vertically or horizontally [23]. Prolonged forward resting posture of the tongue has been shown to be associated with open bite; however, whether the open bite is cause or effect is not well established.

8.4 Breaking the habit

Breaking a digit-sucking habit is a challenge. Children have the natural desire and necessity to put their thumbs or fingers into their mouths, and sometimes that is seen even before birth. At the beginning, the habit can provide a great deal of pleasure, comfort, and warmth for the child. But later, it can very well lead to a habit that is hard to break. While it may appease anxieties and tediousness, the habit may also lead to a more complex malocclusion.

As discussed earlier, nonnutritive sucking habits up to 3 years of age are normal, but persistence of these habits beyond age 3 significantly increases the probability of developing undesirable dentoalveolar characteristics at the end of the deciduous dentition stage.

8.4.1 How and when should a clinician intervene?

When the fact is brought to the attention of a clinician, the first recommendation is to understand the personality of the child, the type of relationship within the family, and the frequency and aggressiveness of the habit. Depending on the duration, direction, and frequency of the habit, the dentoalveolar complex responds in different ways.

After noting all of these important variables, it is time to have a frank conversation with the child, mostly done in front of the parents but without their active participation. It is necessary to build a strong relationship of trust between yourself, the clinician, and the child.

8.4.2 The Araújo approach

The Araújo approach starts with simple questions like: *Which thumb/finger do you like to suck? Do you do it all the time? Do you also do it in school?* Normally, when we ask the last, the child immediately says, *"Of course not,"* and at this time, we say we probably know why and basically whisper in the child's ear, *"Because you feel embarrassed to do it in front of your peers, right or wrong?"* Normally, the question is followed by a positive nod. This initial conversation is usually a very positive way to establish confidence and trust with the child.

The second round of questions starts with *"Do you know the damage that that little guy (thumb/finger) can cause to your mouth?"* It is recommended to show open-bite models of horrendous malocclusions. *"Do you want to stop the habit?"; "Do you want us, me and your parents, to help you?"; "Would you like to be the winner or the loser in this battle?"* Then we talk about how weak that thumb/finger looks and how strong the child is, and we next introduce the protocol:

1) Constantly remind the child that he or she wants to win that battle. We have developed a sticker to help the child remember to say NO to thumb/finger sucking (Figure 8.2a). We ask them to put the stickers all over the place and also give them a poster with the same image for their bedroom wall. For girls, we normally ask the mother to polish the nail of the specific thumb/finger, preferably in red, and we tell the child to repeat to herself, *"I'm gonna beat you"* every time they see that red nail polish (Figure 8.2b). For boys, the protocol is the same, but instead of nail polish, we ask them to draw little eyes on the thumb/finger to be beaten, similar to the ones shown in Figure 8.2c. A key to success is the motto, *"I'm gonna beat you."*

2) At home, we ask the parents to watch the child closely, and if he or she starts to suck the thumb/finger to remind them with gentle words like, *"You asked me to remind you if you were sucking your thumb/finger,"* instead of *"Take your thumb/finger out of your mouth!"*

3) At bedtime, the child comes to mom or dad to ask them to tape their *"guardian"* to the thumb/finger to help with the process during the night, and little eyes are also drawn on the tongue depressor stick used for the occasion (Figure 8.2c). The words *"I'm going to beat you"* are already part of their subconscious behavior.

4) Last, and most important, an alginate impression is made of the thumb/finger to be beaten, plaster is poured, and the fabrication of the **trophy** is completed by adding the base and final polishing (Figure 8.3a–d). When the patient finally wins his or her battle, the trophy delivery ceremony occurs with photos and accolades, and then the child can take it home. This experience may be the first major self-conquered battle in the child's life.

In conclusion, before other means such as appliances with spurs, blue grass appliances, or other mechanical means are implemented to solve a digit habit, the Araújo approach is recommended, as described above. When successful, the experience not only solves the destructive habit, but it also creates a magnificent bond between the patient and the clinician.

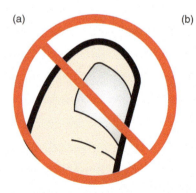 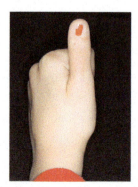 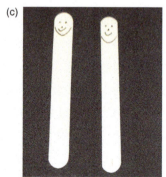

Figure 8.2 (a–c) Reminders for habit control.

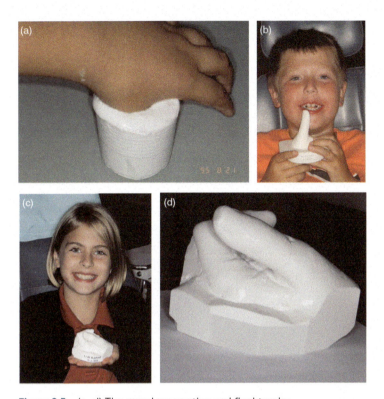

Figure 8.3 (a–d) The award preparation and final trophy.

8.5 Treatment

The cause of an anterior open bite is multifactorial and can be attributed to a combination of skeletal, dental, and soft-tissue effects. Although there is much disagreement on the etiology of an anterior open bite, there is a consensus that malocclusions with an open bite are difficult to treat successfully and to retain properly. Some studies have reported that open bites treated by conventional orthodontic appliances, molar intrusion with temporary skeletal devices (TADs), and/or orthognathic surgery significantly relapse posttreatment [24–26]. Moreover, the existence of persistent deleterious oral habits increases the degree of difficulty of orthodontic treatment, and in cases of persistent open bites, relapse is more likely to occur after orthodontic treatment.

In the correction of an open bite, the success of the treatment depends on the adaptation of the tongue to the new occlusion. Orthodontic appliances are not recommended for correcting an open bite in deciduous dentition. In this scenario, the issue is likely to self-correct if sucking ceases during this stage, as normal lip and cheek pressures will soon restore the teeth to their typical positions. However, if the open bite is a result of a skeletal discrepancy of the maxilla in hyperdivergent patients, spontaneous correction might not occur. Therefore, to address the tooth displacements that arise, orthodontic treatment might be required, with the optimal time to commence such treatment being during the mixed dentition phase.

Multiple treatment strategies have been proposed to correct the anterior open bite and improve masticatory function. Myofunctional therapy, functional orthodontic appliances, vestibular shields, and tongue cribs with or without spurs have been applied with varying success [27–31]. In mixed dentition, besides the orthopedic approaches described in Chapter 6, the most important step in correcting an open bite associated with abnormal habits is to eliminate the habits with patient/parent counseling, behavior-modification techniques, and speech therapy when necessary, frequently associated with orthodontic therapy.

Among all the different orthodontic therapies, tongue spurs have been proven to be efficient, based on the theory that the modification of tongue behavior and function is able to correct the anterior open bite and increase the stability of the treatment result [30, 32]. Spurs were first described in 1927 as a therapeutic approach for faulty tongue posture [33]. The idea was to trigger a nociceptive reflex that would initiate a learning process, in this case, the neuromuscular establishment of a new physiological tongue rest posture and swallowing mode. Previous electromyography studies showed that spikes can stimulate the sensory nerve endings of the tip of the tongue, leading to a new neural arrangement and a new motor engram, and consequently, to a new posture and position of the tongue [34, 35]. It has been suggested that this new tongue pattern may be imprinted permanently in the brain, which could explain the permanent change in tongue posture and the increased stability of the open-bite correction [36].

Figures 8.4–8.6 show a correction of the anterior open bite in a patient who only wore mandibular lingual spurs for 12 months.

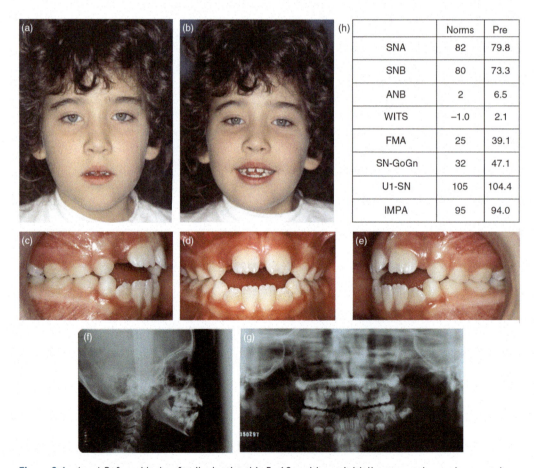

Figure 8.4 (a–g) Referred by her family dentist, this 5y 10m girl was initially seen, and records were taken as seen on the top. A thumb habit was reported. (h) Pre-treatment cephalometric numbers indicate a hyperdivergent facial pattern.

	Norms	Pre
SNA	82	79.8
SNB	80	73.3
ANB	2	6.5
WITS	−1.0	2.1
FMA	25	39.1
SN-GoGn	32	47.1
U1-SN	105	104.4
IMPA	95	94.0

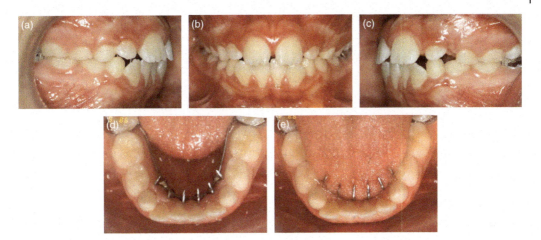

Figure 8.5 (a–e) After the initial steps of making the patient conscious of her self-damaging habit, she was given lower spurs and after 12 months, the bite was close. (center).

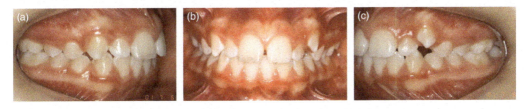

Figure 8.6 (a–c) The patient 2 years later, prephase II.

Furthermore, the psychological effects and the relative effectiveness of tongue spurs and other different types of treatment for children with oral habits have been investigated, and the tongue spurs were the most effective means of arresting the habits [37]. Psychological treatment and other orthodontic appliances alone had no significant effect on arresting the habit. Although tongue spur therapy has many positive results, the use of this appliance has faced resistance from patients, parents, speech pathologists, and psychologists as well as some orthodontists. This aversion is linked to the idea that this device may be a source of irritation, generate discomfort, violate the patient's space, and not be well tolerated by patients and parents.

However, it has been demonstrated that tongue spur therapy is well accepted by patients and parents [38]. This positive result seems to be closely related to how truly informed they were. The study indicated that the predominant functional issues associated with the use of tongue spurs are difficulties in speech and chewing. However, these discomforts are temporary and last only up to 10 days. Moreover, the patients' and parents' reactions to tongue spur therapy seem to be similar to or even better than the studies of other functional and fixed orthodontic appliances when evaluated [39–41].

Two successful early interventions are shown in Figures 8.7–8.13.

8.1 Section I: Habit control: the role of function in open-bite treatment

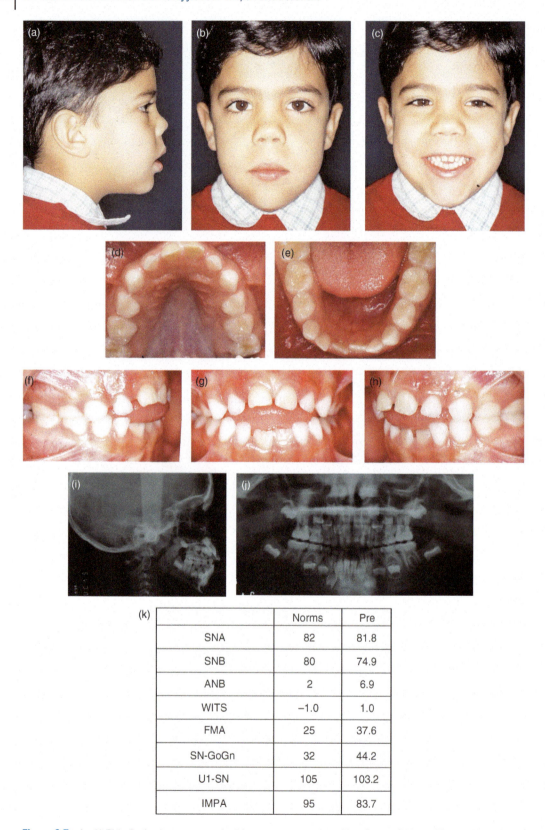

Figure 8.7 (a–k) This 5y 6m boy presented with a very severe open bite due to digit sucking.

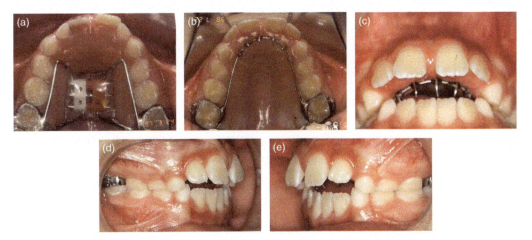

Figure 8.8 (a–e) The Araújo protocol was applied, the maxilla was expanded with a Haas expander, and then the spurs were placed on the maxilla.

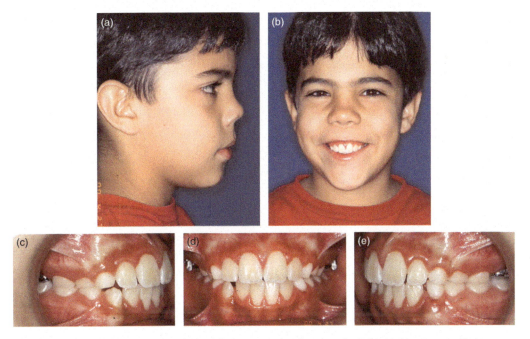

Figure 8.9 (a–e) The patient after 1 year of treatment, showing that the habit had been controlled.

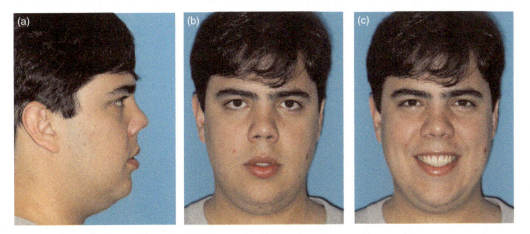

Figure 8.10 (a–h) The patient 18 years later.

8.1 Section I: Habit control: the role of function in open-bite treatment

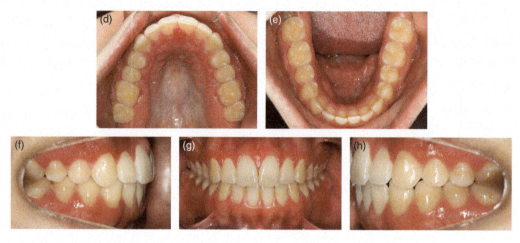

Figure 8.10 (Continued)

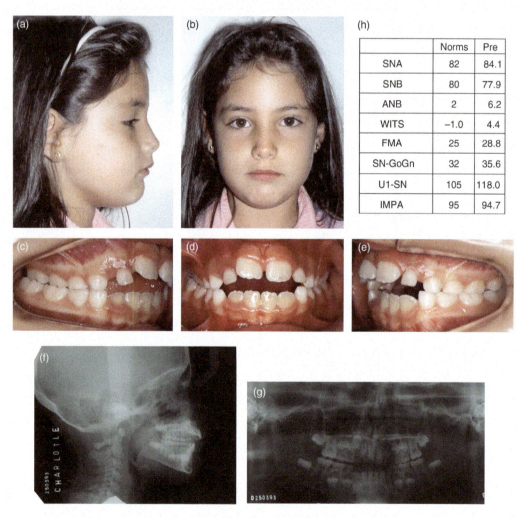

Figure 8.11 (a–h) Six-year-old girl with a severe digit sucking habit.

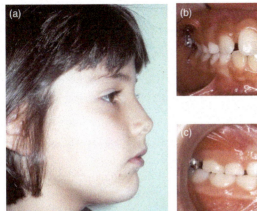
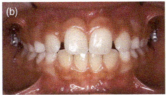
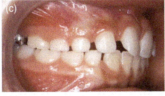
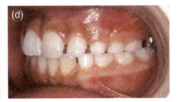

Figure 8.12 (a–d) The results after 15 months of treatment with high-pull headgear along with tongue spurs.

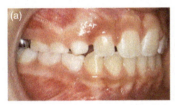
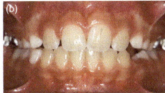
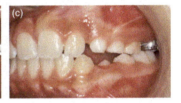

Figure 8.13 After 20 months of treatment.

References

1 Wood W, Neal DT. A new look at habits and the habit-goal interface. *Psychol Rev* 2007;**114**(4):843–63.
2 Nowak AJ, Warren JJ. Infant oral health and oral habits. *Pediatr Clin N Am* 2000;**47**(5):1034–66.
3 Brodie AG. On the growth pattern of the human head from the third month to the eighth year of life. *Am J Anat* 1941;**68**:209–62.
4 Nahoum HI. Vertical proportions and the palatal plane in anterior open-bite. *Am J Orthod* 1971;**59**:273–82.
5 Cangialosi TJ. Skeletal morphologic features of anterior open bite. *Am J Orthod* 1984;**85**:28–36.
6 Cozza P, Baccetti T, Franchi L, et al. Sucking habits and facial hyperdivergency as risk factors for anterior open bite in the mixed dentition. *Am J Orthod Dentofacial Orthop* 2005;**128**:517–9.
7 Ferrillo M, Pandis N, Fleming PS. The effect of vertical skeletal proportions on overbite changes in untreated adolescents: a longitudinal evaluation. *Angle Orthod* 2024;**94**(1):25–30. doi: 10.2319/042823-310.1.
8 Adair SM, Milano M, Lorenzo I, Russell C. Effects of current and former pacifier use on the dentition of 24- to 59-month-old children. *Pediatr Dent* 1995;**17**:437–44.
9 Borrie FR, Bearn DR, Innes NP, Iheozor-Ejiofor Z. Interventions for the cessation of non-nutritive sucking habits in children. *Cochrane Database Syst Rev* 2015;**2015** (3):CD008694. doi: 10.1002/14651858. CD008694.pub2.

10. Adriano LZ, Derech CD, Massignan C, et al. Anterior open bite self-correction after cessation of non-nutritive sucking habits: a systematic review. *Eur J Orthod* 2023;**45**(3):235–43. doi: 10.1093/ejo/cjac054.

11. Ogaard B, Larrson E, Lindsten R. The effect of sucking habits, cohort, sex, intercanine arch widths, and breast or bottle feeding on posterior crossbite in Norwegian and Swedish 3-year-old children. *Am J Orthod Dentofacial Orthop* 1994;**106**:161–6.

12. Lindner A, Modeer T. Relation between sucking habits and dental characteristics in preschool children with unilateral cross-bite. *Scand J Dent Res* 1989;**97**:278–83.

13. Schmid KM, Kugler R, Nalabothu P, et al. The effect of pacifier sucking on orofacial structures: a systematic literature review. *Prog Orthod* 2018;**19**(1):8. doi: 10.1186/s40510-018-0206-4.

14. Warren JJ, Bishara SE. Duration of nutritive and nonnutritive sucking behaviors and their effects on the dental arches in the primary dentition. *Am J Orthod Dentofacial Orthop* 2002;**121**:347–56.

15. Larsson E. The prevalence and aetiology of prolonged dummy and finger-sucking habits. *Eur J Orthod* 1985;**7**:172–6.

16. Katz CR, Rosenblatt A, Gondim PP. Nonnutritive sucking habits in Brazilian children: effects on deciduous dentition and relationship with facial morphology. *Am J Orthod Dentofacial Orthop* 2004;**126**:53–7.

17. Logemann JA. *Manual for the videofluorographic study of swallowing.* 2nd edn. Austin, TX: Pro-ed, 1993.

18. Kahrilas PJ, Lin S, Logemann JA, et al. Deglutitive tongue action: volume accommodation and bolus propulsion. *Gastroenterology* 1993;**104**:152–62.

19. Fujiki T, Takano-Yamamoto T, Noguchi H, et al. A cineradiographic study of deglutitive tongue movement and nasopharyngeal closure in patients with anterior open bite. *Angle Orthod* 2000;**70**(4):284–9.

20. Dixit UB, Shetty RM. Comparison of soft-tissue, dental, and skeletal characteristics in children with and without tongue thrusting habit. *Contemp Clin Dent* 2013;**4**(1):2–6.

21. Hanson ML, Barnard LW, Case JL. Tongue-thrust in pre-school children. *Am J Orthod* 1969;**56**:60–9.

22. Peng CL, Jost-Brinkmann PG, Yoshida N, et al. Comparison of tongue functions between mature and tongue-thrust swallowing: an ultrasound investigation. *Am J Orthod Dentofacial Orthop* 2004;**125**:562–70.

23. Proffit WR, Henry W. *Contemporary orthodontics.* St. Louis, MO: Mosby, Inc, 2000.

24. Lopez-Gavito G, Wallen TR, Little RM, Jondeph DR. Anterior openbite malocclusion: a longitudinal 10-year postretention evaluation of orthodontically treated patients. *Am J Orthod* 1985;**87**:175–86.

25. González Espinosa D, de Oliveira Moreira PE, da Sousa AS, et al. Stability of anterior open bite treatment with molar intrusion using skeletal anchorage: a systematic review and meta-analysis. *Prog Orthod* 2020;**21**(1):35. doi: 10.1186/s40510-020-00328-2.

26. Denison TF, Kokich VG, Shapiro PA. Stability of maxillary surgery in openbite versus nonopenbite malocclusions. *Angle Orthod* 1989;**1**:5–10.

27. Huang GJ, Justus R, Kennedy DB, Kokich VG. Stability of anterior openbite treated with crib therapy. *Angle Orthod* 1990;**60**:17–24.

28. Smithpeter J, Covell D Jr. Relapse of anterior open bites treated with orthodontic appliances with and without orofacial myofunctional therapy. *Am J Orthod Dentofacial Orthop* 2010;**137**(5):605–14. doi: 10.1016/j.ajodo.2008.07.016.

29. Klocke A, Korbmacher H, Hahl-Nieke B. Influence of orthodontic appliances on myofunctional therapy. *J Orofac Orthop* 2000;**61**:414–20.

30. Justus R. Correction of anterior open bite with spurs: long-term stability. *World J Orthod* 2001;**2**:219–31.

31 Shapiro PA. Stability of open bite treatment. *Am J Orthod Dentofacial Orthop* 2002;**121**:566–8.

32 Graber MT. The "three M's". Muscles, malformation and malocclusion. *Am J Orthod* 1963;**49**:418–50.

33 Rogers AP. Open bite cases involving tongue habits. *Int J Orthod* 1927;**13**:837.

34 Schwestka-Polly R, Engelke W, Hoch G. Electromagnetic articulography as a method for detecting the influence of spikes on tongue movement. *Eur J Orthod* 1995;**5**:411–7.

35 Yashiro K, Takada K. Tongue muscle activity after orthodontic treatment of anterior open bite: a case report. *Am J Orthod Dentofactial Orthop* 1999;**115**:660–6.

36 Meyer-Marcotty P, Hartmann J, Stellzig Eisenhauer A. Dentoalveolar open bite treatment with spur appliances. *J Orofac Orthop* 2007;**68**(6):510–21.

37 Haryett RD, Hansen FC, Davidson PO, Sandilands ML. Chronic thumb-sucking: the psychologic effects and the relative effectiveness of various methods of treatment. *Am J Orthod* 1967;**8**:569–85.

38 Araújo EA, Andrade I Jr, et al. Perception of discomfort during orthodontic treatment with tongue spurs orthodontics. *Orthodontics (Chic.)* 2011;**12**(3):260–7.

39 Surge HG, Klages U, Zentner A. Pain and discomfort during orthodontic treatment: causative factors and effects on compliance. *Am J Orthod Dentofacial Orthop* 1998;**6**:684–91.

40 Sergl HG, Zentner A. A comparative assessment of acceptance of different types of functional appliances. *Eur J Orthod* 1998;**5**:517–24.

41 Johnson PD, Cohen DA, Aiosa L, et al. Attitudes and compliance of pre-adolescent children during early treatment of Class II malocclusion. *Clin Orthod Res* 1998;**1**:20–8.

8.2

Section II: Eruption deviations

Bernardo Q. Souki, DDS, MSD, PhD[1] and Eustáquio A. Araújo, DDS, MDS[2]

[1] *Department of Dentistry, Pontifical Catholic University of Minas Gerais, Belo Horizonte, Brazil*
[2] *Department of Orthodontics, Center for Advanced Dental Education, Saint Louis University, St. Louis, MO, USA*

8.6   Eruption deviations

The migration of the teeth from their sites of development within bone to their functional position within the oral cavity is complex, and the mechanisms are not fully understood [1, 2]. There is evidence that tooth eruption is too complex to be associated with a single functioning tissue and that genetic and environmental factors may impact the process. Theories have been postulated, and these indicate that almost every tissue in or near an erupting tooth is essential to the process [1]. Thus, the root growth changes in the periodontal ligament, the proliferation of dental pulp, dentin formation, and contraction of the *gubernaculum dentis* (soft tissue connection between the enamel organ and oral epithelium) have all been considered essential to the process [3].

In the daily practice of orthodontics and pediatric dentistry, clinicians frequently deal with eruption deviations in growing patients. It has been claimed that the early diagnosis of eruption deviation is important in order to start treatment at the optimal time and to minimize future complications [4]. Most of the disorders related to dental eruption occur during the transitional stage. Knowing the major eruption deviations that can occur during occlusal development and how to deal with them is essential for the effective clinical management of preventive and interceptive orthodontic monitoring (PIOM), presented in Chapter 2.

Eruption deviations might be classified as: 1) delayed tooth eruption (DTE), 2) changes in the sequence of eruption of teeth, 3) ectopic eruption, and 4) tooth ankylosis.

DTE: The most probable age for each group of primary and permanent teeth eruption is well established for boys and girls from diverse ethnicities. When the eruption time deviates by more than 2 years from the expected mean eruption time for a specific tooth (chronologic norm of eruption) and the root formation is quite adequate for its eruption (⅔ of its final length), the clinician should search for any factor adversely affecting normal tooth eruption. The emergence of permanent teeth occurs earlier in girls [5], and the difference between eruption times is, on average, 4–6 months. Earlier eruption of permanent teeth in girls is attributed to earlier onset of maturation [5]. However, genetic, ethnic, and individual factors might also influence eruption [3]. As discussed in Chapter 4, genetics also plays an important role in tooth development. Generalized tooth developmental delay

---

Recognizing and Correcting Developing Malocclusions: A Problem-Oriented Approach to Orthodontics,
Second Edition. Edited by Eustáquio A. Araújo and Peter H. Buschang.
© 2025 John Wiley & Sons, Inc. Published 2025 by John Wiley & Sons, Inc.

is frequently seen in patients with syndromes as well as a familial pattern. Various mechanisms have been suggested to explain DTE in relation to genetic disorders. Defects in bone resorption, alterations in the cellular cementum, and the presence of supernumerary teeth might be responsible for DTE associated with syndromes. The presence of a gene that controls tooth eruption has also been suggested, and its "delayed onset" might be responsible for DTE in "inherited retarded eruption." Physical obstruction is also a common local cause of DTE related to a single tooth. Supernumerary teeth, odontomas, and deficient arch length are the most frequent physical obstructions associated with DTE. Mucosal barrier, scar tissue, and tumors may also be related to DTE [6].

Changes in the eruption sequence: Deviations in the eruption sequence of deciduous teeth are frequent but are rarely indicative of eruption disturbance. Permanent teeth, however, present a consistent eruption sequence and deviations from its normality can be indicative of a disturbance with clinical significance. Changes in the sequence of eruption of permanent dentition might be responsible for arch length shortening and intraarch space problems. Clinicians should be aware of the most favorable sequence of eruption of permanent teeth (see Chapter 5) and carefully monitor the various stages of occlusal development. Supervised extraction of deciduous teeth with adequate space management may help normalize the eruption sequence.

Ectopic eruption: This is a disturbance in which the tooth does not follow its natural course. It is very rare in the deciduous dentition. In the permanent dentition, however, ectopic eruption is highly prevalent. The most frequently affected teeth are the maxillary first permanent molars and canines, followed by the mandibular canine, mandibular second premolar, and the maxillary lateral incisors. Due to arch length discrepancy and posterior crowding, second and third permanent molars may also assume an ectopic direction of eruption. Correction of an ectopically erupting tooth is critical for the development of a stable occlusion, and it is an important component of interceptive orthodontic treatment. The clinician can choose from various effective treatment modalities to successfully manage ectopically erupting permanent teeth.

Ankylosis: Tooth ankylosis is characterized by the fusion of bone and cementum and it is considered a progressive anomaly of tooth eruption that usually has a profound effect on the occlusion. Submerged teeth refer to a clinical condition whereby, after eruption, teeth become ankylosed and lose their ability to maintain the continuous eruptive potential as the jaws grow. Deciduous teeth become ankylosed far more frequently than permanent ones. The ratio can be up to 10:1 with mandibular teeth ankyloses being twice as common as maxillary ankylosis. It seems as if the site of tooth ankylosis is also well defined, since nearly all ankylosed teeth are either deciduous or permanent molars. Treatment depends upon whether the ankylosed tooth is deciduous or permanent, the time of onset, the time of diagnosis, and the location of the affected tooth.

A systematic review [7] on the ankylosed primary molars concluded that: they ...

> often manifest with mild to moderate progressive infraocclusion. Conservative monitoring of ankylosed primary molars is recommended. The clinician should consider extraction if the permanent successor has an altered path of eruption, if the ankylosed primary molar is severely infraoccluded with the adjacent teeth tipping to prevent the successor from erupting, or both. The ankylosed molar often exfoliates spontaneously within six months; however, when exfoliation is more delayed, arch-length loss, occlusal disturbance, hooked roots or impaction of permanent successors may occur. Ankylosed primary molars initially should be

monitored closely for up to six months. If they do not exfoliate spontaneously, they should be removed because arch-length loss, alveolar bone defects, impacted permanent successors and occlusal disturbances often occur when the removal is delayed.

In the recent years, it has been proposed that infraoccluded teeth should be considered a category under "primary failure of eruption (PFE)" [8].

PFE is regarded as an eruption defect, manifesting as a complete failure of eruption or cessation of initial eruption with no obvious local or systemic causative factor. It is a poorly understood condition, associated with tooth eruption failure, but evidence suggests a strong genetic basis. Unfortunately, attempts to implement orthodontic movements to manage an affected tooth will likely be unsuccessful.

8.7 Eruption deviation and PIOM: what are the most frequent eruption disturbances in each stage of dental development?

During the development of the occlusion, some eruption disturbances are more likely to be present in each of the stages of dental development. Stage 1 is represented by the eruption of the deciduous dentition. We will present possible disturbances from stages 2 to 7.

8.7.1 Stage 2 – Completion of deciduous dentition

During the maturity of the deciduous dentition period (3–5-year-old), eruption deviations are rare. However, clinicians must be aware that tooth ankylosis can be present, and depending on the time of the onset, it may represent a real threat to an adequate arch development. Early onset of deciduous molar ankylosis (before 5 years old) deserves special attention. In severe cases, with clear indication of vertical bone loss, the ankylosed teeth should be extracted and a space maintainer installed. Usually, the early infra-occluded deciduous molar favors the loss of arch length. Adequate space management must be offered in order to allow the eruption of succedaneous permanent tooth (Figure 8.14).

8.7.2 Stage 3 – Eruption of the first permanent molars

The maxillary first permanent molar ectopic eruption, which has been widely described in the literature, shows a variable prevalence of 2–6%, depending on the studied population. Harrison Jr. and Michal [9] proposed a classification for the ectopic eruption of first permanent molars. The *jump* type (when a self-correction is established) presents a higher incidence (Figure 8.15a), while the *hold* type (when there is no self-correction) is less frequent (Figures 8.15b and 8.16).

PFE of permanent mandibular first molar (Figures 8.17 and 8.18) is a rare condition (<0.05%). When it occurs, the prognosis is poor. Ankylosis is very likely to develop. Most of the cases require extraction of the infraoccluded tooth since orthodontic movement may not be possible, and alternative techniques such as surgical luxation are rarely capable of creating a new scenario despite isolated reports of success [10].

8.7.3 Stage 4 – Eruption of the permanent incisors

Delayed eruption of maxillary incisors can have a major impact on dental and facial aesthetics. Yaqoob et al. [11] published an updated guideline on the management of unerupted maxillary incisors, with an extensive bibliography on the topic. The most common causes of delayed incisor eruption include an abnormal tooth-to-tissue ratio (Figure 8.19), the presence of supernumerary teeth (Figures 8.20 and 8.21), and gingival fibrosis (Figure 8.22).

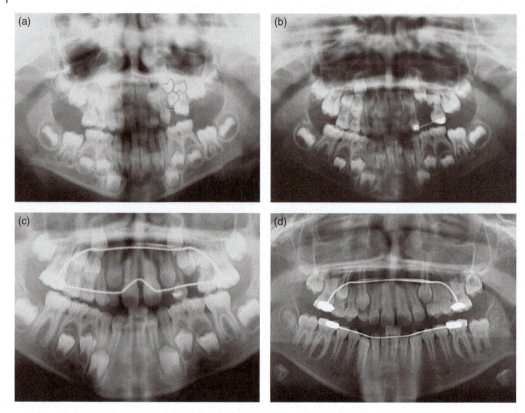

Figure 8.14 (a) Stage 2 girl (4y 6m) presented with an infraoccluded left deciduous maxillary first molar with primary failure of eruption (PFE). Observe that succedaneous first premolar was displaced upward and that arch length was reduced. (b) At 12 months after space regaining and extraction of the left maxillary deciduous first molar, a better position of the first premolar can be observed. (c) Patient at 7y 6m showed the first premolar in a better position. (d) At age 12, the first premolar erupted symmetrically with the contralateral tooth.

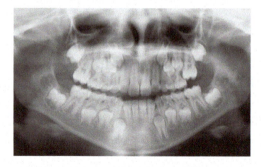

Figure 8.15 Ectopic eruption of both permanent maxillary first molars. The right-side molar presented the *jump* type, while the left side presented the *hold* type. Observe the resorption in the root of both deciduous maxillary second molars.

8.7.4 Stage 5 – Eruption of the mandibular canines and the first premolars

Permanent mandibular canines can assume a deviant eruption pattern. Careful monitoring is necessary to define any intervention. Figures 8.23 and 8.24 show the examples of inadequate and adequate management of ectopic eruption of permanent mandibular canines. First premolars can also assume an ectopic eruption pattern and panoramic radiographic monitoring can help the clinicians to implement treatment. Most of the time it indicates the extraction of deciduous molars

8.7 Eruption deviation and PIOM | 243

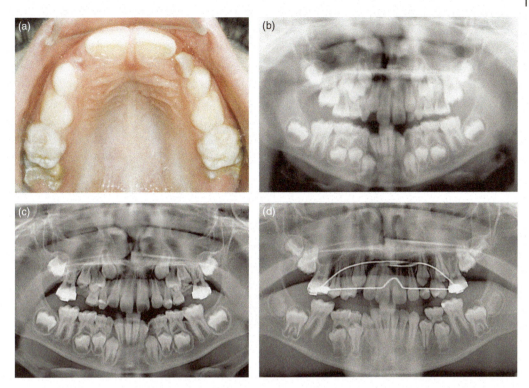

Figure 8.16 (a) An 8-year-old girl presented with a bilateral ectopic eruption of permanent maxillary first molars. (b) Extreme resorption of the maxillary deciduous second molars cementum and dentin. (c) At 8 months after the deciduous maxillary second molars extraction, followed by the permanent maxillary first molars distalization with a headgear, a Class I molar relationship was achieved. (d) Space maintenance with fixed palatal appliances. Right maxillary second premolar erupted passively in the available space. Left maxillary second premolar became blocked and needed fixed orthodontic mechanics to be aligned.

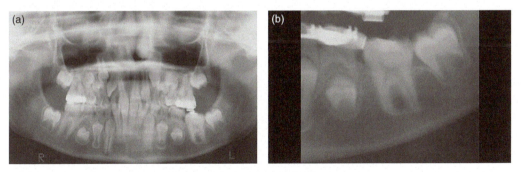

Figure 8.17 (a) A 7-year-old girl presented with a submerged mandibular left first permanent molar. Previous orthodontic treatment aimed its extrusion by means of intermaxillary elastics. However, only extrusion of the maxillary left molars was observed. No orthodontic movement of the mandibular infraoccluded molar could be detected. (b) Luxation followed by 18 months of intraarch orthodontic mechanics was tried. As no tooth movement could be observed, extraction of the ankylosed permanent molar was requested. (c) Adjacent permanent mandibular second molar erupted with marked mesial angulation. (d, e) Permanent second molar was orthodontically uprighted. Treatment plan included the space management for the prosthetic replacement of the extracted permanent molar.

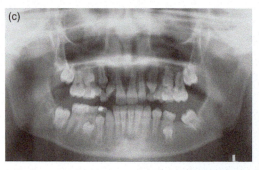
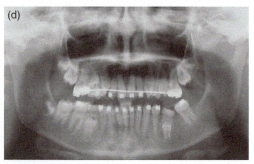
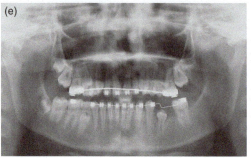

Figure 8.17 (Continued)

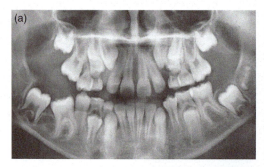
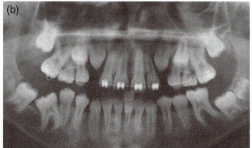
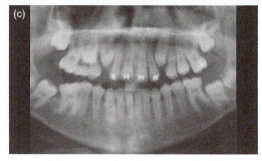

Figure 8.18 (a) An 8y 3m boy presented a PFE of the permanent mandibular right first molar. A panoramic baseline radiograph showed a submerged tooth. Ankylosis of the permanent first molar was diagnosed and tooth extraction was indicated. The patient's parents refused to extract it and asked for a noninvasive control. Phase I orthodontic treatment was implemented in the maxillary arch to manage space and occlusion guidance. (b) At 18 months after the beginning of orthodontic treatment, the adjacent permanent mandibular second molar showed radiographic signs of eruptive migration over the submerged tooth. A new extraction referral was given to the patient. The prognosis for a situation like that is poor. The patient's parents still refused to extract it. (c) At 12 months later, the panoramic radiograph showed the unlikely improvement of the submerged tooth position.

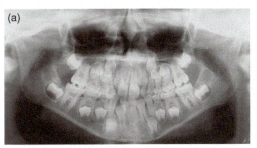
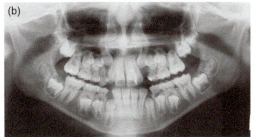

Figure 8.19 (a) An 8-year-old girl presented severe negative space discrepancy. Permanent mandibular incisors had no available space to fully erupt. The left permanent mandibular lateral incisor was blocked. (b) At 12 months after the extraction of the deciduous mandibular cuspids, the mandibular permanent incisors erupted and aligned adequately. An active lip-bumper was used to avoid arch perimeter loss.

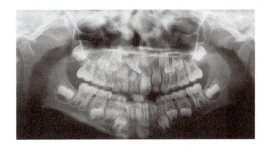

Figure 8.20 No signs of eruption of the right permanent maxillary central incisor 10 months after the eruption of the contralateral permanent maxillary central incisor. The panoramic radiography of this 7y 9m boy showed the presence of a supernumerary tooth, blocking the normal eruption.

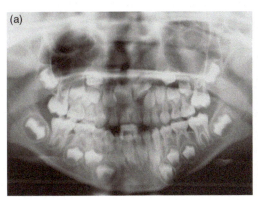
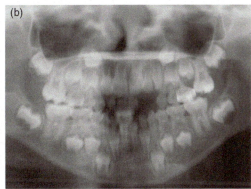

Figure 8.21 (a) Panoramic radiography of a 5y 9m girl showing the presence of supernumerary deciduous and permanent maxillary left lateral incisors. Permanent maxillary left central incisor was ectopically displaced in comparison with the contralateral central incisor. The patient also presented ectopic eruption of the permanent maxillary left first molar. The extraction of the two left deciduous maxillary lateral incisors (normal series and supernumerary) was performed, aiming to accelerate the eruptive process of the succedaneous permanent lateral incisors and the improvement of the eruption of the ectopic central incisor. (b) At 12 months after the extraction of the left deciduous lateral incisors, an improvement in the position of the left permanent maxillary central incisor was noted. The maxillary deciduous central incisors were not extracted. (c) At age 7y 9m, the supernumerary permanent maxillary lateral incisor had not yet been extracted. The similarity in the anatomy of the two left permanent lateral incisors (normal series and supernumerary) in the radiographic examination made the indication of early extraction more difficult. The decision on which teeth to extract was postponed up to the full eruption of these teeth, when the clinical inspection of the anatomy and color would help in the extraction indication. (d) At age 9, after the eruption of the two left permanent lateral incisors, the decision was to extract the most medial one. The decision was based on the crown's color. (e) At 24 months after the extraction of the supernumerary permanent lateral incisor (11 years old), no spontaneous mesial migration of the permanent maxillary left lateral incisor was observed. (f) At age 12, the left permanent maxillary lateral incisor was orthodontically moved. The maxillary cuspids were surgically exposed and orthodontic traction was implemented. (g) After 22 months of orthodontic treatment, mandibular second molars were uprighted, and spaces were closed. Artistic bends for the improvement of the maxillary incisors were indicated.

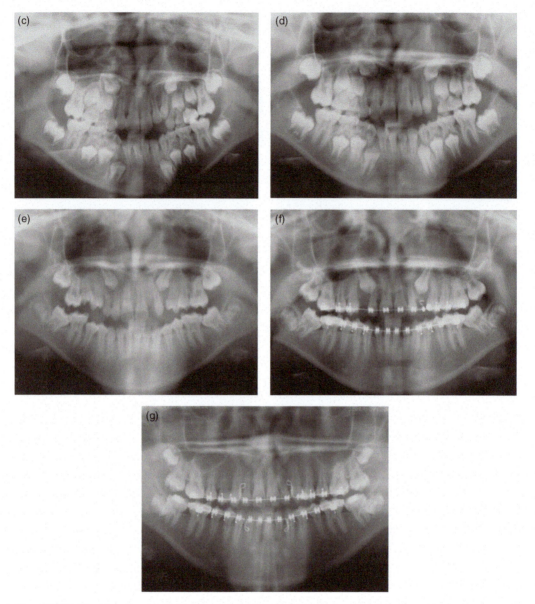

Figure 8.21 (Continued)

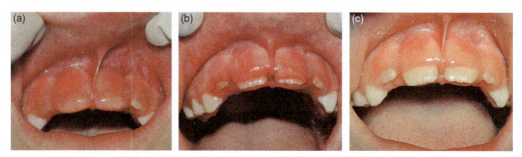

Figure 8.22 (a) A 9y 10m girl with delayed eruption of the maxillary incisors. Palpation showed a localized gingival fibrosis. Deciduous maxillary incisors had exfoliated 16 months earlier, but the permanent successors were "blocked" by gingival fibrosis. Radiographic examination showed adequate root formation. No other mechanical obstruction was observed. There was a great psychosocial concern due to the delayed eruption. (b) Ulectomy was performed. (c) At 10 days after the surgical approach, the incisors showed active eruption.

8.7 Eruption deviation and PIOM | 247

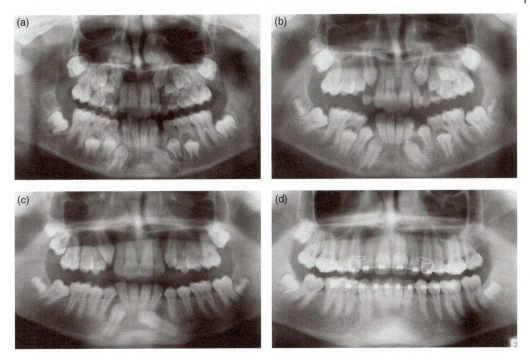

Figure 8.23 (a) Severe negative space discrepancy in the mandibular arch of an 8-year-old boy. Deciduous mandibular cuspids had been extracted early to allow the eruption and alignment of the permanent incisors. However, at that time, no space management procedures with the purpose of preserving arch length were implemented for this patient. (b) At age 9, the mandibular permanent left cuspid showed a marked mesial inclination, but no active orthodontic treatment was proposed in the expectation of a spontaneous self-correction of the cuspid ectopic eruption. (c) At age 11, the mesial migration of the mandibular left cuspid got worse. As severe negative space discrepancy and incisors protrusion was observed, the extraction of the first premolars, followed by orthodontic treatment, was indicated. At that stage, the family refused the premolar extractions. (d) At 12 months later, the left permanent mandibular cuspid was in an even worse position. It was then decided to extract the permanent left mandibular cuspid, the first premolar on the mandibular right side, and the maxillary first premolars. Full braces therapy was necessary to achieve good intercuspation and space closure.

and arch length management. Clinicians, however, might be alerted that delayed premolars formation is not unusual and that long-term monitoring may be the best approach (Figure 8.25).

8.7.5 Stage 6 – Eruption of the second premolars

Agenesis of the second premolars is a frequent finding in orthodontic patients. Also a delayed crown and root formation is not rarely found (Figure 8.26).

8.7.6 Stage 7—Eruption of maxillary canines and second molars

Deviation of the eruption path of the maxillary canines is a condition that orthodontists, pediatric dentists, and general practitioners face in the daily basis. Late diagnosis can lead to irreversible loss (Figure 8.27), but even severely displaced maxillary canines may be orthodontically moved into an adequate position (Figures 8.28 and 8.29). Clinicians must also be aware of the risk of impaction of permanent second molars (Figures 8.30 and 8.31).

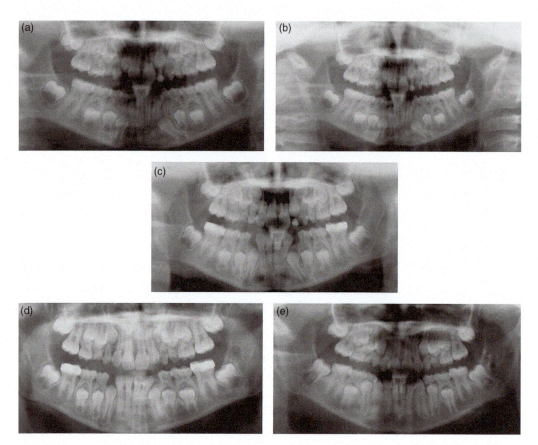

Figure 8.24 (a) A 7-year-old girl presented with the permanent mandibular left cuspid with an increased mesial inclination on the panoramic radiograph. (b) At 6 months later the adjacent permanent lateral incisor presented an increased distal inclination of the crown. The pediatric dentist requested a new panoramic radiograph, which showed that the left mandibular cuspid had moved toward the left permanent lateral incisor's root. (c) At 4 months after the deciduous mandibular cuspids' extraction and the use of an active lip-bumper the improvement in the eruption pattern of the left permanent cuspid could be seen. (d) After 8 months of orthodontic treatment, the left permanent mandibular cuspid is much more symmetric in comparison with the contralateral right side. (e) At age 10, both permanent mandibular cuspids have erupted. Early orthodontic management of the eruption deviation was effective.

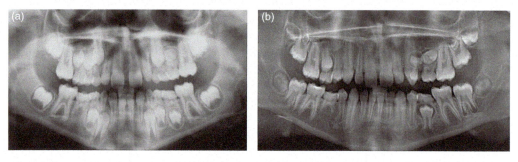

Figure 8.25 (a) Panoramic view of a 9-year-old boy showing the absence of the germs of the right mandibular second premolar and maxillary left first premolar. (b) At 4 years later, age 13, it was observed that the left maxillary first premolar had started to develop, but a significant delay was evident. (c) At age 15, the left maxillary first premolar still presented a significant delay in development. The extraction of this tooth was postponed, since orthodontic treatment would be combined with prosthodontics. This treatment was strongly rejected by the patient's parents. Agenesis of the right permanent mandibular second premolar was evident. (d) At age 18, both left maxillary premolars erupted with adequate crown and root anatomy. The final treatment plan included comprehensive orthodontic mechanics, aiming at space closure on the mandibular right side, to a final Class III molar relationship on the right side. Temporary anchorage devices (TADs) were used to assist in the mandibular space closure with adequate control of the midline. The family was satisfied because no prosthetic replacement was necessary.

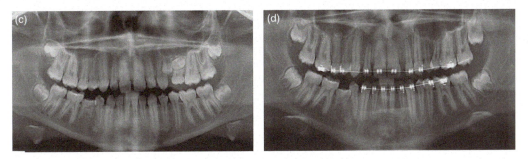

Figure 8.25 (Continued)

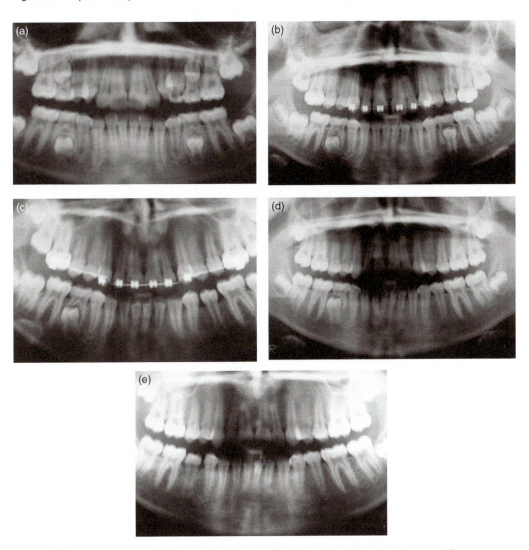

Figure 8.26 (a) Panoramic radiograph of an 11-year-old girl showing delayed and asymmetric development of the mandibular second premolars. (b) At age 13, the mandibular left second premolar showed a significant improvement in the root formation, while the contralateral second premolar showed some improvement but still delayed root formation. (c) At age 14, the mandibular left second premolar erupted. The mandibular right showed a better root formation but was still far from the active eruptive phase. (d) At age 15, the mandibular right second premolar presented half of the root formation and it was in active eruptive process. (e) Finally, at age 17, the right mandibular second premolar erupted. Observe that its apex was still opened.

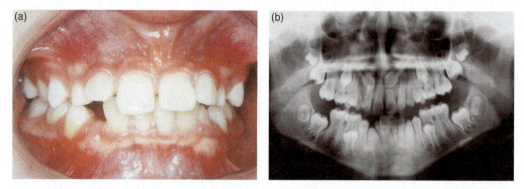

Figure 8.27 (a, b) Intraoral frontal view and panoramic radiography of an 11-year-old boy with ectopic maxillary canines. The asymmetric position of the permanent maxillary lateral incisors indicates possible deviations. The permanent right lateral incisor had compensated for the ectopic eruptive path of the permanent maxillary canines and developed a distal and labial crown movement ("ugly-duckling"). On the left side, however, the permanent central incisor was significantly resorbed.

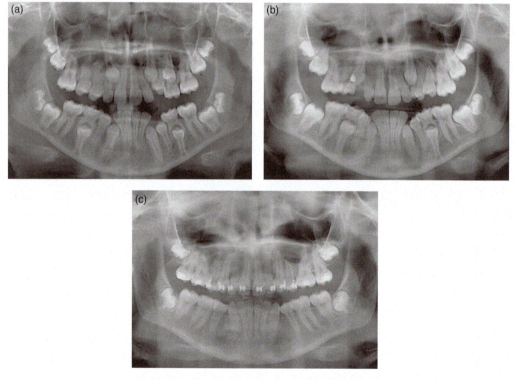

Figure 8.28 (a) An 11-year-old girl presented with severe negative space discrepancy and right permanent maxillary canine in an ectopic position. (b, c) The treatment plan included the extraction of four first premolars and orthodontic traction of the ectopic left maxillary canine. Right maxillary first premolar was extracted first, and then the traction of the ectopic canine was performed with a removable appliance. The extraction of the remaining first premolars was done only after the canine traction was completed.

8.7 Eruption deviation and PIOM | 251

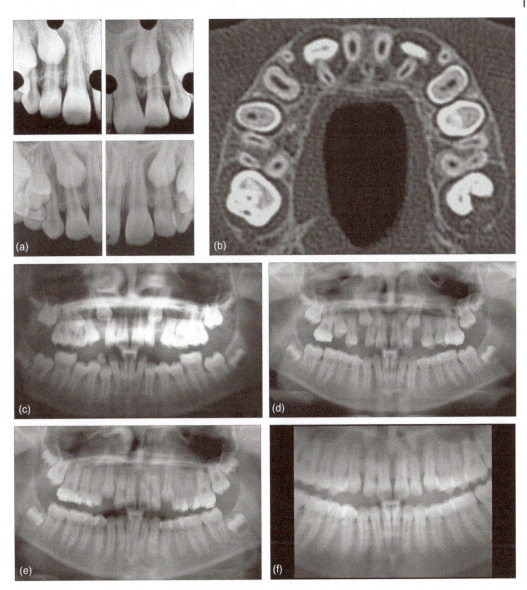

Figure 8.29 (a, b) Periapical radiograph and computed tomography of an 11-year-old girl showing the ectopic position of the permanent maxillary canines. The deciduous maxillary first molars and canines were extracted, and the patient submitted to rapid maxillary expansion. (c) A 12 months after the extractions, a spontaneous improvement in the position of the maxillary canines could be noted. At this moment, a cervical headgear was prescribed to improve the arch length and gain additional space for the eruption of the maxillary canines. (d) After 8 months of headgear use, at the age of 12y 8m, an additional improvement could be seen in the position of the maxillary canines. (e, f) Spontaneous eruption of both permanent maxillary canines was achieved after 30 months of interceptive treatment.

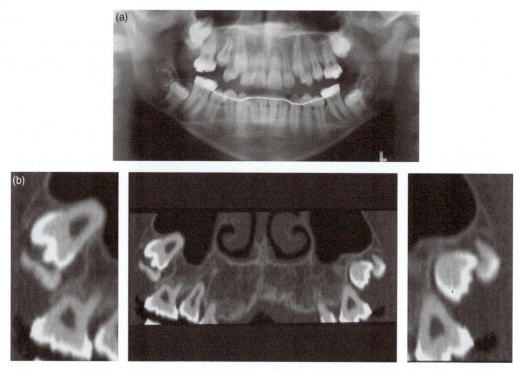

Figure 8.30 (a) Panoramic radiograph of an 11-year-old boy suggested that a radiopaque mass was interfering with the eruption of the right permanent maxillary second molar. No evident blockage of the left permanent maxillary second molar was identified. (b) The computed tomography (CT) acquired in the same month, however, showed that the germs of the maxillary third molars were blocking the eruption of the adjacent second molars bilaterally. Investigation on the delayed eruption of permanent maxillary second molars should include an evaluation of the adjacent third molar position. A new CT scan examination might be considered later on, to evaluate the third molars.

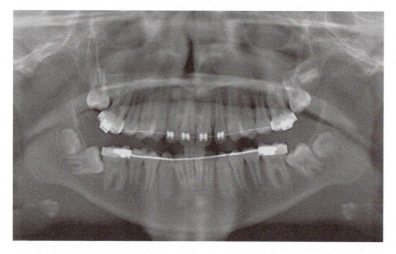

Figure 8.31 Permanent mandibular second molar impaction associated with the orthodontic space management with a lower lingual holding arches (LLHAs). Orthodontic appliances intended to maintain mandibular arch perimeter in the mixed dentition may increase the probability of eruption disturbances of the mandibular second molars. Clinicians should monitor these patients carefully [12].

References

1. Marks SC, Schroeder HE. Tooth eruption: theories and facts. *Anat Rec* 1996;**245**: 374–93.
2. Wise GE, King GJ. Mechanisms of tooth eruption and orthodontic tooth movement. *J Dent Res* 2008;**87**:414–34.
3. Nanci A. *Ten Cate's oral histology: development, structure, and function*. 8th edn. St. Louis, MO: Elsevier Mosby, 2013.
4. Loriato LB, Machado AW, Souki BQ, Pereira TJ. Late diagnosis of dentoalveolar ankylosis: impact on effectiveness and efficiency of orthodontic treatment. *Am J Orthod Dentofacial Orthop* 2009;**135**:799–808.
5. Gron AM. Prediction of tooth emergence. *J Dent Res* 1962;**41**:573–85.
6. Peedikayil FC. Delayed tooth eruption. *e-J Dent* 2011;**1**:81–6.
7. Tieu LD, Walker SL, Major MP, Flores-Mir C. Management of ankylosed primary molars with premolar successors: a systematic review. *J Am Dent Assoc* 2013;**144**:602–11.
8. Ahmad S, Bister D, Cobourne MT. The clinical features and etiological basis of primary eruption failure. *Eur J Orthod* 2006;**28**:535–40.
9. Harrison LM Jr, Michal BC. Treatment of ectopically erupting permanent molars. *Dent Clin N Am* 1984;**28**:57–67.
10. Smith CP, Al-Awadhi EA, Garvey MT. An atypical presentation of mechanical failure of eruption of a mandibular permanent molar: diagnosis and treatment case report. *Eur Arch Paediatr Dent* 2012;**13**:152–6.
11. Yaqoob, O. et al. Management of unerupted maxillary incisors. Available at: https://www.researchgate.net/publication/238754282_Management_of_unerupted_maxillary_incisors
12. Rubin RL, Baccetti T, McNamara JA Jr. Mandibular second molar eruption difficulties related to the maintenance of arch perimeter in the mixed dentition. *Am J Orthod Dentofacial Orthop* 2012;**141**:146–52.

8.3

Section III: Strategies for managing missing second premolar teeth in the young patient

David B. Kennedy, BDS, LDS (RCSEng), MSD, FRCD(C)

Faculty of Dentistry, University of British Columbia, Vancouver, BC, Canada

This section will deal with how the frequency of congenitally missing teeth differs by location of teeth, gender, and geographic region [1]. The frequency range of missing teeth is 3.2–7.6% with the most commonly missing tooth (excluding third molars) being the mandibular second premolar, followed by the maxillary lateral incisor and then the maxillary second premolar [1]. The prevalence in females is 1.37 times higher than in males [1]. Continental differences demonstrate a reduced frequency for North American Caucasians and an increased frequency for both Europeans and Australians [1]. Of all subjects with missing teeth, 83% have either one or two permanent teeth missing [1]. Kokich and Kokich have described methods of managing pontic spaces for subsequent implant restorations in adults [2]. However, this section will review the response of the second deciduous molar when the underlying second premolar is absent, and alternatives for management in the young child.

8.8 General concepts

Comprehensive diagnostic records evaluate the patient in all planes of space, establishing a problem list, leading to treatment alternatives and informed consent [3]. The status of the deciduous molar crown, roots, restorative status, and alveolar support in conjunction with its level to the occlusal plane are factors needing consideration [4]. When a young patient presents with congenitally absent teeth, the clinician should ask some questions to decide whether the deciduous tooth should be retained versus extracted with either space opening, or managed space closure [5]. These questions are [5]: What would you do if the absent tooth were present? Can this malocclusion be satisfactorily treated with an extraction and space closure approach? What is the expected longevity of the deciduous molar?

Patients with minimal crowding, deep overbites, retrusive incisors, decreased anterior lower facial height, and flat mandibular plane angles are usually best treated by nonextraction [5]. Therefore, in such patients, second deciduous molars should be retained for as long as possible, provided there is good root structure and absence of infraocclusion [5]. Interproximal reduction of the retained mandibular second deciduous molar approximates the mesiodistal width closer to that of the absent second premolar [2]. This strategy is limited by the size of the pulp and the curvature of the deciduous second molar roots and their proximity to the adjacent first permanent molar

---

Recognizing and Correcting Developing Malocclusions: A Problem-Oriented Approach to Orthodontics,
Second Edition. Edited by Eustáquio A. Araújo and Peter H. Buschang.
© 2025 John Wiley & Sons, Inc. Published 2025 by John Wiley & Sons, Inc.

and premolar [5]. Failure to reduce the mesiodistal width of the retained deciduous molar results in a cusp-to-cusp, end-on or half-cusp Class II molar relationship despite a Class I canine occlusion [5] (Figure 8.32). An alternative strategy is to leave space in the upper arch, which maintains both a Class I molar and canine (Figure 8.33). Patients who exhibit greater amounts of crowding with either molar or midline asymmetries, protrusive dentitions, bimaxillary protrusion, shallow overbites, anterior open bites, and increased facial height are often best treated with extractions and space closure.

When the decision is made to retain the missing second premolar space, care must be taken in the management of second deciduous molars [5]. Failure to adhere to proper principles disrupts either the occlusion or the ridge area of the missing tooth, leading to future restorative compromise [5]. By contrast, if the decision is made to close the missing tooth space, a major goal will be to place the incisors in the correct position [5]. Failure to do so may result in excessive incisor retraction compromising facial esthetics.

8.9 Longevity of the second deciduous molar, resorption, and infraocclusion

The clinician must consider the anticipated longevity of the retained deciduous molar and whether it has become infraoccluded [5]. The retained deciduous molar may fail because of restorative problems, root resorption, or progressive infraocclusion [5]. When young children present with extensive restorative dentistry in a second deciduous molar with no successor, its longevity must be questioned.

8.9.1 Resorption

Rune and Sarnas [4] reported on the longevity of 123 retained deciduous second molars without successors, where the decision was made to retain the deciduous molars. Of the maxillary deciduous second molars, 26% were lost to resorption and none to infraocclusion. Approximately, half of the retained mandibular deciduous molars showed progressive root resorption over the 5-year mean observation period. However, in a similar study, the degree of root resorption was unchanged in 23 of 26 second deciduous molars with a 15-year observation period [6]. As a result, the deciduous

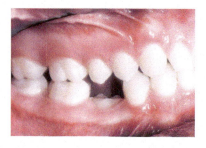

Figure 8.32 Retained infraoccluded deciduous molars compromise occlusion, alveolar support, and challenges restorative buildup.

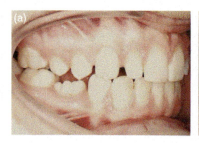 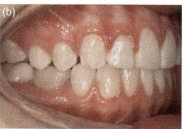

Figure 8.33 Spaces left in the maxillary arch allow Class I molar and canine with restorative buildup of retained deciduous molar. (a) Before buildup. (b) After buildup.

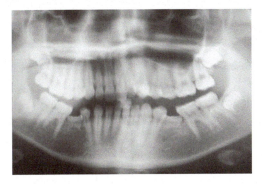

Figure 8.34 Panoramic X-ray shows the effects of infraoccluded deciduous molars with adjacent tooth tipping, space loss, and root resorption.

second molar lasted up to 15 years beyond normal anticipated exfoliation [6].

Bjerklin and Bennett [7] reported that from ages 10 to 20, there was a tendency for all 59 retained second deciduous molars to exhibit mild progressive root resorption (Figure 8.34). Sletten et al. [8] reported negligible root resorption in adults (age 36–48) who had retained second deciduous molars and absent second premolars. Their sample had a less than expected incidence of retained maxillary deciduous second molars compared to mandibular teeth, similar to Rune and Sarnas [4]; they implied that mandibular deciduous molars may be more durable than their maxillary counterparts [4, 6, 8]. These studies [4, 6–8] likely reflect the retained second deciduous molars that had a good prognosis and were the "survivors," as the decision had been made to retain these teeth. They give orthodontists the reassurance that, if the retained second deciduous molars reach adulthood without root resorption or infraocclusion, then they can be expected to last decades or at least the anticipated survival time of a fixed bridge [9].

8.9.2 Infraocclusion

The association of infraoccluded retained second deciduous molars and missing permanent successors has been reported [4, 6, 7, 10–12]. More mandibular second deciduous molars showed infraocclusion (31%) than maxillary second deciduous molars (0%) when underlying premolars were absent [4]. Bjerklin and Bennett reported the frequency of infraocclusion of 59 retained second deciduous molars to be 45%; however, 55% showed insignificant infraocclusion over a 10-year follow-up period [7]. Ankylosis is best diagnosed with a triad of submergence, a dull sound to percussion, and an oblique radiographic angular bone level compared to adjacent teeth [2]. This oblique defect indicates that adjacent teeth are erupting and the retained deciduous molar is submerging [2].

Infraocclusion becomes magnified with skeletal growth due to compensatory eruption of adjacent teeth. Therefore, the earlier that ankylosis and infraocclusion occurs, the greater potential there is for problems [12–15]. Space loss occurred from tipping of the teeth adjacent to the infraoccluded deciduous molar with the space loss being greater than that normally lost by the leeway space [13]. The teeth adjacent to infraoccluded deciduous molars tipped significantly [14] (Figure 8.34) and showed reduced vertical eruption [14]. In unilateral cases, the midline was deflected toward the side of the ankylosis and the infraoccluded deciduous molar [14].

The further that an ankylosed deciduous molar becomes infraoccluded, the more challenging is its surgical removal. This compromises the alveolar bone level both vertically and buccolingually for future prosthetic replacement (Figures 8.32 and 8.34). Today's patients frequently exhibit low decay rates resulting in the preferred long-term restorative option for replacing missing teeth to be an implant-supported crown. Therefore, every effort must be made to avoid compromised bone in the future implant site [5].

8.10 The alveolar ridge in extracted deciduous molars

When mandibular deciduous molars without successors are extracted, three-quarters of all buccal lingual ridge loss occurred within the first 3 years with minimal loss occurring after that time [16]. Despite this bone loss, there was adequate bone for future implant placement [16]. Therefore, when managing these cases from the mixed dentition to completion, infraocclusion should not extend to the point where bone support is compromised by extensive surgical removal (Figures 8.32 and 8.34). Intervention is warranted before the occlusal surface of the deciduous second molar drops below the maximum convexity of the adjacent teeth. The vertical alveolar ridge is usually adequate for implant placement, because compensatory eruption of adjacent teeth coincident with skeletal maturation carries the interproximal bone occlusally (Figures 8.36–8.38).

8.11 Overall dental health and cost

Long-term studies on periodontal health in patients where the missing second premolar spaces are closed, versus keeping them open for either bridge work or implant supported crowns, are not available. However, patients with missing lateral incisors who had spaces left open for bridge work exhibited poorer periodontal health than patients who had the missing maxillary lateral incisor space closed by bringing the canine adjacent to the central incisor [17, 18]. These results remained, despite advances in restorative dentistry over the 20-year time period between these two studies [17, 18]. Therefore, the less restorative dentistry that the patient experiences in terms of bridge work may lead to improved periodontal health based upon the missing lateral incisor studies [17, 18].

When a space closure treatment plan is selected, the patient incurs the cost of the orthodontic treatment alone. When spaces are left open and the second deciduous molar either has been lost or is to be lost, and replaced prosthetically, the patient incurs the cost of the orthodontic treatment, any preprosthetic procedures, the restorative replacement, and future maintenance of the restorations. As the number of congenitally absent teeth increases, so does the cost of potential restorative replacement in addition to any preprosthetic orthodontic work [1, 5]. Therefore, where possible, consideration should be given to space closure treatment plans for reasons of improved periodontal health and reduced overall costs. Furthermore, space closure treatment plans are complete when retainers are placed.

8.12 Case histories

Various case histories demonstrate the treatment options available for managing young growing patients with missing second premolars.

Retain deciduous molar: disk and buildup as needed – In a nonextraction treatment plan, deciduous molars should be retained with interproximal reduction to make the tooth width similar to that of the absent second premolar (Figure 8.35a). When there is minimal infraocclusion, secondary to ankylosis and limited anticipated future growth, restorative buildup of the occlusal surface maintains proximal contact integrity and prevents both supraeruption of the opposing dentition and tilting of the adjacent teeth (Figure 8.35b). Short-term buildup can be done with composite resin (Figure 8.35b). More durable restorative buildup with on lays or crowns (Figure 8.33) should be deferred until the long-term prognosis of the retained deciduous molar has been established.

Extract retained deciduous molar maintain the space and restore prosthetically – When a nonextraction approach is indicated, but there is significant ankylosis, infraocclusion, and/or loss of root structure of the deciduous molar, the deciduous molar(s) should be extracted and the space proportioned for future prosthetic replacement as shown in Figures 8.36–8.38.

Leaving the ankylosed deciduous molar in place invites future compromise in the alveolus of the restorative site. Pretreatment records

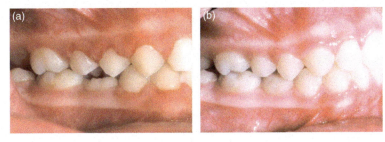

Figure 8.35 (a) Mildly infraoccluded retained deciduous molar has had mesial distal width reduced. (b) Restorative buildup maintains interproximal integrity and occlusal table.

(Figure 8.36) demonstrated minimal crowding and infraocclusion of the retained mandibular second deciduous molars, which had no underlying second premolars, deep overbite, and retrusive incisor position. A nonextraction treatment plan was selected. The infraoccluded deciduous molars were extracted at age 10 before infraocclusion became too extensive, and a lingual arch space maintainer was placed. Nonextraction treatment with fixed appliance was used in the permanent dentition followed by implant-supported crowns (Figures 8.37

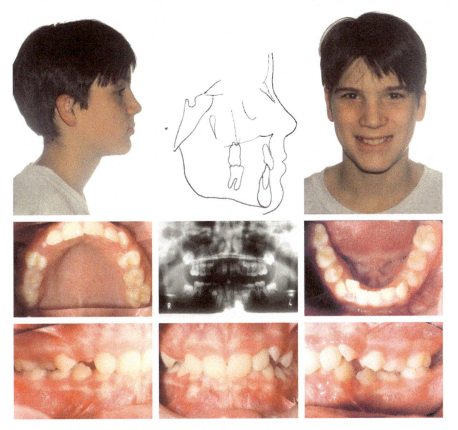

Figures 8.36–8.38 Class I deep bite malocclusion with absent mandibular second premolars; second primary molars were extracted with space left open for restorations. 8.36) Pretreatment records. 8.37) Posttreatment records. 8.38) Implant supported crowns.

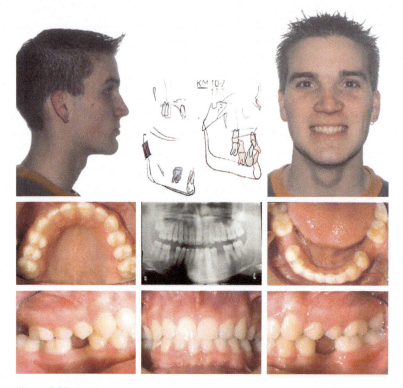

Figure 8.37

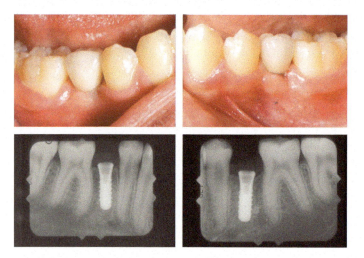

Figure 8.38

and 8.38). Despite extraction of the deciduous molars, the alveolar ridge was not compromised for the implant, because compensatory eruption of adjacent teeth brings the interproximal bone occlusally. In the nongrowing individual, the best restorative option in a patient with a low decay rate is an implant-supported crown (Figure 8.38). Prior to debanding, radiographs were taken to ensure that there was adequate space and satisfactory root angulation to accommodate implant placement. Collaboration between the orthodontist and the restorative dentist confirmed satisfactory pontic widths and coordination of debanding, retention, and restorative care. Cessation of facial growth was confirmed by serial lateral cephalometric radiograph superimposition before implant placement. In a growing individual, a temporary intermediate restoration could be a Maryland bridge, a removable partial denture, or a bonded wire retainer. An alternative treatment plan for this patient would have been to place temporary anchorage devices in the mandibular arch to allow molar protraction treating to a Class III molar and Class I canine. Unfortunately, this treatment plan leaves the maxillary second molar with no antagonist, inviting supraeruption.

Extract second deciduous molar and close the spaces in the early permanent dentition – In Class I crowded malocclusions, second deciduous molars can be extracted when second premolars are absent and spaces closed. Other premolars may require extraction to maintain symmetry as appropriate. Figure 8.39 shows a Class I mildly crowded malocclusion with an absent mandibular left second premolar. Incisor position was slightly procumbent, and the mandibular plane angle was steeper than average. All second premolars were extracted except in the mandibular left quadrant where the deciduous second molar without a successor was removed. Space closure was managed with minimal incisor retraction, as shown in the final records (Figure 8.40); this was helped by a steep mandibular plane angle which encouraged permanent molar mesial movement, as shown in the superimposition (Figure 8.40).

Extract deciduous molars in the mixed dentition and close the spaces/modified serial extraction – Patients who exhibit crowding and missing teeth can be treated with a modified serial extraction plan involving deciduous tooth extraction in the quadrant with missing teeth. Figure 8.41 demonstrates a

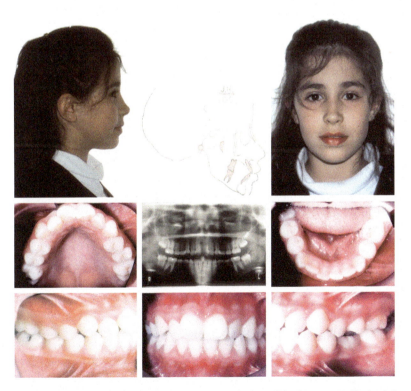

Figures 8.39 and 8.40 Class I crowded malocclusion with absent mandibular left second premolar, treated by extraction of second premolars. 8.39) Pretreatment. 8.40) Posttreatment.

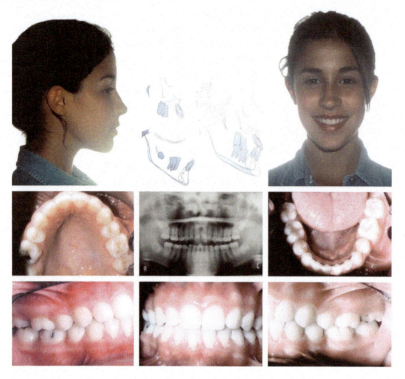

Figure 8.40

Class I mixed dentition crowded malocclusion with congenital absence of the maxillary right second premolar. The overlying maxillary right second deciduous molar was significantly infraoccluded from ankylosis. Also there was a deep overbite and maxillary constriction. Stage 1 treatment goals involved relief of crowding through serial extraction and control of the maxillary right molar position and the maxillary dental midline. The maxillary right deciduous molars were extracted and a Nance space maintainer placed for control of both the maxillary dental midline and the maxillary first permanent molar. In the other three quadrants, first premolars were extracted upon eruption followed by a period of spontaneous dental drifting. During this time, the crowded maxillary right canine and first premolar drifted distally into the deciduous molar extraction spaces and the maxillary midline and right molar were held, as shown in Figure 8.42. Then full fixed appliances with maxillary expansion was used to complete treatment (Figure 8.43).

An alternative use of modified serial extraction can occur in Class II mixed dentition patients, which exhibit crowding and congenitally missing mandibular second premolars as shown in Figure 8.44. In conceptual terms, the plan was to deal with the Class II malocclusion and the crowding with the extraction of maxillary first premolars and the mandibular second deciduous molars, which had no underlying permanent successors; this provides a "camouflage approach" to Class II treatment. While the extractions are usually done in the permanent dentition followed immediately by fixed appliances, they can be done in the mixed dentition with a modification of the extraction timing. In this instance, mandibular second deciduous molars were extracted to encourage forward movement of the mandibular first permanent molar to assist in Class I correction

8.12 Case histories | 263

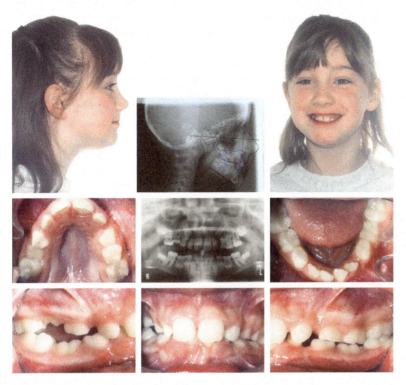

Figures 8.41–8.43 Class I mixed dentition crowded malocclusion with absent maxillary right second premolar. 8.41) Pretreatment. 8.42) After serial extraction of the maxillary right second primary molar and other first premolars. 8.43) Final.

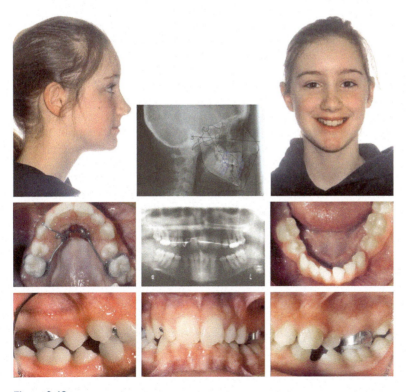

Figure 8.42

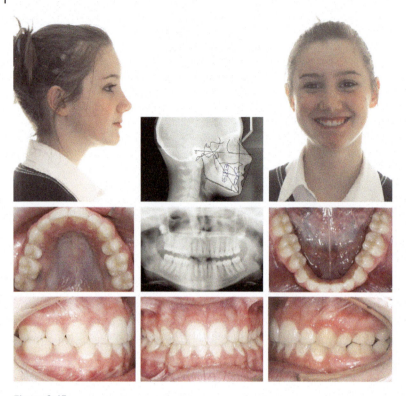

Figure 8.43

(Figure 8.45). Extraction timing in the mandibular arch was adjusted by performing the left extraction first and the right extraction second allowing for spontaneous resolution of the previous midline discrepancy (Figure 8.45); without maxillary extractions the canines remained Class 2. Maxillary first premolar extraction was delayed until fixed appliance treatment to conserve anchorage. After a period of drifting of the mandibular arch, there was significant improvement in the midline, the alignment, and the Class II correction on the permanent molar (Figure 8.45). Stage 2 treatment involved extraction of maxillary first premolars, the provision of a Nance holding arch during maxillary canine retraction and conventional fixed appliances resulting in a Class I finished occlusion (Figure 8.46).

An aggressive extraction sequence involving the removal of second deciduous molars which have no permanent successors has been recommended in the mixed dentition even with minimal or no crowding around age 8 or 9 [19, 20]. The objective is to obtain spontaneous closure of the space with mesial drift of the posterior dentition [19, 20]. Spontaneous space closure after deciduous second molar extraction therapy in Class I non-crowded cases demonstrated a space closure of almost 50% of the deciduous molar extraction space after the first year [21]. At 4-year follow-up, almost 90% of maxillary and 80% of mandibular extraction spaces were closed [21]; this left 0.9 mm of maxillary and 2.0 mm of mandibular space to close [21]. Considering that mandibular second deciduous molars are approximately 9 mm wide, this approach significantly reduces mechanical space closure. Tipping at the extraction sites comes more from the premolar than the molar. Most tipping occurred in the first year after deciduous molar extraction. These noncrowded Class I cases showed space closure with minimal incisor retraction,

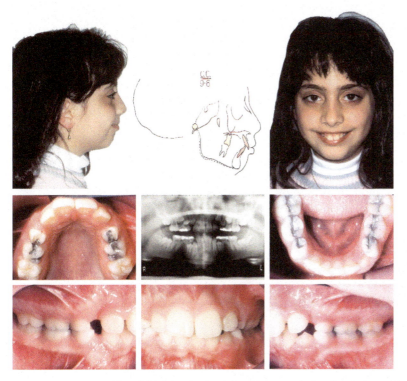

Figures 8.44–8.46 Class II Division 1 mixed dentition crowded malocclusion with absent mandibular second premolars. 8.44) Pretreatment. 8.45) Progress after extraction of mandibular second primary premolars. Note improvement in molar Class II relationship and midline discrepancy. 8.46) Final, after extraction of maxillary first premolar and fixed appliances.

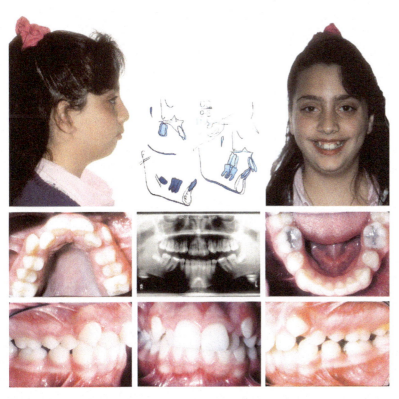

Figure 8.45

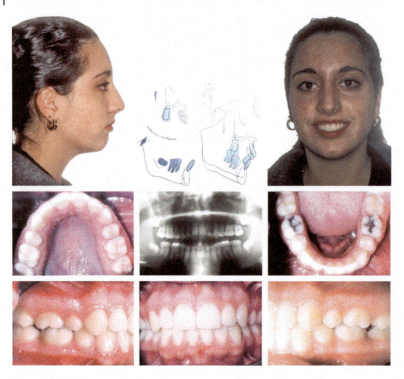

Figure 8.46

indicating that the posterior dentition drifted forwards [21]. Alternatives to this early extraction protocol are mandibular molar protraction with face mask traction [2] or with temporary anchorage devices, both of which increase treatment time and cost.

Space closure treatment plans eliminate the need for future prosthetic work and may reduce the length of time in fixed appliances because of spontaneous extraction space closure. Furthermore, potential negative sequelae to Class II mechanics and incisor retraction are reduced. Disadvantages of this approach are tipping of teeth adjacent to the extraction sites, buccal lingual narrowing of the alveolar ridge, and distal drifting of the mandibular first premolar [21] (Figure 8.48).

Figure 8.45 shows a Class I mixed dentition minimally crowded malocclusion at age 8 with congenital absence of all second premolars. Maxillary second deciduous molars were extensively restored and incisor position was not procumbent. Of interest, the patient's mother had an identical occlusion and had experienced significant problems with her four bridges that were replacing her missing second premolars. She therefore requested a space closure treatment plan for her daughter. All second deciduous molars were extracted at age 8 and there was a 5-year "drifting" period, during which the posterior dentition moved mesially with minimal incisor retraction (Figure 8.47). Progress records shown in Figure 8.48 reveal that the majority of the extraction spaces closed spontaneously with mesial drifting and rotation of the molars. There was also premolar rotation and distal drifting. Tilting of teeth adjacent to the extraction site was more severe in the mandibular arch but there was minimal incisor retraction (Figure 8.48). Then fixed appliances were placed for less than 18 months (Figure 8.49). This aggressive mixed dentition intervention eliminated the potential for future prosthetic

8.12 Case histories

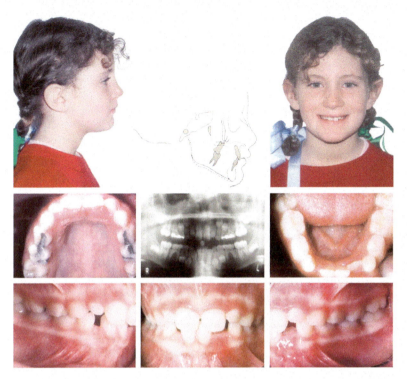

Figures 8.47–8.49 Class I minimally crowded malocclusion. Absent all second premolars; second primary molars were extracted to allow space closure. 8.47) Pretreatment. 8.48) Progress (after 5-year "drifting"). 8.49) Final.

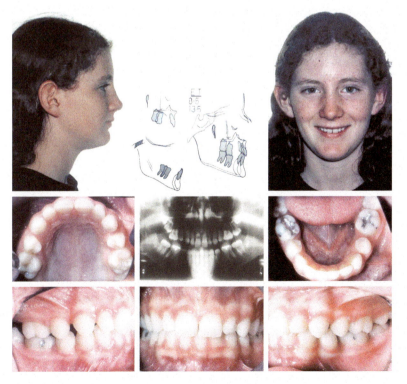

Figure 8.48

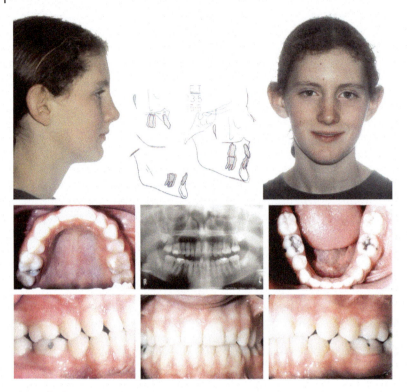

Figure 8.49

replacement of four missing second premolars, resulted in a short orthodontic treatment time, and reduced unfavorable incisor retraction.

Transplant – There are selected instances where transplantation should be considered. One would be a case which exhibits crowding in conjunction with missing teeth [22] (Figure 8.50). To manage crowding, premolar teeth may have to be extracted in one arch. If there are congenitally absent teeth in the opposing arch, consideration can be given to an autogenous tooth transplant [23]. Figure 8.50a shows mandibular crowding with absent maxillary lateral incisors, an absent maxillary right second premolar, and root resorption on the retained maxillary right second deciduous molar. Mandibular first premolars were

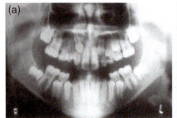
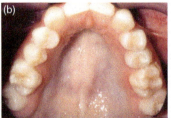
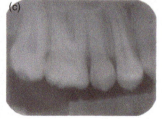

Figure 8.50 Class I crowded. (a) Panoramic X-ray with mandibular crowding and absent maxillary lateral incisors and right second premolars. (b) Mandibular left first premolar transplanted to position maxillary right second premolar. Clinical view. (c) Periapical X-ray of transplant after treatment.

extracted, and the mandibular left first premolar was transplanted to the maxillary right second premolar space at two-thirds root development (Figure 8.50b). After transplantation, there was some pulp canal calcification but continued apical development (Figure 8.50c). Subsequently fixed appliances were used to complete treatment. Autogenous premolar transplants are highly successful over a 10-year period but may carry with them risks of pulp problems and ankylosis [22].

A second transplant option for patients with missing second premolars can involve removal of maxillary premolars (provided that all maxillary premolars are present) and transplanting to the mandibular arch. Figure 8.51 shows that the canines are a half cusp Class II with an absent maxillary and mandibular second premolar, and infraoccluded second deciduous molars. The deciduous second molars were extracted, and a maxillary second left premolar transplanted to the missing mandibular premolar socket (Figure 8.52). Future orthodontics included the closure of all maxillary spaces leaving the patient with a Class I canine and a Class II molar relationship (Figure 8.53). Transplants are best done using premolar teeth at ⅔ to ¾ root development.

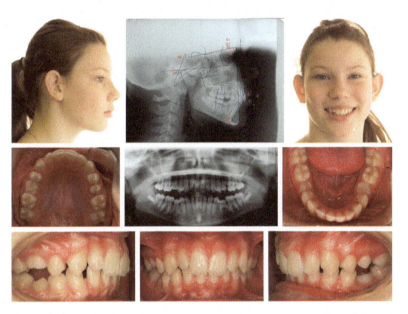

Figures 8.51–8.53 8.51) Pre-treatment records show absent maxillary right, and mandibular left premolars with a Class II canine. 8.52) Radiographs showing the maxillary second left premolar transplanted to the missing mandibular premolar socket. 8.53) Posttreatment records show a Class II molar relationship.

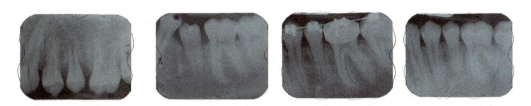

Figure 8.52

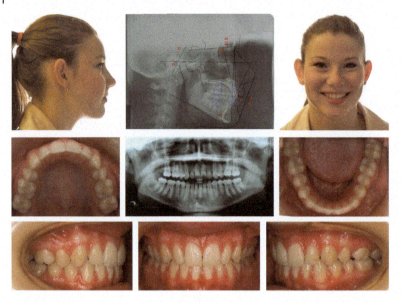

Figure 8.53

8.13 Summary

The frequency and consequences of root resorption and ankylosis of second deciduous molars which have no successors has been reviewed. Various treatment strategies that are available for the young patient are described with case histories. There are two major principles involved with treating growing children who present with absent second premolars. One is to establish the correct space for the missing tooth without compromising the alveolar ridge when a nonextraction approach is selected. The second principle is to ensure that the lower incisor position is not compromised when a space closure extraction treatment plan is selected. Early extraction of deciduous second primary molars frequently helps this goal.

References

1 Polder BJ, Van'thof MA, Van der Linden FPGM, Kuijpers-Jagtman AM. A meta-analysis of the prevalence of dental agenesis of permanent teeth. *Community Dent Oral Epidemiol* 2004;**32**:217–26.

2 Kokich VG, Kokich VO. Congenitally missing mandibular second premolars: clinical options. *Am J Orthod Dentofacial Orthop* 2006;**130**:437–44.

3 Profitt WR, Ackerman JL, Fields HW. Diagnosis and treatment planning in orthodontics. In: *Contemporary orthodontics*. 2nd edn. St. Louis, MO: Mosby, 1993. p. 139–225.

4 Rune B, Sarnas KV. Root resorption and submergence in retained deciduous second molars. *Eur J Orthod* 1984;**6**:123–13.

5 Kennedy DB. Review: Treatment Strategies for ankylosed primary molars. *Eur Arch Pediatr Dent* 2009;**10**:201–10.

6 Hansen K, Kjaer I. Persistence of deciduous molars in subjects with agenesis of the second premolars. *Eur J Orthod* 2000;**22**:239–43.

7 Bjerklin K, Bennett J. The long term survival of lower second primary molars in subjects with agenesis of the premolars. *Eur J Orthod* 2000;**22**:245–55.

8. Sletten DW, Smith BM, Southard KA, et al. Retained deciduous mandibular molars in adults. A radiographic study of long term changes. *Am J Orthod Dentofacial Orthop* 2004;**124**:625–30.
9. Scurrin MS, Bader JD, Shugars DA. Meta-analysis of fixed partial denture survival; prostheses and abutments. *J Prosthet Dent* 1998;**79**:459–64.
10. Ruprecht A, Wright GZ. Ankylosis with and without oligodontia: report of seven cases. *J Can Dent Assoc* 1967;**9**:444–7.
11. Kurol J, Thilander B. Infraocclusion of primary molars with aplasia of the permanent successor. *Angle Orthod* 1984;**54**:283–94.
12. Brearle LJ, McKibben DH. Ankylosis of primary molar teeth. *J Dent Child* 1973;**90**:54–63.
13. Becker A, Karnei-Rèm RM. The effects of infraocclusion part I: tilting of the adjacent teeth and local space loss. *Am J Orthod* 1992;**102**:256–64.
14. Becker A, Karnei-Rèm RM. The effects of infraocclusion part II: the type of movement of the adjacent teeth and their vertical development. *Am J Orthod* 1992;**102**:302–9.
15. Becker A, Karnei-Rèm RM, Steigman S. The effects of infraocclusion part III: dental arch length and midline. *Am J Orthod* 1992;**102**:427–33.
16. Ostler MS, Kokich VG. Alveolar ridge changes in patients with congenitally missing mandibular second premolars. *J Prosthet Dent* 1994;**71**:144–9.
17. Nordquist GG, McNeill RW. Orthodontic vs. restorative treatment of the congenitally absent lateral incisor – long term periodontal and occlusal evaluation. *J Periodontol* 1975;**46**:139–43.
18. Robertsson S, Mohler B. The congenitally missing upper lateral incisor. A retrospective study of orthodontic space closure versus restorative treatment. *Eur J Orthod* 2000;**22**:697–710.
19. Joondeph DR, McNeill RW. Congenitally absent second premolars: an interceptive approach. *Am J Orthod* 1971;**59**:50–66.
20. Lindquist B. Extraction of the deciduous second molar in hypodontia. *Eur J Orthod* 1980;**2**:173–81.
21. Mamopoulou A, Haag U, Schroder U, Hansen K. Agenesis of mandibular second premolars. Spontaneous space closure after extraction therapy: a 4-year follow up. *Eur J Orthod* 1996;**18**:589–600.
22. Jonsson T, Sigurdson TJ. Autotransplantation of premolars to premolar sites. A long-term follow-up study of 40 consecutive patients. *Am J Orthod Dentofacial Orthop* 2004;**125**:668–75.
23. Kennedy DB. Autogenous tooth transplants for the pediatric dental patient: report of three cases. *Pediatr. Dent* 2013;**35**:E113–9.

8.4

Section IV: Principles and techniques of premolar autotransplantation

Ewa M. Czochrowska, DDS, PhD[1] and Paweł Plakwicz, DDS, PhD[2]

[1] Department of Orthodontics, Medical University of Warsaw, Warsaw, Poland
[2] Department of Periodontology, Medical University of Warsaw, Poland

Rehabilitation of growing patients with missing teeth is restricted, since traditional prosthodontic replacements, especially dental implants, are contraindicated before cessation of growth [1]. Alternative solutions include:

- preservation of deciduous teeth
- fixed partial dentures (resin-reinforced composite or ceramic bridges)
- orthodontic space closure
- autotransplantation of teeth.

Each of these options has advantages and disadvantages and it is the responsibility of a multidisciplinary dental team to look for and to select the option that solves most of the patient's needs.

Autotransplantation of teeth is the surgical movement of a tooth from one location to another in the same mouth and may be an attractive option, because it has a potential of providing natural, life-long tooth substitution [2]. The best donor teeth are developing premolars. Those teeth have been documented to undergo a successful healing after surgery in more than 90% of cases [3–5]. Important factors, which contribute to their successful healing, include:

- relatively good surgical access – located in the middle of the dental arch
- favorable morphology – often single, pointed and relatively short roots, which allow for their gentle removal
- subgingival location – often transplanted before eruption.

All these factors reduce the risk of trauma to the donor tooth during the surgery and result in a more predictable outcome when compared to transplantation of other teeth, especially wisdom teeth and impacted canines, which have also been used as donors. Premolars are often extracted for orthodontic reasons and therefore their transplantation might be incorporated in the overall treatment plan possibilities.

The size of a donor tooth can be assessed from intraoral radiographs, but a cone-beam computed tomography (CBCT) offers the possibility of improved accuracy of morphologic evaluation in more demanding cases including premolar transplantation to a previously traumatized anterior maxilla. The CBCT may also aid in producing a replica of a donor tooth that can be used in the preparation of the recipient site [6].

Typical orthodontic indications for premolar transplantation in growing patients include [7] the following.

Recognizing and Correcting Developing Malocclusions: A Problem-Oriented Approach to Orthodontics,
Second Edition. Edited by Eustáquio A. Araújo and Peter H. Buschang.
© 2025 John Wiley & Sons, Inc. Published 2025 by John Wiley & Sons, Inc.

8.14 Class II malocclusion with congenitally missing lower second premolars

If no advanced root resorption or caries is present, preservation of healthy primary molars can be considered [8], but often ankylosis and progressing infraocclusion are observed [9]. If pronounced local tooth displacements occur, such as tilting of neighboring teeth, overeruption of opposing teeth, and many others, subsequent implantations may potentially jeopardize the procedure since impairment of the alveolar bone development may be present (Figure 8.54). Patients with Class II malocclusion and congenitally missing lower second premolars, in general, should not undergo orthodontic space closure in the mandibular arch, as this may result in unwanted retraction of mandibular incisors. Temporary anchorage devices can be applied to aid during orthodontic space closure, but this treatment approach demands a very good control of tooth movement, especially in the mandibular arch and can be time-consuming. Therefore, if indications for premolar extraction in the maxillary arch are favorable, those teeth can be autotransplanted to replace congenitally missing mandibular premolars. Orthodontic space closure in the maxillary arch will follow the surgery and produces the most favorable tooth contacts.

8.15 Traumatic loss of upper incisor/s

Missing incisors are probably the most important indication for premolar transplantation in growing patients. Missing an anterior tooth or teeth always generates a great concern for the patient and the parents who immediately seek dental intervention. Orthodontic space closure or tooth transplantation are the only treatment options to replace a missing tooth with a natural, biologic substitute, and they can be successfully applied in instead of indicated for children. Different orthodontic solutions are considered for each of these options [10] and they are related to the indication for dental arch length reduction at the site of the missing tooth (orthodontic space closure) or the need to preserve the space (tooth transplantation). Tooth transplantation requires an available donor tooth and should be part of a comprehensive orthodontic treatment plan. Atraumatic loss of maxillary incisors in patients with a normal Class I occlusion may imply the transferring of a premolar tooth which, otherwise, would not be scheduled for extraction. It becomes an alternative in cases of a great need for substitution of an anterior tooth (Figure 8.55). In these cases, compensatory extraction (Figure 8.55f) or the use of temporary anchorage devices should be considered to obtain a stable occlusion. Preferably, a donor tooth should be selected from another dental arch quadrant other than the one with the missing tooth. Tooth transplantation combined with orthodontic space closure is a viable treatment option in growing patients who have lost more than two maxillary incisors [4].

8.16 Uneven tooth distribution with multiple agenesis

The decision to perform premolar autotransplantation in patients with multiple agenesis is difficult because in those patients the number of available donor teeth is restricted. The best candidates are patients, who present crowding in one part of a dental arch and a missing tooth/teeth at another location and for whom orthodontic space closure is contraindicated. Patients with tooth agenesis in one arch may be considered but no more than two contralateral premolars from a nonaffected arch should be selected as donors. A good example is a young patient with agenesis of maxillary lateral incisors and maxillary second premolars. A possible plan is the autotransplantation of mandibular premolars to substitute missing maxillary premolars followed by orthodontic

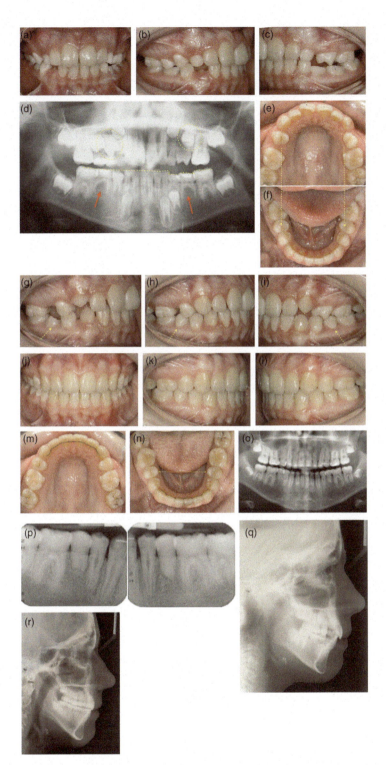

Figure 8.54 A 11y 5m girl was seeking orthodontic treatment (a–d). She had congenitally missing lower second premolars, detected on the panoramic radiograph (d, arrows). Infraocclusion of the primary molars on the left side was noted during her clinical examination. The patient's mother also had congenitally missing lower second premolars and she was concerned about the progressing infraocclusion of her daughter's teeth. Autotransplantation of unerupted upper second premolars (d, circles) was performed to replace missing teeth in the mandible (e, f, arrows). Eruption of the transplanted premolars and spontaneous correction of the dental relationships was seen after 12 months (g) and 18 months (h, i), when the orthodontic treatment was initiated. A stable occlusion and normal tooth contacts were present 1 year after debonding (j–n). No infraocclusion and hard tissue pathology was detected on the post-treatment radiographs (o, p). The patient's profile remained generally unchanged after the treatment (q: before the treatment, r: after the treatment).

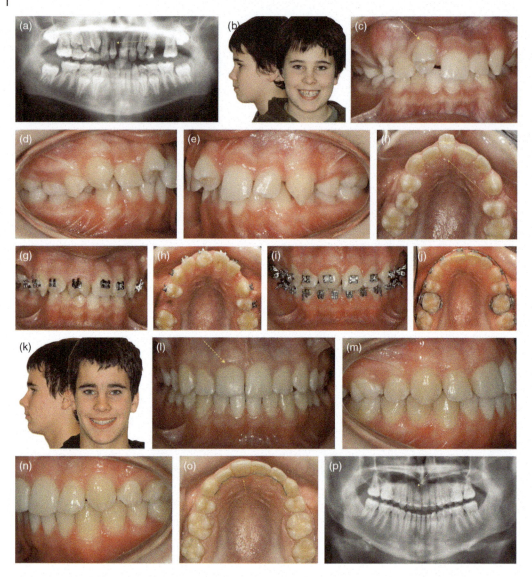

Figure 8.55 An 11-year-old boy had avulsion of his upper right central incisor. The tooth was replanted after 30 min, but 6 months later extensive inflammatory root resorption developed. Transplantation of the unerupted upper left second premolar was performed (a, arrow). After 18 months, the patient started orthodontic treatment (b–e), because the width of the transplanted premolar (arrow) mismatched the neighboring central incisor (f). The transplant was then rotated (g, h) to match the width of the neighboring incisor (i, j). The upper right second premolar was extracted to obtain normal canine relationship. After debonding, good smile aesthetics was obtained and the patient's profile has normalized (k). Stable occlusion and normal tooth contacts were achieved after orthodontic treatment (l–o). The transplanted premolar was reshaped to the incisor's morphology with a composite veneer (l, arrow); however, the width of the transplant at the gingival level was too wide to obtain a perfect match with the neighboring central incisor. No hard tissue pathology was present after the treatment (p).

space closure in the anterior maxilla and in the mandibular arch [2].

Different factors including patient's age, distribution and number of missing teeth, presence and status of primary teeth, occlusion, facial profile, and the patient's wishes must be considered and carefully assessed, individually, before performing tooth transplantation.

8.17 Surgery

When transplanting a premolar with incomplete root formation, it is important to realize that a significant part of the root consists of developing soft tissues that need to be handled gently and with respect during surgery, avoiding trauma and maximizing the potential for undisturbed healing.

8.18 Selection of anesthesia (local vs. general)

Usually, tooth transplantation is performed under local anesthesia, but the type of anesthesia strongly depends on patient's attitude to the surgery, general health conditions, operator's preferences, type and expected duration of surgery and evaluation of patient's cooperation. Communication with the patient during surgery may be very helpful. Transplantations of developing premolars performed in young children often require good communication skills from the operator. In addition, the equipment required for general anesthesia (intubation) and a limited mobility of the patient's head may create difficulties for performing surgery in some areas of the mouth in younger patients. Conversely, the surgery may cause a considerable stress to a young patient, and thus an anxious child can obstruct the procedure and irreversibly compromise the entire treatment plan. A number of consultations before the surgery with the patient and the parents will help reach the most appropriate decisions including the type of anesthesia selection.

The duration of surgery depends on the stage of root development of the donor tooth, its position in the dental arch and the required surgical preparation and location of the recipient site. Previous experience of the operating team is also an important factor. Generally, maxillary premolars are easier to be removed than mandibular premolars, due to a greater amount of surrounding trabecular bone and a thinner alveolar buccal plate in the maxilla. The more superficial the position of the donor tooth – for example, just below a loose primary molar – and the more anterior the donor tooth in the mouth, the shorter the time required for its removal. If preparation of the recipient site is straightforward, for example, when nonankylosed primary molars or a traumatized incisor are present before the surgery, then the time of the surgery usually does not exceed 90 min. An excessive osteotomy, particularly in the anterior maxilla, can be challenging for the patient and may necessitate general anesthesia.

8.19 Premolar to premolar transplantation

The surgery starts at the donor site assessing whether the donor tooth can be removed from the alveolar bone without trauma to cementum and Hertwig's epithelial root sheath (first stage). If a deciduous molar is present at the donor site, it is then extracted. The first incision (intrasulcular) is made along the gingival margin and is followed by a vertical incision and release of a flap on the buccal side of the adjacent tooth at the donor site. The labial cortical plate covering the donor tooth is carefully demarcated with a bur under saline irrigation. The remaining bone adjacent to the donor tooth is gently removed with an elevator to prevent any damage to the root (Figure 8.56a). If a gentle removal of a donor is estimated to be possible, the preparation of a recipient site is started (second stage). The presence of a primary molar (even if ankylosed) at the

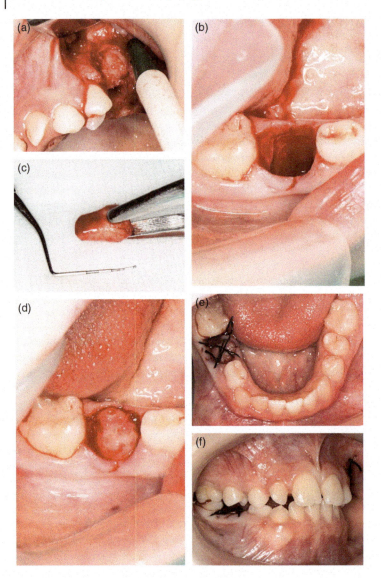

Figure 8.56 An 11-year-old girl with congenitally missing lower second premolars – at the first stage of surgery (at the donor site), the mucoperiosteal flap was elevated and the buccal bone removed with a bur and elevators to uncover the unerupted, developing upper left second premolar (a). At the second stage (at the recipient site), the lower right primary second molar was extracted and the tooth socket was deepened and reshaped to accommodate the donor tooth (b). After gentle elevation, the donor tooth was removed from its crypt with forceps (c) and immediately transferred to the prepared artificial socket in the mandible (third stage of surgery) (d). The tooth was stabilized to adjacent gingiva with sutures crossing its occlusal surface and the dental follicle (e). The final position of the transplant was at the level of gingiva to avoid occlusal contacts (f).

recipient site helps to maintain an adequate size and shape of the alveolus and the width of the keratinized gingiva. Therefore, those teeth must be kept until the time of surgery. A number of surgical burs, from a small size to a finishing conical bur resembling the shape of the root are used in the preparation of the new socket (Figure 8.56b) that must accommodate the donor tooth with a surplus space of 1 mm around its root. After preparation of the recipient site the donor tooth is gently elevated and removed from the alveolar bone with the dental follicle attached (third stage) (Figure 8.56c). It is important to avoid any contact with the donor's root since direct injury to the cementum may lead to ankylosis after transplantation. The donor is then positioned and checked for its accurate accommodation in the prepared artificial socket (Figure 8.56d). If further adjustment of the recipient bed is required, then the donor tooth is kept in saline to protect it from drying out. The tooth is stabilized with sutures, which cross the occlusal surface and cover the dental follicle and adjacent gingiva (Figure 8.56e). No semirigid or rigid fixation is required. The final vertical position of the transplanted tooth usually corresponds to its initial position at the donor site. Occasionally, it is more occlusal at the recipient site but the occlusion must be checked to ensure that no contacts are present (Figure 8.56f).

8.20 Premolar to anterior maxilla transplantation

There are various clinical scenarios resulting from trauma to anterior maxilla. Traumatized incisors with an active inflammation as well as ankylosed incisors with a restricted development of the alveolar bone may result from previous trauma. In patients with concomitant tooth and alveolar bone loss, extended bone defects and soft tissue scars are usually present at the recipient site (Figure 8.57a). As a consequence, the width and height of the alveolar bone may not be adequate to accommodate a donor tooth (Figure 8.57b). Due to an existing buccal bone defect and soft tissue dehiscence created during surgical preparation, the socket may sometimes be partially open on the labial side (Figure 8.57c). In such cases, the apical part of the root of the transplanted premolar is placed within the trabecular bone, while the coronal part of the root extends labially through the alveolar bone and is covered only by the repositioned mucoperiosteal flap (Figure 8.57d). Therefore, premolars transplanted to the anterior maxilla may require more rigid stabilization that can be achieved using a thin wire bonded with composite resin to adjacent teeth. It improves the stability and helps to keep the transplanted teeth out of occlusion.

8.21 Postoperative instructions

The patient is advised to follow standardized postoperative instructions that include: appropriate antibiotics (usually amoxicillin – 500 mg three times daily), nonsteroid anti-inflammatory drugs, ice packs, refraining from tooth brushing at the surgical sites, gentle rinsing with 0.12–0.2% chlorhexidine gluconate, avoidance of chewing and using a soft diet for 7 days. All sutures are removed after 10–14 days.

8.22 Follow-up

After the removal of sutures, transplanted teeth are examined clinically and radiographically after 1, 3, 6 months and then annually, if possible, to confirm uneventful healing.

The clinical examination comprises the evaluation of the periodontal tissues, which includes measurements of pocket depths, clinical attachment levels, and width of keratinized gingiva, assessment of plaque accumulation and detection of any signs of inflammation. Tooth mobility must also be assessed and includes a percussion test for the presence of ankylosis (high, metallic sound). Electric pulp testing (EPT) of the transplanted tooth can be helpful to monitor pulp healing, but its recordings might be reduced for a period after surgery. The natural, contralateral tooth should serve as a control, but if not available, a neighboring, unaffected tooth can serve as a reference. No significant differences between transplanted premolars with developing roots and their controls have been reported in the literature, which confirms successful healing after this type of tooth transplantation.

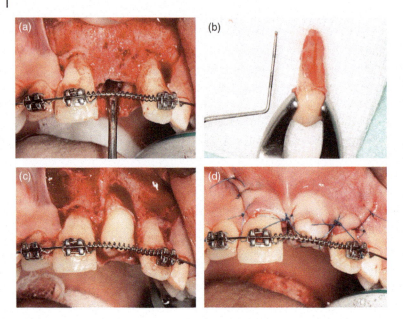

Figure 8.57 A 10-year-old boy after traumatic loss of the upper left central incisor – at the recipient site, the labial cortical bone defect was present after previous avulsion of the upper left central incisor (a). The preparation of the recipient site in the anterior maxilla (the second stage of surgery) was performed after initial uncovering of the donor tooth, which enabled its gentle removal. It also helped to avoid resorption of the alveolar process at the recipient site, if the removal of the donor was not possible. After gentle elevation, the semierupted lower right second premolar was transferred to the prepared recipient site at the gingival level (b). The buccal bone dehiscence resulted from the initial bone defect and surgical preparation of the artificial socket (c). The root of the transplanted premolar and the bone dehiscence were covered with repositioned flap, which was stabilized using sutures (d).

Intraoral radiographs are usually used to monitor healing of hard tissues after transplantation and, occasionally, CBCT examination may be performed to confirm formation of alveolar bone around transplanted teeth in cases with initial extensive alveolar bone loss and the need for more advanced orthodontic adjustments.

After transplantation of teeth with developing roots, the following features must be observed to confirm successful outcome.

8.23 Pulp healing

In teeth with open apices at transplantation, pulp revascularization starts shortly after surgery as a result of in growth of newly formed blood vessels from the connective tissue through the apical part of the root [11]. After a few months, the pulp tissue of the transplanted teeth is reduced in cells and blood vessels and a newly formed tissue that resembles bone or cementum occupies most of the original pulp cavity. Radiographically, it appears as progressive pulp obliteration (Figure 8.54p) which is a common finding after transplantation of developing teeth [2, 4] and should be detected after a few months on the intraoral radiographs. Lack of pulp obliteration might indicate a pulp necrosis, which can be confirmed by pulp tests. If pulp necrosis occurs after transplantation, then the transplant requires endodontic treatment, which by contrast is always performed after transplantation of mature teeth. Teeth with ½ to ¾ of the final root length at the time of surgery are the preferred donors [3, 12], and pulp necrosis is seldom observed in those teeth (Figures 8.54 and 8.55). Teeth with shorter roots and open apex have a better chance for revascularization and are easier accommodated at the recipient site.

8.24 Periodontal healing

If no damage to the root surface occurs during surgery, then establishment of normal periodontal ligament takes place and the transplant erupts (Figures 8.54g–i) [13]. The progress of eruption depends on the stage of root development at the time of surgery and usually tooth eruption is seen 2–6 month after surgery [14]. Teeth transplanted at a nearly stage of root development require more time to erupt in accordance with their normal development [15]. Absence of eruption after surgery might indicate ankylosis which may be later confirmed with a lack of response to orthodontic traction. If ankylosis occurs, sometimes another donor tooth is available, offering the possibility for a second transplantation. Normal healing can be expected, even if the first transplantation was unsuccessful. If no other donors are available, then observation of the ankylosed transplant must be considered. In this situation, the final outcome depends on the remaining growth of the alveolar process and the progress of root ankylosis, which varies from patient to patient.

8.25 Root growth

Further root growth is to be expected after transplantation of teeth and depends on the initial stage of root development [16]. Usually, these teeth develop slightly shorter roots compared to contralateral controls (Figures 8.54p and 8.55p) [4, 5] but this has no clinical consequences. Final root length of the transplanted tooth is usually reached within 2 years after surgery [17]. Sometimes, root growth does not continue after transplantation which is noted on teeth that were transplanted at earlier stages of root formation – less than half of the root length at the time of surgery.

8.26 Reshaping to incisor morphology

When a premolar is transplanted to replace a traumatized or lost maxillary incisor, it has to be reshaped to the incisor morphology. If during surgery, it was not possible to place the donor tooth at the optimal position in relation to neighboring incisors the orthodontic adjustment after transplantation significantly improves its position for a satisfactory reshaping (Figures 8.55g–j) [18]. Usually, a provisional composite buildup is performed not earlier than 6 months after transplantation with no or minimal grinding of the enamel surface. Overhanging margins must be avoided to protect periodontal tissues. Veneers are the preferred solution as they have the best potential for optimal aesthetics regarding reshaping to the incisor morphology and optimal color match (Figure 8.55l). Porcelain veneers also have the best periodontal compatibility with the natural enamel. Since veneers require some enamel grinding, they should be postponed until at least 2 years after transplantation.

Generally, complications after transplantation are seen during the first year after surgery [3, 16]. As tissue healing after transplantation takes time, it is important to postpone orthodontic movement of the transplanted tooth, if required, for at least 12 months after surgery.

8.27 Alveolar bone after autotransplantation

Positive changes of the volume of the alveolar bone can be expected after successful autotransplantation of developing teeth. The bone grows progressively during spontaneous eruption of the transplants. Maintenance of the alveolar bone was reported in the retrospective study of developing premolars transplanted to replace missing teeth in the anterior maxilla [19]. Similarly, numerous case observations reported the formation of the new alveolar bone during healing and eruption of transplanted developing teeth ([20] and later [21]). Recently, an umbrella review confirmed a distinctive advantage of bone induction related to autotransplantation of teeth [22].

References

1. Thilander B, Ödman J, Lekholm U. Orthodontic aspects of the use of oral implants in adolescents: a 10-year follow-up study. *Eur J Orthod* 2001;**23**(6):715–31.
2. Czochrowska EM, Stenvik A, Bjercke B, Zachrisson BU. Outcome of tooth transplantation: survival and success rates 17–41 years post treatment. *Am J Orthod Dentofacial Orthop* 2002;**121**(2):110–9.
3. Andreasen JO, Paulsen HU, Yu Z, et al. A long-term study of 370 autotransplanted premolars. Part II: tooth survival and pulp healing subsequent to transplantation. *Eur J Orthod* 1991;**12**(1):14–24.
4. Czochrowska EM, Stenvik A, Album B, Zachrisson BU. Autotransplantation of premolars to replace maxillary incisors: a comparison with natural incisors. *Am J Orthod Dentofacial Orthop* 2000;**118**(6):592–600.
5. Plakwicz P, Wojtowicz A, Czochrowska EM. Survival and success rates of autotransplanted premolars: a prospective study of the protocol for developing teeth. *Am J Orthod Dentofacial Orthop* 2013;**144**(2):229–37.
6. Keightley AJ, Cross DL, McKerlie RA, Brocklebank L. Auto-transplantation of an immature premolar, with the aid of cone beam CT and computer-aided prototyping: a case report. *Dent Traumatol* 2010;**26**(2):195–9.
7. Zachrisson BU, Stenvik A, Haanæs HR. Management of missing maxillary anterior teeth with emphasis on autotransplantation. *Am J Orthod Dentofacial Orthop* 2004;**126**(3):284–8.
8. Bjerklin K, Al-Najjar M, Kårestedt H, Andrén A. Agenesis of mandibular second premolars with retained primary molars: a longitudinal radiographic study of 99 subjects from 12 years of age to adulthood. *Eur J Orthod* 2008;**30**(3):254–61.
9. Hvaring CL, Øgaard B, Stenvik A, Birkeland K. The prognosis of retained primary molars without successors: infraocclusion, root resorption and restorations in 111 patients. *Eur J Orthod* 2014;**36**(1):26–30.
10. Stenvik A, Zachrisson BU. Orthodontic closure and transplantation in the treatment of missing anterior teeth. An overview. *Endod Dent Traumatol* 1993;**9**(2):45–52.
11. Skoglund A, Tronstad L, Wallenius KA. A microangiographic study of vascular changes in replanted and autotransplanted teeth of young dogs. *Oral Surg Oral Med Oral Pathol* 1978;**45**(1):17–28.
12. Kristerson L. Autotransplantation of human premolars. A clinical and radiographic study of 100 teeth. *Int J Oral Surg* 1985;**14**(2):200–13.
13. Paulsen HU, Andreasen JO. Eruption of premolars subsequent to autotransplantation. A longitudinal radiographic study. *Eur J Orthod* 1998;**20**(1):45–55.
14. Paulsen HU, Shi XQ, Welander U, et al. Eruption pattern of autotransplanted premolars visualized by radiographic colorcoding. *Am J Orthod Dentofacial Orthop* 2001;**119**(4):338–45.
15. Plakwicz P, Czochrowska EM. The prospective study of autotransplanted severely impacted developing premolars: periodontal status and the long-term outcome. *J Clin Periodontol* 2014;**41**(5):489–96.
16. Andreasen JO, Paulsen HU, Yu Z, Bayer T. A long-term study of 370 autotransplanted

premolars. Part IV: root development subsequent to transplantation. *Eur J Orthod* 1991;**12**(1):38–50.

17 Myrlund S, Stermer EM, Album B, Stenvik A. Root length in transplanted premolars. *Acta Odontol Scand* 2004;**62**(3):132–6.

18 Czochrowska EM, Stenvik A, Zachrisson BU. The esthetic outcome of autotransplanted premolars replacing maxillary incisors. *Dent Traumatol* 2002;**18**(5):237–45.

19 Plakwicz P, Andreasen JO, Górska R, et al. Status of the alveolar bone after autotransplantation of developing premolars to the anterior maxilla assessed by CBCT measurements. *Dent Traumatol* 2021 Oct;**37**(5):691–8. doi: 10.1111/edt.12680.

20 Plakwicz P, Czochrowska EM, Milczarek A, Zadurska M. Vertical bone growth following autotransplantation of the developing maxillary third molar to replace a retained mandibular permanent molar: a case report. *Int J Periodontics Restorative Dent* 2014 Sep–Oct;**34**(5):667–71.

21 Plakwicz P, Wojtaszek J, Zadurska M. New bone formation at the site of autotransplanted developing mandibular canines: a case report. *Int J Periodontics Restorative Dent* 2013 Jan–Feb;**33**(1):13–20.

22 Cremona M, Bister D, Sherriff M, Abela S. Prognostic factors, outcomes, and complications for dental autotransplantation: an umbrella review. *Eur J Orthod* 2024 Jan 1; **46**(1):cjad067. doi: 10.1093/ejo/cjad067.

8.5

Section V: Dental trauma: revisiting posttrauma protocols and long-term follow-ups

Eustaquio A. Araújo, DDS, MDS and Gabriel Miranda, DDS, MS

Department of Orthodontics, Saint Louis University, St. Louis, MO, USA

The importance of a multidisciplinary approach across different areas of dentistry to achieve high-quality treatment is unquestionable. This topic has been described several times in the literature, in orthodontics [1, 2], periodontics, prosthodontics as well as in maxillofacial surgery. It is consistently part of a treatment planning in order to create a list of problems, priorities, and solutions leading to a more predictable outcome for final results [3]. Another key area that significantly influences our profession is endodontics [4]. Unfortunately, it is sometimes overlooked as some inexperienced clinicians may consider it of less importance. Definitely, it is a misconception.

The current literature shows various studies evaluating the role of endodontics into the orthodontic field [4–8]. One enlightening systematic review [7] combined the most frequent questions of orthodontists regarding endodontics:

- Orthodontic movement and pulp cell viability
- Comparison of resorption between vital and treated teeth during the orthodontic treatment.
- Movement of endodontically treated teeth.
- Dental trauma and its relation to orthodontic treatment.

Even though some reviews were written in the late 90ths, many of those topics remain under discussion, with new questions, answers, and emerging perspectives [6, 9]. In relation to this chapter, the authors believe that dental trauma and its management is probably one of the most crucial topics for those looking into learning more about the management of developing malocclusions.

8.28 An overview of dental trauma

According to Lam et al., dental trauma can be defined as "an impact injury to the teeth and/or other hard and soft tissues within and around the vicinity of the mouth and oral cavity" [10]. This condition, sometimes underestimated, has been proven to affect a significant part of the world population [11]. The World Health Organization considers it as a public health issue [12], as confirmed by a comprehensive review that examined studies on trauma from 1996 to 2016. This study revealed that dental traumatic injuries (DTI) have affected one billion living individuals [11]. The prevalence of this condition is estimated to be 15–30% [13].

Recognizing and Correcting Developing Malocclusions: A Problem-Oriented Approach to Orthodontics, Second Edition. Edited by Eustáquio A. Araújo and Peter H. Buschang.
© 2025 John Wiley & Sons, Inc. Published 2025 by John Wiley & Sons, Inc.

A study looking at a Brazilian sample of 1.210 school children found a prevalence of 12.6% [14], which increased with age. A more recent systematic review investigated dental injuries in emergency dental services. A population of 209.099 individuals 21 years old or younger was assessed, obtaining a prevalence of 24% [15]. Sex differences also demonstrated significant variations in the prevalence, with boys being more affected than girls [14–16].

Trauma in the primary and permanent dentitions lead to different outcomes. The International Association of Dental Traumatology and the American Academy of Pediatric Dentistry developed some guidelines for traumatic injuries [17]: enamel fracture/enamel dentin fracture/ crown fracture with exposed pulp/crown-root fracture/root fracture/alveolar fracture/concussion/subluxation/extrusive luxation/lateral luxation/intrusive luxation and finally avulsion. They all lead to different approaches and interventions. It has been reported that upper incisors are the most affected group of teeth, and luxation was the most common outcome [18].

Several causes of trauma have been reported: sports activities, playing, fights, and traffic crashes [12, 18]. Among them, falling has been the most common one (56%) [18], which agrees with the findings of another systematic review that also describe that falling at home is the most common of the traumatic injuries [19].

8.29 Orthodontic treatment and dental trauma

Following the review of some basics on prevalence and occurrence of traumatic injuries, there are still questions on how these meaningful highlights might affect a daily orthodontic practice. To address its importance, it is necessary to reassess a crucial topic in dental trauma – the predisposing factors of a traumatic injury.

The literature reports that an inadequate lip coverage [12, 14], Angle's Class II malocclusion, facial convexity [12], and overjet over 3 mm certainly increase the risk of trauma [13]. A 2020 longitudinal study evaluated a school sample and revealed that increased overjets have the most significant impact on the risk of traumatic injuries [16].

Considering all these predisposing factors and correlating them with what we observe in our daily practice, an interesting question arises. How many patients per day come to our offices with these characteristics? How can your role as an orthodontist improve or modify these predisposing factors and create a protective protocol for the young patients? These questions serve as the starting point for orthodontists to focus on preventing dental trauma through proper education for families and schools. Such prevention not only decreases financial burdens for the patient's family but also mitigates negative psychological effects during the teen years [20].

The sequence of cases below will review, illustrate, and discuss different situations/patients.

The first boy was admitted at the Orthodontic Department of the Center for Advanced Dental Education (CADE), Saint Louis University, at the age of 9y 11m. By analyzing his facial and intraoral pictures, it may be observed a typical example of a patient with various predisposing factors for trauma: facial convexity, lack of lip coverage, increased overjet, and Angle Class II with protrusive incisors (Figure 8.58).

The second patient joined the same orthodontic program at the age of 9y 10m. Her pictures reveal a similar pattern to the first one, perhaps with a higher degree of severity. Her cephalometric measurements further support this indicating a pronounced proclination of upper incisors (U1-SN -127.5/ U1-NA 40.8/ U1-NA 9.2 mm), well above the norms (U1-SN -105.1/U1-NA 22/U1-NA 4.0 mm) (Figure 8.59).

This chapter does not aim to address the decision-making process of treating a Class II in one or two phases. However, it has been consistently demonstrated on the literature that proposing treatment in the early dentition

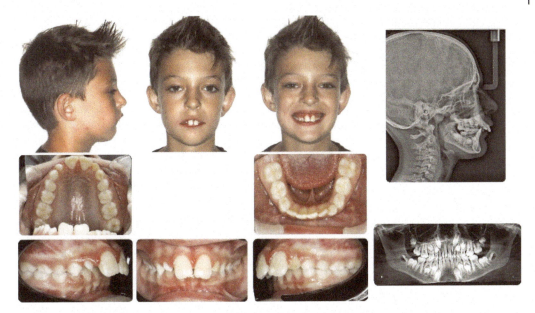

Figure 8.58 Predisposing factors for dental traumatic injuries.

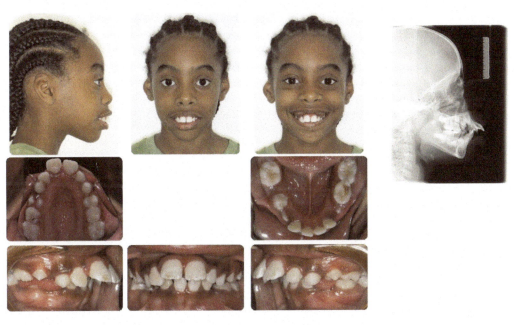

Figure 8.59 Predisposing factors for dental traumatic injuries.

when the patient has an excessive overjet [21] is the appropriate choice. O'Brien and coworkers conducted a Cochrane systematic review on early treatment and found that decreases in the overjet are related to a reduction in risk of trauma. Therefore, it can be consider an indication for Class II treatment [22].

The following patient is also a good example of the protective role provided by orthodontics. She was admitted to CADE at the age of 8y 10m

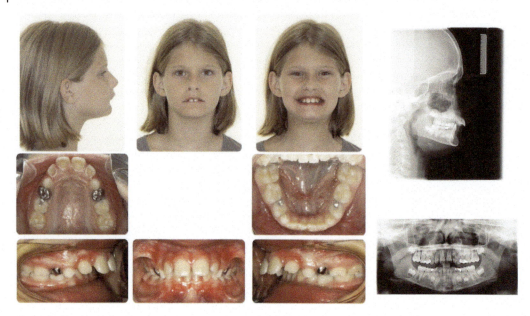

Figure 8.60 Predisposing factors for dental traumatic injuries.

with a main complain of an inability to close the lips together and bullying. Similarly, to the first and the second patients, she exhibits all the predisposing factors for a dental trauma: excessive overjet, absence of lip coverage, lip biting, convex profile, and dental Class II. Given those facts, and with the support of the literature, it was decided to start a phase I treatment (Figure 8.60).

After the completion of Phase I, with and AdvanSync and a 2 by 4, a considerable improvement can be noticed on her overjet, inclination of upper incisors, and molar classification. There was an improvement from a convex to a straighter and more pleasant profile as well, and her chief complaint was addressed (Figure 8.61).

Looking at the two different treatment time points, the positive effects that a well-planned phase I treatment can bring into the patient's life are undeniable. The orthodontic treatment transformed her emotionally and moved her to another level, from an individual with increased risk of being affected by a severe trauma, to a low/moderate risk. The importance of this transformation goes beyond the trauma itself, considering the potential consequences throughout teenage years. It has been reported that a traumatic injury may also have a relevant financial, physiological and behavioral consequences for patients and family[20].

The patient bellow presented the predispose factors but did not have the chance to be treated in the proper time. Figure 8.62 shows the early loss – avulsion – of a central incisor, which imposed complicated clinical decisions.

8.30 Managing traumatized teeth and preserving bone width – The decoronation approach

It would be ideal to be able to alert and treat patients with increased risk for trauma in the mixed dentition. Unfortunately, it is not the reality. Most of the time, patients seek for help only after traumatic injuries have already occurred.

Orthodontists, in general, receive a good education and demonstrate considerable knowledge of trauma cases and endodontics is mandatory in multidisciplinary cooperation.

8.30 Managing traumatized teeth and preserving bone width – The decoronation approach | 289

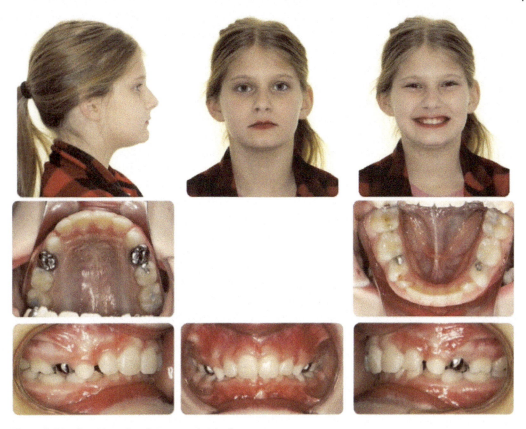

Figure 8.61 Postphase I and decreased risk of trauma.

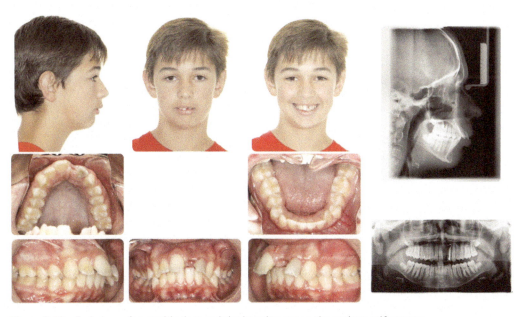

Figure 8.62 Early loss of central incisor and the impairment on the patient self-esteem.

Collaborating with an endodontist allows an adequate interdisciplinary treatment plan and better decision-making. This intercommunication between different areas leads to a more predictable outcome for the treatment.

Trauma may lead to different consequences. A thorough diagnosis must include a good history (when and how it happened), first interventions (who did it), the time of the intervention, how it was performed, its severity, ranging from a simple enamel fracture to more complicated situations such as avulsions, and the patient's biological response.

Ankylosis is described as one of the most severe consequences leading to serious outcomes depending on the age of the patient. Growth is a major factor. The younger the patient, the more he/she must be followed. Ankylosis in growing patients usually lead to a surgical removal of the tooth or a coronectomy attempting to preserve a good condition for a later implant. Is important to note that the extraction of an ankylosed tooth is not an easy procedure, even for an experienced surgeon. It often results in alveolar bone volume loss, consequently complicating the prognosis for future prosthetic rehabilitation.

One alternative to the surgical removal is the aforementioned decoronation technic. This procedure, developed and described in 1984 by a Sweden group led by Barbo Malmgren, clearly indicates the better time to perform it. It aims to overcome the deleterious effects that extracting an ankylosed tooth could bring to the alveolar bone. In addition, it addresses the esthetic damage that a tooth in infraposition could cause if the patient/dentist chose not to intervene until the crown had fallen off [23]. Studies also indicate that the more severe the level of infraposition, the more complex the future rehabilitation process [17, 23, 24].

The decoronation procedure is simple to execute. Initially, a mucoperiosteal flap is opened around the ankylosed tooth. The entire crown is then removed at the level of the cementum-enamel junction using a diamond drill. Following that, all filling material present inside the root canal is removed, and intense saline irrigation is performed to allows the root canal system to be filled with blood. Following this, the root surface is reduced to 2 mm below the bone level and the flap is simply sutured [25, 26].

Figure 8.63a–c shows 19-months follow-up of a patient treated with decoronation. The youngster was 8y 3m when admitted at CADE for interceptive treatment; however, he was involved in a trampoline accident. The initial objectives were to reduce his overjet, improve the Class II relation, and reduce the overbite.

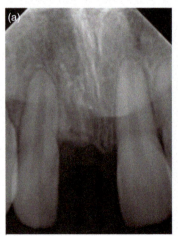 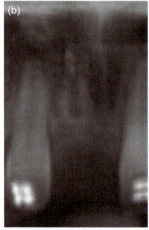 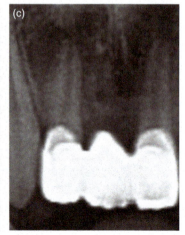

Figure 8.63 (a–c) Decoronation follow-up (8, 11, 19 months).

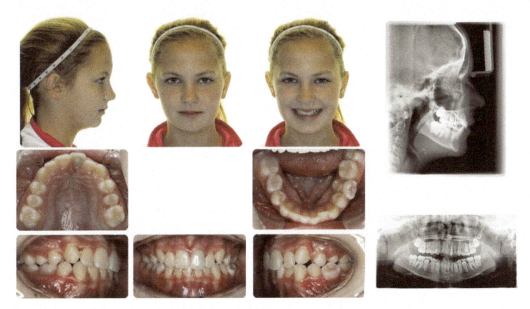

Figure 8.64 Initial facial, intraoral, and cephalometric features.

Unfortunately, right at the beginning of the phase I, he experienced an avulsion on the UR1; a reimplantation was performed by a General Dentist and a subsequent ankylosis occurred. Decoronation was the chosen treatment, the periapical follow-up illustrates turnover of cementum into alveolar bone and the preserved bone volume. The General dentist elected to restore it with a Maryland bridge.

Figure 8.64 presents the case of a girl, who reported a trauma and became a clear example of how the decoronation technic can be helpful in maintaining the alveolar bone width for a future implant placement. This girl was admitted to CADE at the age of 11y 11m, presenting a convex profile due to a retrusive mandible, symmetrical and proportional face, and adequate gingival display. The intraoral examination showed a Class II molar and canine relationship on the left side and Class I on the right side. Her cephalometric measurements were all within normal limits. The upper left central had a previous history of trauma due to a fall in her house, aligning with what the literature states as the most common cause for DTI.

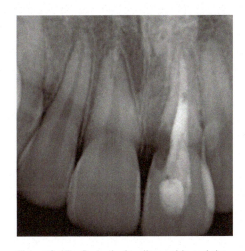

Figure 8.65 Periapical radiographic and the external root resorption.

Before initiating any procedure, the endodontic department was contacted to evaluate the case. A periapical radiograph (Figure 8.65) revealed that an external resorption was underway, suggesting a future extraction of the tooth. Subsequent discussions focused on determining the most appropriate treatment – whether immediate extraction or another viable solution. Considering the patient's age,

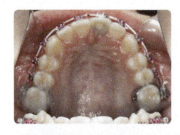
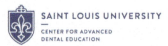
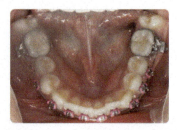
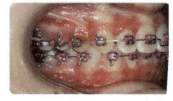
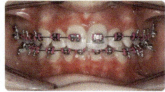
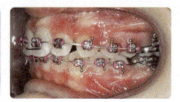

Figure 8.66 Intraoral pictures, 6 months follow-up.

potential psychosocial issues that may arise as she was too young for an implant, the decision was to postpone any definite decision until she was older. The risk of alveolar bone loss during and after the extraction associated with a close interaction with endodontics made it possible to retain the tooth for as long as possible during the orthodontic treatment.

The decoronation technic, originally developed for ankylosed teeth, is also a good option for this case and was the chosen treatment, thereby preserving alveolar bone. It was agreed with the endodontic department to periodically take periapical X-rays monitoring the resorption during the orthodontic treatment. It was decided that no force would be exerted on this element during treatment. The patient was very cooperative and followed all the instructions. As the orthodontic treatment was close to be completed, it was decided by the two departments that upon completion of the treatment, the decoronation procedure would be performed, allowing the patient some extra time to keep her original tooth in the month. The correction of the mild dental Class II would be addressed by taking advantage of growth, the e-space, and the use of light Class II elastics when necessary. The family agreed with the plan and the treatment progressed successfully.

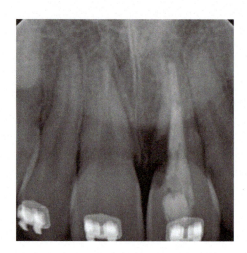

Figure 8.67 Periapical X-ray, 6 months follow-up.

The 6-month progress pictures illustrate a better anteroposterior position of the left canine and molar, with the leveling and alignment of the upper and lower arch in progress (Figure 8.66). It is important to note a bypass on the UL1 to avoid applying any force to this tooth. A new periapical X-ray was taken and assessed by the orthodontic-endodontic team. It was decided that tooth was still viable to stay in the mouth for some more time (Figure 8.67).

8.30 Managing traumatized teeth and preserving bone width – The decoronation approach

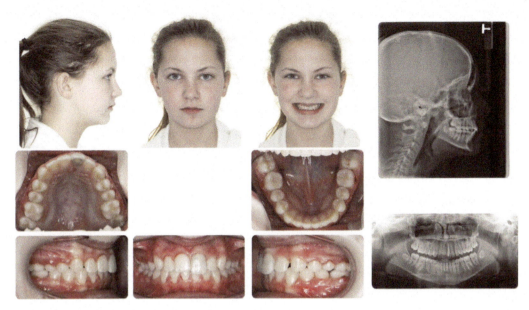

Figure 8.68 Records at the debond.

After 1y 8m of treatment, the patient was ready for the debond appointment (Figure 8.68). Facial pictures demonstrate a slight improvement on the convexity of the profile. It was possible to maintain the proportion of her facial thirds as well as the incisal display. Cephalometric numbers were within the normal limits. Dentally, she was a Class I molar and canine on both left and right sides. At this point, it was necessary to emphasize the importance of keeping the UL1 in place during this time. Thanks to the multidisciplinary effort, this young girl was able to go through her initial teen years with her tooth in position, leading to a good quality of life and her psychosocial behavior.

As after the bracket removal, the young girl was taken to the endodontic department, evaluated the decoronation procedure was done at that time. Her crown was preserved and used as a provisional tooth attached to a Hawley appliance (Figure 8.69a–c). Figure 8.70a,b shows the radiographic aspects before and immediately after decoronation. One month later, the patient was scheduled for the first periapical follow-up of the decoronated tooth area. It is possible to note that the surrounding bone area is stable with no signs of periapical lesion or any bone loss. Some degree of root remodeling can also be observed (Figure 8.71).

A provisional Maryland bridge was later installed to preserve esthetics until the appropriate time for the implant placement (Figure 8.72). The literature suggests that the complete resorption of the root will vary based on the individual biological response of each patient, ranging from 1 to 10 years [27]. However, the same article introduces an important concept: there is no need to wait until the root is fully transformed in bone to place the implant. In fact, if the procedure was completed following all the guidelines to avoid any contamination, the remaining root may be considered normal bone and the placement of the implant can occur.

In this specific case, the periodontics team had reservations about placing the implant due to her early age and maintained continuous follow-up appointments.

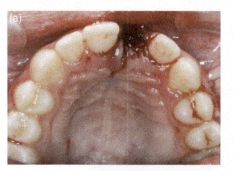
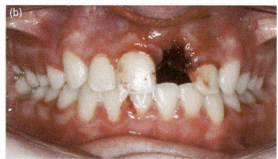
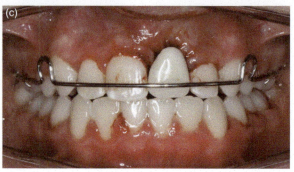

Figure 8.69 (a–c) Records at decoronation.

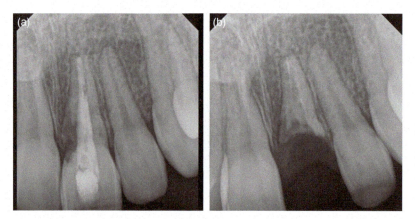

Figure 8.70 (a, b) Records at decoronation.

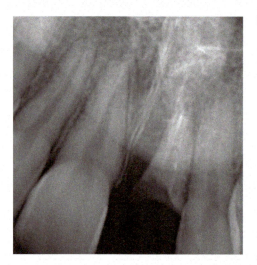

Figure 8.71 One-month postdecoronation.

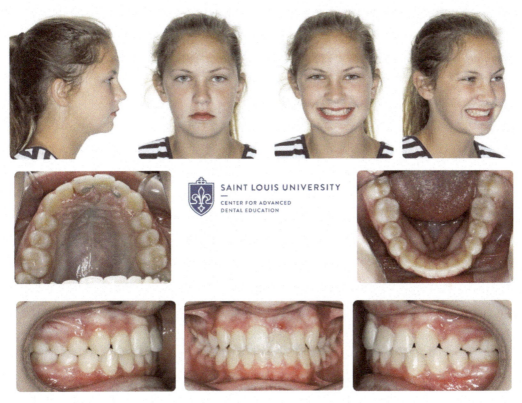

Figure 8.72 Maryland bridge delivery.

Figure 8.73a–d shows the periapical X-rays for 1 month, 5 months, 2 years, and 3 years postdecoronation. It is noteworthy how the bone was preserved not only on the horizontal dimension but also vertically. This preservation was crucial for her future rehabilitation.

Figure 8.74 illustrates the 5-year retention. The patient returned with the implant successfully placed in the region of the UL1. It was placed when she turned 19 years old (sic). She reported that the surgeon had no issue performing the implant and **no** bone grafting was needed. It is possible to note on the panoramic X-ray (Figure 8.75) an adequate bone volume. The frontal intraoral picture shows an even gingival margin. This scenario could have been different if the decoronation procedure had not been performed.

8.31 Final considerations

Orthodontics holds the ability to promote changes that possibly no other area of dentistry may be able to. In this chapter, the authors address how, as health professionals, it is possible to effectively intervene on a very prevalent condition that can lead to many financial and psychological problems for a growing patient – traumatic injuries. By incorporating phase I treatment strategies to reduce overjet and improve lip coverage, our profession takes a proactive attitude in preventing dental trauma.

In this concluding section, it must be emphasized the importance of an integrated treatment plan involving general dentistry, orthodontics, endodontics, and periodontics.

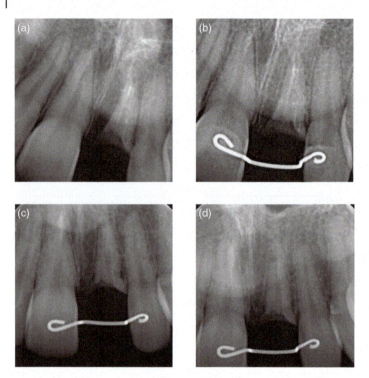

Figure 8.73 (a–d) 1 month; 5 months; 2 years, and 3 years postdecoronation.

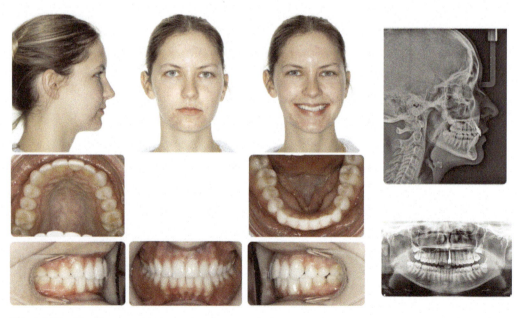

Figure 8.74 Five-year retention records.

Figure 8.75 Panoramic X-ray – 5-year retention records.

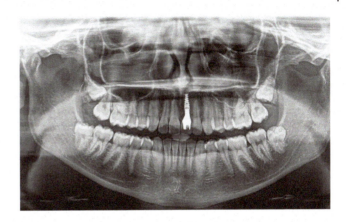

This collaborative effort ensures a more predictable and successful outcome for the patient while minimizing the likelihood of "unpleasant surprises." The integrated approach also opens various options, as exemplified by the decoronation technique discussed on this article.

References

1 Ng DY, Wong AYC, Liston PN. Multidisciplinary approach to implants: a review. *N Z Dent J* 2012 Dec;**108**(4):123–8.
2 Matsumoto MAN, Stuani MBS. Tooth transposition: a multidisciplinary approach. *Dent Press J Orthod* 2018 Jan;**23**(1):97–107.
3 Gkantidis N, Christou P, Topouzelis N. The orthodontic-periodontic interrelationship in integrated treatment challenges: a systematic review. *J Oral Rehabil* 2010 May 1;**37**(5):377–90.
4 Consolaro A, Miranda DAO, Consolaro RB. Orthodontics and endodontics: clinical decision-making. *Dent Press J Orthod* 2020 May;**25**(3):20–9.
5 Kindelan SA, Day PF, Kindelan JD, et al. Dental trauma: an overview of its influence on the management of orthodontic treatment. Part 1. *J Orthod* 2008 Jun;**35**(2):68–78.
6 Consolaro A, Consolaro RB. Orthodontic movement of endodontically treated teeth. *Dent Press J Orthod* 2013;**18**(4):2–7.
7 Hamilton RS, Gutmann JL. Endodontic-orthodontic relationships: a review of integrated treatment planning challenges. *Int Endod J* 1999 Sep;**32**(5):343–60.
8 Parashos P. Endodontic-orthodontic interactions: a review and treatment recommendations. *Aust Dent J* 2023 Jun;**68**(Suppl 1):S66–81.
9 Owtad P, Shastry S, Papademetriou M, Park JH. Management guidelines for traumatically injured teeth during orthodontic treatment. *J Clin Pediatr Dent* 2015;**39**(3):292–6.
10 Lam R. Epidemiology and outcomes of traumatic dental injuries: a review of the literature. *Aust Dent J* 2016 Mar;**61**(Suppl 1):4–20.
11 Petti S, Glendor U, Andersson L. World traumatic dental injury prevalence and incidence, a meta-analysis-one billion living people have had traumatic dental injuries. *Dent Traumatol* 2018 Apr;**34**(2):71–86.
12 Zaleckiene V, Peciuliene V, Brukiene V, Drukteinis S. Traumatic dental injuries: etiology, prevalence and possible outcomes. *Stomatologija* 2014;**16**(1):7–14.
13 Petti S. Over two hundred million injuries to anterior teeth attributable to large overjet: a

meta-analysis. *Dent Traumatol* 2015 Feb;**31**(1):1–8.
14. Goettems ML, Torriani DD, Hallal PC, et al. Dental trauma: prevalence and risk factors in schoolchildren. *Community Dent Oral Epidemiol* 2014 Dec;**42**(6):581–90.
15. da Silva Lima TC, Coste SC, Fernandes MIAP, et al. Prevalence of traumatic dental injuries in emergency dental services: a systematic review and meta-analysis. *Community Dent Oral Epidemiol* 2023 Apr;**51**(2):247–55.
16. Schatz JP, Ostini E, Hakeberg M, Kiliaridis S. Large overjet as a risk factor of traumatic dental injuries: a prospective longitudinal study. *Prog Orthod* 2020 Nov 9;**21**(1):41.
17. Malmgren B, Andreasen JO, Flores MT, et al. Guidelines for the management of traumatic dental injuries: 3. Injuries in the primary dentition. *Pediatr Dent* 2017 Sep 15;**39**(6):420–8.
18. Antipovienė A, Narbutaitė J, Virtanen JI. Traumatic dental injuries, treatment, and complications in children and adolescents: a register-based study. *Eur J Dent* 2021 Jul;**15**(3):557–62.
19. Azami-Aghdash S, Ebadifard Azar F, Pournaghi Azar F, et al. Prevalence, etiology, and types of dental trauma in children and adolescents: systematic review and meta-analysis. *Med J Islam Repub Iran* 2015;**29**(4):234.
20. Kaur P, Singh S, Mathur A, et al. Impact of dental disorders and its influence on self esteem levels among adolescents. *J Clin Diagn Res* 2017 Apr;**11**(4):ZC05–8.
21. Araújo EA, McCray J, Miranda GFPC. Growth: sometimes a friend, sometimes an enemy. *Semin Orthod* 2023 Jun 1;**29**(2):119–36.
22. Thiruvenkatachari B, Harrison J, Worthington H, O'Brien K. Early orthodontic treatment for Class II malocclusion reduces the chance of incisal trauma: results of a Cochrane systematic review. *Am J Orthod Dentofac Orthop* 2015 Jul;**148**(1):47–59.
23. Malmgren B, Cvek M, Lundberg M, Frykholm A. Surgical treatment of ankylosed and infrapositioned reimplanted incisors in adolescents. *Scand J Dent Res* 1984 Oct;**92**(5):391–9.
24. Einy S, Kridin K, Kaufman AY, Cohenca N. Immediate post-operative rehabilitation after decoronation. A systematic review. *Dent Traumatol* 2020 Apr;**36**(2):141–50.
25. Araújo EA, Miranda GFPC. Management of ankylosed teeth using the decoronation technique: integrative literature review and case report. *Dent Press J Orthod*;**28**(4):e23spe4.
26. Malmgren B. Ridge preservation/decoronation. *J Endod* 2013 Mar;**39** (3 Suppl):S67–72.
27. Consolaro A, Ribeiro Júnior PD, Cardoso MA, et al. Decoronation followed by dental implants placement: fundamentals, applications and explanations. *Dent Press J Orthod* 2018 Jan;**23**(1):24–36.

8.6

Section VI: Sleep-disordered breathing (SDB) in the growing child

Juan Martin Palomo, DDS, MDS[1] and Luciane M. de Menezes, PhD[1,2]

[1] Department of Orthodontics, Case Western Reserve University, Cleveland, OH, USA
[2] Pontifical Department of Orthodontics, Catholic University of Rio Grande do Sul, Porto Alegre/RS, Brazil

Sleep-disordered breathing(SDB) is a continuum condition in which the patient is not able to intake the ideal amount of air during sleep. SDB is considered a public health concern due to the increasing number of children under 12 affected, around 5–25% [1]. There are different levels of severity of SDB, ranging from primary snoring to obstructive sleep apnea (OSA), which can lead to complete airway obstruction. SDB is a common problem during childhood, with variable consequences [2], and should be managed as soon as possible, to reduce its negative consequences on the child's health.

Sleep is fundamental for a child's development [1] as it has the potential to modulate brain activity [3]. The quality of sleep can affect the child's attention, behavior, cognitive functioning, emotional regulation, and physical health.

Sleep apnea is a common disorder that causes frequent pauses in breathing during sleep and can be classified as central sleep apnea (CSA) or OSA. Both promote breathing interruptions. In CSA, the breathing disruptions are due to a lack of communication between the brain and the muscles involved in breathing. In OSA, there is partial upper airway obstruction (hypopnea) and/or intermittent complete obstruction (apnea) that disrupts normal ventilation during sleep. These breathing interruptions dramatically reduce the quality of sleep in children, leading to potentially serious health consequences that include cardiovascular, metabolic, growth, development, and cognitive impairments.

Sleep can be divided into two phases: rapid eye movement (REM) sleep and nonrapid eye movement (NON-REM) sleep. Both phases are important for a child to recover from a day's activity and develop physically and neurologically [1]. REM sleep is essential for the brain to recover and to maintain and establish new neuronal connections during development [4]. The NON-REM sleep functions as a restorative phase, as the brain is very quiet and muscle tone returns [1]. Children should have at least 4–6 cycles of sleep per night. The average sleep time needed, according to each age is presented in Table 8.1.

8.32 The need for sleep

It is only during sleep that the body rests and restores. During sleep, growth hormones are released, which help renew body tissues and

Table 8.1 The average sleep needs according to each age.

Age	Sleep needs (hours a day)
0–3 months	14–18
4–12 months	12–16
1–2 years	11–14
3–5 years	10–13
6–12 years	9–12
13–18 years	8–12
19–64 years	7–9
Above 65 years	7–8

form new red blood cells. Parathormone, responsible for calcium in the blood, reaches its peak during sleep. Deep sleep helps the body mobilize its defenses against illness. During sleep, cerebral fluids flow in and out, cleaning the brain of toxins. Without any sleep, toxins build up and can cause death in about 200 hours. In case of limited sleep, these toxins accumulate and eventually result in death.

8.33 Diagnosis and management of sleep-disordered breathing (SDB) and obstructive sleep apnea (OSA) in children

The development of SDB in children involves an intricate and multifaceted origin, characterized by a complex interplay of various contributing factors. The diagnosis and management of SDB in a child usually involve a multidisciplinary team of healthcare professionals, including pediatricians, sleep specialists, otolaryngologists, and dentists. Pediatric dentists and orthodontists play a crucial role in identifying and managing these issues, as they may be the first point of contact for parents concerned about their child's snoring or other signs of sleep-disordered breathing. Early detection and intervention can help prevent or minimize the dental and skeletal consequences associated with breathing disturbances.

The diagnosis of pediatric SDB is a process of several steps. The first is to diagnose the child's breathing disorder through a comprehensive medical and dental history as well as a thorough physical examination of the head and neck. The definition and criteria used for the diagnosis of OSA in adults do not apply to OSA in developmental age. Depending on the child's symptoms and medical history specific tests may be ordered as imaging tests, nasal endoscopy, or even a sleep study.

Validated questionnaires are used as screening tools to identify children who may be at high risk of having OSA and who may need further evaluation. The most commonly used questionnaires for OSA risk assessment in children are summarized in Table 8.2, with their sensitivity and specificity, and are the following:

- **Pediatric sleep questionnaire (PSQ):** The PSQ is a 22-item questionnaire that assesses snoring, breathing pauses, sleepiness, and other symptoms of OSA in children. It has been validated in children aged 2–18 years, and a score of 0.33 or higher is considered positive for OSA.
- **Sleep-related breathing disorder (SRBD) scale:** The SRBD scale is a 22-item questionnaire that assesses snoring, mouth breathing, choking, and other symptoms of OSA in children. It has been validated in children aged 2–17 years, and a score of 0.33 or higher is considered positive for OSA.
- **Obstructive sleep apnea-18 (OSA-18) questionnaire:** The OSA-18 is an 18-item questionnaire that assesses the quality of life and symptoms related to OSA in children. It has been validated in children aged 2–18 years, and a score of 60 or higher is considered positive for OSA.
- **Berlin questionnaire:** The Berlin questionnaire is a 10-item questionnaire that assesses snoring, fatigue, and other

8.33 Diagnosis and management of sleep-disordered breathing (SDB) and obstructive sleep apnea (OSA) in children

Table 8.2 Summary of some of the risk assessment questionnaires for OSA in children, with its key features.

Questionnaire	Range values	Age range (years)	Sensitivity[a] (%)	Specificity[b] (%)
Pediatric Sleep Questionnaire (PSQ)	Positive if the score is 0.33 or higher	2–18	87	43
Sleep-related breathing disorder (SRBD) scale	Positive if the score is 0.33 or higher	2–17	78	80
Obstructive sleep apnea-18 (OSA-18) questionnaire	Positive if the score is 60 or higher	2–18	76	61
Berlin questionnaire	Positive if high risk in two or more categories	2–18	86	77

[a] Sensitivity measures how well the test identifies people who have the condition.
[b] Specificity measures how well the test identifies people who do not have the condition.

symptoms of OSA. It has been validated in children aged 2–18 years, and a score of high risk in two or more categories is considered positive for OSA.

Currently, there is no universally accepted tool that uses history and clinical examination alone to diagnose pediatric OSA [5]. The gold standard test for diagnosing OSA in children is polysomnography (PSG), which is a type of sleep study. The PSG is a comprehensive non-invasive exam that measures various physiological parameters, including brain waves, eye movements, muscle activity, heart rate, oxygen levels, and breathing patterns. PSG can detect the presence and severity of OSA as well as provide information about the type and frequency of breathing disturbances during sleep.

There are two main types of PSG: in-lab PSG and home sleep apnea testing (HSAT).

In-lab PSG involves spending the night in a sleep laboratory or center, where the child is monitored with multiple sensors and monitoring devices. The data collected during the test includes information on sleep stages, respiratory events, movement disorders, and other physiological parameters. The disadvantages of the in-lab PSG are its cost, time-consuming exam, labor-intensive, and sometimes not readily available.

HSAT is a simplified version of PSG that can be done in the child's own home, using a portable monitoring device that typically includes sensors to measure breathing movements, oxygen levels, and heart rate. HSAT is less expensive and more convenient than PSG, but it may be not as accurate.

The PSG gives information on the number and duration of partial or complete obstructions of the airway, generating a number called the apnea-hypopnea index (AHI).

The AHI is used to indicate the severity of sleep apnea and classifies the OSA into mild, moderate, or severe (Table 8.3) [6]. AHI represents the number of apnea and hypopnea events per hour of sleep. To be considered an event, the apneas (pauses in breathing) must last for at least 10 s and be associated with a decrease in blood oxygenation of at least 4%.

Table 8.3 Summary of values for classification of obstructive sleep apnea (OSA) in children and adults, according to the apnea-hypopnea index (AHI) [6].

OSA Risk	Mild	Moderate	Severe
Child	$1 \leq AHI < 5$	$5 \leq AHI < 10$	$AHI \geq 10$
Adult	$5 \leq AHI < 15$	$15 \leq AHI < 30$	$AHI \geq 30$

To determine the AHI, one adds the total number of apnea/hypopnea events and divides it by the total number of minutes of actual sleep time, then multiply it by 60. An adult with less than five events per hour is considered within normal limits, but a child is considered to have OSA when there is at least one event per hour [1]. It is important to point out that the severity of OSA in children may be influenced by factors such as age, sex, obesity, craniofacial abnormalities, and underlying medical conditions. Before puberty, both sexes show similar risk for OSA, but after puberty, males are more affected than females [1]. Obesity is another strong predictor of OSA in children.

Other diagnostic tests that may be used to evaluate the risk assessment of OSA in children are as follows:

Nasal endoscopy: A procedure in which a small, flexible tube with a camera on the end is inserted into the child's nose to examine the nasal passages and throat for signs of obstruction.

Drug-induced sleep endoscopy (DISE): This exam involves the use of sedative drugs to induce sleep while an endoscope is inserted into the airway to visualize any anatomical obstructions that may be contributing to OSA. DISE can provide valuable information about the location and severity of airway obstructions, which can guide treatment decisions.

Imaging tests: X-rays, computed tomography (CT) scans, magnetic resonance imaging (MRI) scans, and ultrasound (US) can be used to evaluate the structure of the airway and identify any abnormalities that may be contributing to OSA.

8.34 Risk factors for OSA in children

Despite years of research into the causes and consequences of OSA, the early identification of patients who are most at risk remains challenging [7]. Until now, the most common risk factors associated with OSA in children are as follows.

8.34.1 Enlarged tonsils and adenoids

This is known to be the most common cause of OSA in children. When the tonsils and adenoids are enlarged, they can obstruct the airway during sleep and cause breathing difficulties. The most prevalent age for OSA is between 2 and 8 years, due to the tonsils and adenoid size, occupying almost the space of the growing airway [1].

The physical examination has a practical value when evaluating for sleep disorders breathing. The Mallampati classification and the Brodsky scale should be considered when evaluating a patient for OSA, as these factors are [5, 8].

The original Mallampati score is derived from a noninvasive and simple airway classification, used to identify patients at risk for difficult tracheal intubation. This exam requires no special equipment, and it is performed as part of a routine clinical assessment, by asking the patient to open his/her mouth widely, while protruding the tongue, without emitting sounds. The Modified Mallampati score is similar, but obtained without protruding the tongue, and has been used to predict OSA (Figure 8.76). A higher Mallampati classification is often correlated with anatomical features that contribute to the narrowing or collapse of the upper airway, a common characteristic of OSA. Therefore, the Modified Mallampati classification serves as a valuable clinical tool for predicting and assessing the risk of OSA in individuals.

The tonsil size can be graded with the Brodsky scale, according to its occupancy of the oropharyngeal: Grade 0 – tonsils removed or within the tonsillar fossa; Grade 1 – tonsils occupying less than 25% of the oropharyngeal width; Grade 2 – tonsils occupying 25–50% of the oropharyngeal width; Grade 3 – tonsils occupying 50–75% of the oropharyngeal width,

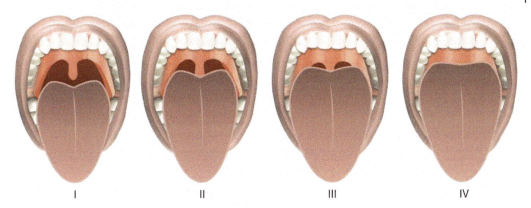

Figure 8.76 Scores of the modified Mallampati classification that can be used during the physical examination when evaluating for sleep disorders breathing (Class I: soft palate, uvula, and pillars are visible, Class II: soft palate and uvula are visible, Class III: only the soft palate and base of the uvula are visible, Class IV: only the hard palate is visible) (Font: Dental Study App [15]).

Grade 4 – tonsils occupying 75–100% of the oropharyngeal width (Figure 8.77).

Adenoid and tonsil hypertrophy contributes to the narrowing of the retro-palatal area, which has the smallest cross-sectional area and is, therefore, the most frequent site of obstruction [9]. When this occurs, tonsils and adenoids emerge as primary contributors to SDB, and the recommended intervention is adenotonsillectomy – a surgical procedure involving the extraction of both adenoids and tonsils. Figure 8.78 underscores the pivotal role of a clinical examination, particularly employing the Brodsky scale, in assessing the obstructive impact attributed to tonsils.

Adenotonsillectomy stands out as one of the most frequently conducted surgeries in children, typically carried out under general anesthesia within a hospital setting. While risks are infrequent, it is crucial to acknowledge that complications related to general anesthesia and post-surgery bleeding cannot be overlooked. In addition, it is noteworthy that individuals with chronic obstruction may persist in breathing primarily through the mouth, even post-removal of causative factors, due to maintaining a mouth-breathing habit. Persistent OSA after adenotonsillectomy occurs in more than 25% of the cases [10]. Lingual tonsil hypertrophy is also suggested in the pathogenesis of

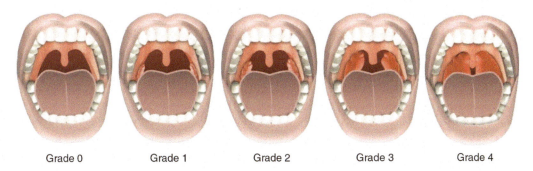

Figure 8.77 Tonsils' scores according to Brodsky scale: Grade 0 – tonsils removed or within the tonsillar fossa; Grade 1 – tonsils occupying less than 25% of the oropharyngeal width; Grade 2 – tonsils occupying 25–50% of the oropharyngeal width; Grade 3 – tonsils occupying 50–75% of the oropharyngeal width, Grade 4 – tonsils occupying 75–100% of the oropharyngeal width (Font: Dental Study App [15]).

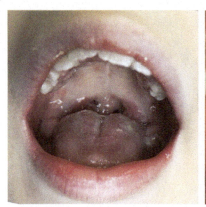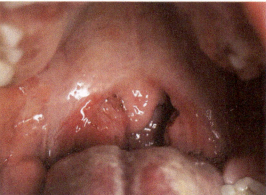

Figure 8.78 Images showing the mouth of a 9-year-old boy exhibiting prominent tonsillar enlargement, classified as Grade 4 on the Brodsky scale. Observe the enlarged tonsils that occupy 75–100% of the oropharyngeal width. In addition to this, a buccal breathing pattern is evident, associated with dryness and cracking of the lips.

pediatric OSA [9]. Nose obstructions are a common cause of persistent OSA and should be also assessed. Multidisciplinary treatment is also beneficial for children with persistent OSA [9].

8.34.2 Obesity

Obesity is becoming an increasingly common and important risk factor for pediatric OSA, mainly in the second childhood (6–9 years) and during adolescence. Overweight or obese children are more likely to develop OSA [11]. Excess fat in the neck can put pressure on the airway and make it more difficult to breathe during sleep. Body mass index (BMI), a scale that defines obesity by taking body weight and height as well as higher waist circumference are strong predictors for OSA in children [1]. Regardless of a child's gender, a healthy BMI puts them between the 5th and 85th percentiles when compared with their peers.

Nutritional counseling is a necessary part of the multidisciplinary care for children who are obese with persistent OSA [10].

Various factors may contribute to the child's weight, including family history, mental health issues, socioeconomic status, and lifestyle habits. It is important to encourage healthy eating habits and regular physical activity to help prevent obesity.

8.34.3 Allergies and respiratory infections

Allergies and respiratory infections emerge as significant risk factors for OSA, contributing to inflammation and swelling in the nasal passages and throat. This inflammatory response threatens the integrity of the airway – a lengthy, collapsible tube comprising soft tissues that necessitates continuous support from upper airway dilator muscles to remain open. The intricate neuromuscular control of these muscles can be disrupted by chronic inflammation and other diseases, ultimately diminishing the diameter of the airway.

The repercussions extend beyond the realm of OSA, impacting overall sleep quality and potentially leading to disruptions and disturbances. Individuals with a history of allergies or recurrent respiratory infections may find themselves at a higher risk for developing OSA, highlighting the importance of early detection and intervention.

In cases where nasal obstruction, whether from allergies or anatomical abnormalities, is identified as the root cause of obstruction, a comprehensive evaluation and treatment by an otolaryngologist are imperative. Treatment options may vary ranging from surgical interventions to weight management (especially in cases where obesity is a contributing factor) and the management of underlying medical conditions like asthma or allergies. In this case, nasal corticosteroid sprays may be prescribed to reduce inflammation and improve airflow.

A strong correlation exists between OSA and asthma. For this reason, it is highly advised for individuals with asthma who fall within the moderate-to-severe range or prove challenging to manage to undergo screening for OSA and seek suitable treatment [12]. Healthcare providers should perform early detection, diagnosis, and intervention for OSA in individuals with asthma. This approach aims to mitigate the progression of airway remodeling and the decline in lung function [12].

In some cases, the complexity of addressing both structural and functional aspects of the airway necessitates a multidisciplinary approach. Collaborative efforts between otolaryngologists, pulmonologists, and other specialists become crucial in providing adequate care. Moreover, patient education is pivotal, enabling individuals to help recognize and manage underlying conditions to mitigate the risk of OSA. This includes focusing on lifestyle modifications, such as weight management, to complement the overall treatment strategy. In essence, a thorough understanding of the interplay between allergies, respiratory infections, and OSA is crucial for developing effective and personalized intervention strategies.

8.34.4 Structural abnormalities and craniofacial anomalies

Some children may exhibit structural anomalies in the facial, jaw, or airway regions, which can significantly contribute to the onset of OSA. Changes in the dimensions, location, and structure of the mandible and tongue can result in the thickening of the retro-palatal region, a commonly observed site of obstruction in pediatric patients [9], and may elevate the susceptibility of a child to developing OSA. In addition, children diagnosed with specific syndromes, such as Down syndrome, are at an increased risk of OSA. This heightened risk can be attributed to factors such as relative macroglossia, mid-face hypoplasia, and hypotonia, common findings within these individuals.

8.35 Consequences of SDB in children

When the airway is obstructed, children tend to breathe through their mouths instead of their noses. While it is normal for a person to breathe through the mouth in certain situations, such as during exercise or when the nasal passages are congested, chronic mouth breathing can lead to several negative consequences. One of the main consequences of mouth breathing is a reduction in the amount of air that is filtered, warmed, and moistened as it passes through the nasal passages. The consequences can vary and may include impaired attention and concentration, reduced quality of life, increased risk for cardiovascular disease, physiologic dysfunction, growth impairment, obesity, depression, increased risk of respiratory infections, dry mouth, bad breath, and other oral health issues.

The criteria for diagnosing OSA in adults do not apply to OSA in developmental age. While in adults, an obstructive event must persist for a minimum duration of 10 seconds, in children, the obstructive event duration is characterized by the absence of at least two respiratory acts. In addition, central events in children last 20 s or longer or at least the duration of two breaths if associated with an arousal or oxygen desaturation of $\geq 3\%$. Furthermore, the lower functional residual capacity, characteristic of the pediatric age, can result in significant oxyhemoglobin desaturations even after brief apneic episodes. Excessive daytime sleepiness in children is a symptom of OSA less common than in adults. Robust evidence establishes a connection between SDB in children and a range of behavioral modifications encompassing somatization, depression, aggressiveness, emotional regulation, school performance, hyperactivity, inattention, vigilance, and sustained and selective attention [11].

The impact of OSA on cognitive functions extends beyond adulthood, exhibiting a more pronounced effect on children. This influence on a malleable brain structure can have irreversible effects on neuro-psychic development, learning capacities, and social interactions [11]. When untreated or treated late, OSA can affect different organs. There is a higher risk of developing metabolic syndromes and cardiovascular consequences and a detrimental effect on skeletal growth. The repercussions highlight the importance of timely and comprehensive intervention for optimal health outcomes.

A prevalent shift toward mouth breathing, as opposed to nasal breathing, can potentially impact the posture of the head and jaws. This alteration can influence tongue position, leading to consequences for growth and culminating in various dental and health issues. These complications encompass increased overjet, anterior or posterior crossbite, open bite, and a retrognathic mandible. Timely intervention becomes imperative to address these underlying factors contributing to malocclusion, aiming to prevent its onset or further exacerbation.

Skeletal and dental consequences of SDB in children depend on its duration, frequency, and intensity. These skeletal and dental consequences can have a significant impact on the child's health and well-being, including their ability to breathe, sleep, eat, and speak properly. The most common skeletal and dental consequences of SDB in children are described below and illustrated in Figures 8.79–8.83:

Long face syndrome or "adenoid face": Breathing disturbances can cause the face to present an elongated facial type (dolichocephalic). As a consequence of the breathing disturbance, the mouth stays open for an extended amount of time with lip incompetence, and the tongue does not rest on the palate, resulting in overeruption of the posterior teeth, a narrow maxilla (high-arched palate, with a "v" shape upper arch). It can cause teeth crowding and posterior crossbite. The nasal apertures may be small and atonic, showing a lack of nasal breathing.

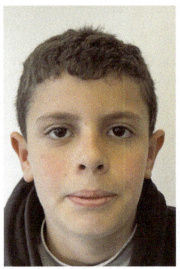 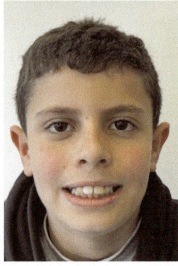 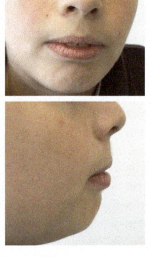

Figure 8.79 Ten-year-old boy exhibiting characteristics of habitual mouth-breathing. Observe the retrognathic mandible with a posterior positioning of the lower jaw. This anatomical aspect contributes to difficulty in achieving proper lip sealing. The images reveal signs of dryness and cracking of the lips, potential oral consequences associated with chronic mouth breathing.

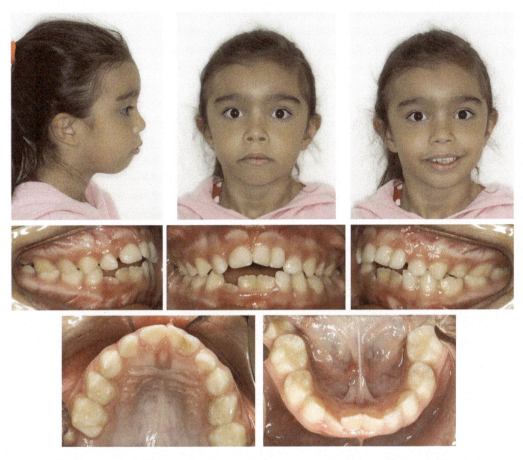

Figure 8.80 Images of a 5.10-year-old girl presenting a convex profile, retrognathic mandible, transverse maxillary deficiency, and anterior open bite associated with SDB. The patient sought dental treatment due to the presence of upper left primary double teeth.

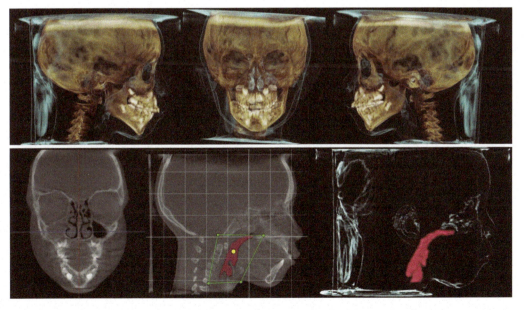

Figure 8.81 Tomographic images of the 5.10-year-old girl showing the class II malocclusion with a vertical skeletal pattern, mucosal thickening of the maxillary sinuses, hypertrophic adenoids, and reduced airway. Adenotonsillectomy was indicated by the ENT (ear, nose, and throat doctor).

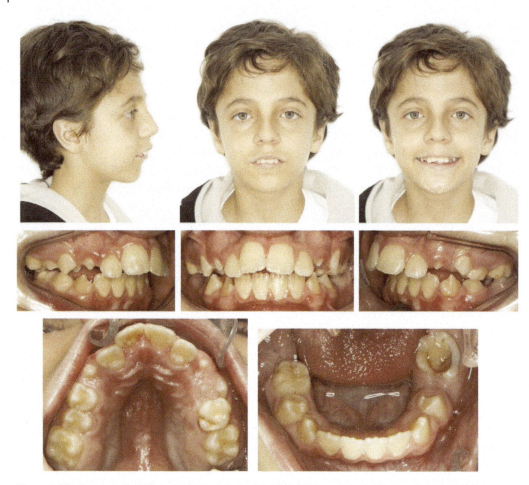

Figure 8.82 Images of an 11-year-old boy presenting SDB and long face syndrome characteristics, with his mouth opened and lip incompetent. Observe the class II malocclusion with a predominant vertical pattern, protruded maxilla, ogival palate, proclination of the upper incisors, and excessive overjet. A Thurow headgear appliance, to control and restrict the vertical growth of the upper jaw, allowing the lower jaw to catch up is an option for the first-phase treatment, followed by maxillary expansion, after eruption of the upper premolars.

Individuals who habitually breathe through their mouths have a tendency to maintain an open mouth posture at rest, leading to potential dryness or cracking of the lips due to increased saliva evaporation. The upper lip may appear more relaxed or dropped, while the lower lip might exhibit signs of tension or strain, especially when efforts are made to keep the mouth closed. Achieving a complete lip seal may be challenging, contributing to increased air escape and oral dryness. Prolonged mouth breathing can also influence facial muscle development, potentially resulting in noticeable changes in the appearance of the lips and surrounding areas.

- **Open bite:** Breathing disturbances can also result in an open bite, a malocclusion characterized by a lack of overlap between the upper and lower incisors, which can cause difficulties with speech and eating.
- **Exaggerated overjet:** This characteristic is due to upper incisors' proclination and retropositioned lower incisors, consequences of lip incompetence, and the buccal breathing habit.

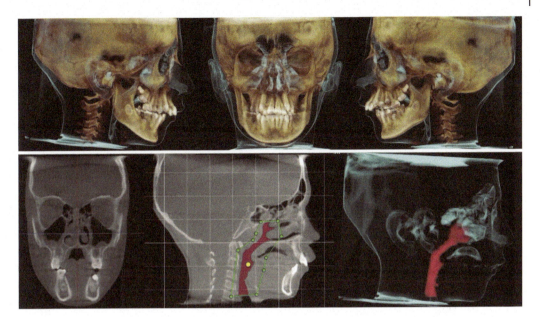

Figure 8.83 Tomographic images of the 11-year-old boy showing the class II malocclusion, vertical skeletal pattern, protruded maxilla, proclination of the upper incisors, and excessive overjet. A mucosal thickening of the maxillary sinuses and reduced airway were observed. An appointment for evaluation with an ENT doctor was recommended.

- **Retrognathic mandible:** Breathing disturbances can also cause a retrognathic mandible, with the mandible and lower jaw set too far back, resulting in an underbite and increased mandibular plane.

8.36 Treatment options for the dental and skeletal consequences of SDB in children

Early detection and intervention can help prevent or mitigate the dental and skeletal consequences of SDB, allowing for normal growth in children. To effectively address the dental and skeletal consequences of SDB in children, a multifaceted approach is often employed. Pediatricians, Pediatric dentists, and Orthodontists play a crucial role in identifying and managing these issues, as they are often the first point of contact for parents concerned about their child's health. A meticulous evaluation of the causal factors underlying a medical condition is pivotal in devising an effective and tailored treatment plan. In the context of pediatric SDB, comprehending the specific triggers contributing to dental and skeletal consequences is imperative. Whether it be anatomical abnormalities, respiratory patterns, or other etiological factors, a nuanced understanding allows for the implementation of precise interventions, addressing the unique needs of each child. This strategic approach not only corrects the evident consequences but also contributes to long-term health outcomes, fostering normal growth and development.

It is important to highlight that the existing scientific literature does not endorse orthodontic interceptive treatment as the elective approach for managing OSA in growing patients [13]. Orthodontic treatment with oral appliances can be prescribed to correct the malocclusion associated with SDB. Maxillary expansion appliances with palatal cribs are commonly indicated in cases where a narrow maxilla, posterior crossbite, and anterior open bite are observed. Dentofacial Orthopedics may come into play, focusing on guiding facial growth and development through specific orthodontic appliances to modify jaw growth and position. In addition, a comprehensive orthodontic treatment plan, encompassing braces, aligners, and other appliances, can be indicated to correct dental and skeletal abnormalities.

Myofunctional therapy, centered on targeted exercises to enhance oral muscle function, may also be necessary, depending on the cause and severity of the obstruction and malocclusion, and should be determined by qualified healthcare professionals, as an integral part of the treatment plan. Speech therapy may be recommended to address articulation and speech challenges arising from the effects of SDB on oral structures.

Concurrently, surgical interventions, such as adenotonsillectomy, play a role in alleviating airway obstruction by removing enlarged adenoids and tonsils.

The use of continuous positive airway pressure (CPAP) therapy, a machine that uses mild air pressure to keep the airway open during sleep, is less common in children, but it may be considered in selected cases. CPAP is a reasonable treatment option for children with obesity and persistent OSA [10]. The use of CPAP is associated with a significant reduction in co-morbidities related to OSA.

Ultimately, the selection and integration of these treatment options are contingent upon a thorough evaluation and a tailored approach to manage the dental and skeletal consequences associated with SDB in children. There is no accepted prophylactic or preventative treatment for OSA. Treatment should only be provided after a positive diagnosis.

8.37 New technologies: the use of apps and devices for SDB and OSA in children

While there are some apps designed to monitor and analyze sleep patterns, including snoring and potential signs of sleep apnea, their reliability for detecting OSA in children may be limited. The accuracy of consumer-grade sleep apps for OSA detection in children is uncertain, as these apps may not have undergone rigorous scientific validation specifically for pediatric populations.

There is a need for sufficient validation data and established clinical practice guidelines, even though some of these devices have obtained FDA clearance for use in children. Despite the regulatory clearance, the lack of comprehensive validation and guidance has contributed to hesitancy in their application. Recognizing the evolving landscape shaped by emerging technologies, the American Academy of Sleep Medicine (AASM) is presently revisiting and updating its position paper on pediatric OSA testing [14]. This initiative seeks to address the current gaps and adapt to the advancements in pediatric sleep medicine.

8.38 Conclusion

SDB is a prevalent issue affecting a significant portion of the pediatric population. Left untreated, it not only diminishes the quality of life but also gives rise to severe health consequences. Sleep apnea manifests differently in children than adults, underscoring the importance of professional evaluation for accurate diagnosis. If there are concerns regarding a child's sleep patterns or potential sleep apnea, consultation with a pediatrician or a sleep specialist is highly recommended. These experts conduct comprehensive assessments, delve into the child's medical history, and may recommend extensive sleep studies in a controlled medical setting. Early detection and timely intervention in sleep disorders among children play a crucial role in preventing or mitigating the associated health repercussions and the adverse effects stemming from breathing disturbances.

References

1 Perez, C.V. (2021). Sleep-disordered breathing in children. In: *Handbook of clinical techniques in pediatric dentistry*, 301–312. John Wiley & Sons, Ltd. Available at: https://onlinelibrary.wiley.com/doi/abs/10.1002/9781119661085.ch27. Accessed October 5, 2024.

2 Ophoff D, Slaats MA, Boudewyns A, Glazemakers I, Van Hoorenbeeck K, Verhulst SL. Sleep disorders during childhood: a practical review. *Eur J Pediatr* 2018 May;177(5):641–8. doi: https://doi.org/10.1007/s00431-018-3116-z.

3 Lokhandwala S, Spencer RMC. Relations between sleep patterns early in life and brain development: a review. *Dev Cogn Neurosci*. 2022 Aug;56:101130. doi: https://doi.org/10.1016/j.dcn.2022.101130.

4 Bathory, E. and Tomopoulos, S. (2017). Sleep regulation, physiology and development, sleep duration and patterns, and sleep hygiene in infants, toddlers, and preschool-age children. *Curr Probl Pediatr Adolesc Health Care* 47 (2): 29–42.

5 Kumar HV, Schroeder JW, Gang Z, Sheldon SH. Mallampati score and pediatric obstructive sleep apnea. *J Clin Sleep Med* 2014 Sep 15;10(9):985–90. doi: https://doi.org/10.5664/jcsm.4032.

6 Palomo JM, Piccoli VD, Menezes LM. Obstructive sleep apnea: a review for the orthodontist. *Dental Press J Orthod*. 2023 Apr 14;28(1):e23spe1. doi: https://doi.org/10.1590/2177-6709.28.1.e23spe1.

7 Nuckton, T.J., Glidden, D.V., Browner, W.S. et al. (2006). Physical examination: Mallampati score as an independent predictor of obstructive sleep apnea. *Sleep* 29 (7): 903–908.

8 Friedman M, Hamilton C, Samuelson CG, Lundgren ME, Pott T. Diagnostic value of the Friedman tongue position and Mallampati classification for obstructive sleep apnea: a meta-analysis. *Otolaryngol Head Neck Surg* 2013 Apr;148(4):540–7. doi: https://doi.org/10.1177/0194599812473413.

9 Gulotta G, Iannella G, Vicini C, Polimeni A, Greco A, de Vincentiis M, Visconti IC, Meccariello G, Cammaroto G, De Vito A, Gobbi R, Bellini C, Firinu E, Pace A, Colizza A, Pelucchi S, Magliulo G. Risk factors for obstructive sleep apnea syndrome in children: state of the art. *Int J Environ Res Public Health* 2019 Sep 4;16(18):3235. doi: https://doi.org/10.3390/ijerph16183235.

10 Chang JL, Goldberg AN, Alt JA, Mohammed A, Ashbrook L, Auckley D, Ayappa I, Bakhtiar H, Barrera JE, Bartley BL, Billings ME, Boon MS, Bosschieter P, Braverman I, Brodie K, Cabrera-Muffly C, Caesar R, Cahali MB, Cai Y, Cao M, Capasso R, Caples SM, Chahine LM, Chang CP, Chang KW, Chaudhary N, Cheong CSJ, Chowdhuri S, Cistulli PA, Claman D, Collen J, Coughlin KC, Creamer J, Davis EM, Dupuy-McCauley KL, Durr ML, Dutt M, Ali ME, Elkassabany NM, Epstein LJ, Fiala JA, Freedman N, Gill K, Gillespie MB, Golisch L, Gooneratne N, Gottlieb DJ, Green KK, Gulati A, Gurubhagavatula I, Hayward N, Hoff PT, Hoffmann OMG, Holfinger SJ, Hsia J, Huntley C, Huoh KC, Huyett P, Inala S, Ishman SL, Jella TK, Jobanputra AM, Johnson AP, Junna MR, Kado JT, Kaffenberger TM, Kapur VK, Kezirian EJ, Khan M, Kirsch DB, Kominsky A, Kryger M, Krystal AD, Kushida CA, Kuzniar TJ, Lam DJ, Lettieri CJ, Lim DC, Lin HC, Liu SYC, MacKay SG, Magalang UJ, Malhotra A, Mansukhani MP, Maurer JT, May AM, Mitchell RB, Mokhlesi B, Mullins AE, Nada EM, Naik S, Nokes B, Olson MD, Pack AI, Pang EB, Pang KP, Patil SP, Van de Perck E, Piccirillo JF, Pien GW, Piper AJ, Plawecki A, Quigg M, Ravesloot MJL, Redline S, Rotenberg BW, Ryden A, Sarmiento KF, Sbeih F, Schell AE, Schmickl CN, Schotland HM, Schwab RJ, Seo J, Shah N, Shelgikar AV, Shochat I, Soose RJ, Steele TO, Stephens E, Stepnowsky C, Strohl KP, Sutherland K,

Suurna MV, Thaler E, Thapa S, Vanderveken OM, de Vries N, Weaver EM, Weir ID, Wolfe LF, Woodson BT, Won CHJ, Xu J, Yalamanchi P, Yaremchuk K, Yeghiazarians Y, Yu JL, Zeidler M, Rosen IM. International consensus statement on obstructive sleep apnea. *Int Forum Allergy Rhinol*. 2023 Jul;13(7):1061–482. doi: https://doi.org/10.1002/alr.23079.

11 Lo Bue A, Salvaggio A, Insalaco G. Obstructive sleep apnea in developmental age. A narrative review. *Eur J Pediatr* 2020 Mar;179(3):357–65. doi: https://doi.org/10.1007/s00431-019-03557-8.

12 Wang D, Zhou Y, Chen R, Zeng X, Zhang S, Su X, Luo Y, Tang Y, Li S, Zhuang Z, Zhao D, Ren Y, Zhang N. The relationship between obstructive sleep apnea and asthma severity and vice versa: a systematic review and meta-analysis. *Eur J Med Res* 2023 Mar 30;28(1):139. doi: https://doi.org/10.1186/s40001-023-01097-4.

13 Bucci R, Rongo R, Zunino B, Michelotti A, Bucci P, Alessandri-Bonetti G, Incerti-Parenti S, D'Antò V. Effect of orthopedic and functional orthodontic treatment in children with obstructive sleep apnea: a systematic review and meta-analysis. *Sleep Med Rev* 2023 Feb;67:101730. doi: https://doi.org/10.1016/j.smrv.2022.101730.

14 American Academy of Sleep Medicine (AASM). 2023. Available at: https://aasm.org/novel-devices-applications-diagnosing-obstructive-sleep-apnea/ (accessed 5 Nov 2023).

15 DENTAL STUDY APP. [Mobile app]. Play Store. 2015. https://play.google.com/store/apps/details?id=creativedge.dentalstudy&hl=pt_BR&gl=US&pli=1 Accessed October 5, 2024.

8.7

Section VII: Mixed dentition orthodontic mechanics

Gerald S. Samson, DDS

Department of Orthodontics, Center of Advanced Dental Education, Saint Louis University, St. Louis, MO, USA

"Merely hoping that clinical orthodontic treatment will be effective does not mean you will succeed." HT Perry, Jr, DDS, PhD.

The year was 1979 – my first year of orthodontic postgraduate residency at Northwestern Dental School in Chicago, Illinois. Entering the clinic, new postgraduate orthodontic residents found 15 part-time faculty members. It was a black rain of mechanical confusion. Monday, the headgear tube was gingival, Tuesday, it was occlusal, Wednesday, back to gingival, Thursday was surgical orthodontics – no headgear tube – and the Friday, instructor was persuasive when he proclaimed that it made essentially no difference. Within the first 6 months, I asked the department chair, Dr. Harold T Perry, Jr why we were required to learn both 0.018 and 0.022 slot edgewise. Dr. Perry's answer to my question spoke to my professional youth:

> Samson, you are too inexperienced to understand what I am going to tell you, but I'll try to explain. Some things work, some do not, some are effective for a while and then stop working. When treating patients, you will encounter various treatment responses. The first and second approaches to a given problem may not be effective. In fact, in order to be successful you will need to know more than just a few clinical orthodontic techniques. You will need to understand how to mix, match and how to be inventive. You are not learning only orthodontic technique. You are learning how to think.

Then, in his regal fashion, Dr. Perry dismissed me from his office: "When everything works, nothing matters." Lysle E Johnston, DDS, PhD.

Ask yourself this question: during any given day how many patients not responding to orthodontic treatment will it take to upset you? The answer for all of us is the same: "one." Practically, we understand that a daily and hourly perfect score is not realistic. Emotionally, however, when confronted with a lack of response or worse, a real "treatment problem," statistical reality is of little consolation. Every time I collided with this unpleasant chair-side experience, the same reverberation would rattle my mind – that if I had a more complete understanding of applied orthodontic mechanics, this would be less likely to happen. At the very least, it would be less of a struggle to solve treatment problems.

Recognizing and Correcting Developing Malocclusions: A Problem-Oriented Approach to Orthodontics, Second Edition. Edited by Eustáquio A. Araújo and Peter H. Buschang.
© 2025 John Wiley & Sons, Inc. Published 2025 by John Wiley & Sons, Inc.

In the spirit of Dr. Harold T Perry, Jr, the purpose of this section is to stimulate neurosynaptic junctions, allow the flow of acetylcholine, and trigger the reader to *think*.

8.39 Definitions and terminology [1–3]

Center of resistance (Figure 8.84) – CRes is the point on a body (tooth) where a single force would produce translation (similar to the center of mass).

Translation (Figure 8.84) – The movement of a body as a whole, such that the displacements of all points of that body are alike (equal) in magnitude and direction. For example, the angulation of the long axis of a tooth (or a set of teeth) remaining unchanged is necessary for a tooth movement to be translational. Any movement of a body that is not a translation is referred to as a "rotation."

Center of rotation (Figure 8.85) – CRot is the point around which a body appears to have rotated during a *nontranslational* displacement.

Force – Any action or influence that accelerates an object. Force is a *vector*, which means it has *direction and magnitude*.

Moment – The tendency to cause rotation around a point or axis.

Moment of force (Figure 8.86) – M_F, with regard to a line or a point, is the turning effect of the force with respect to that line or point, that is, a tendency to rotate. A tooth that receives a force not acting through the center of resistance "feels" a tendency to rotate, or, a "moment from the applied force."

Couple – Two equal and opposite forces separated by a perpendicular distance. Equal and opposite forces that are not collinear (not in the same line).

Moment of a couple (Figures 8.87 and 8.88) – M_C is the rotational tendency produced by a couple.

Torque (Figure 8.88) – This is the change along the long axis of a body, the "turning moment" of a force or of a set of forces. For example, a "third-order couple" can be created by twisting a wire along its long axis. This will result in crown movement in one direction and root movement in the opposite direction.

Synopsis [1].

All force systems applied to a tooth are composed of single forces and/or couples. The application of a force through the center of resistance of a tooth will result in translation of the tooth. The application of a force to act at points other than through the center of resistance of a tooth will produce different tendencies of tipping and/or rotation. Tooth rotation resulting from the application of a force always creates a simultaneous tendency to move the center of resistance of a tooth in the direction the force is acting. By contrast, the location of a couple on a tooth is irrelevant to the resulting

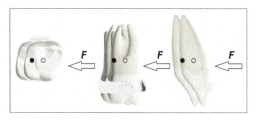

Figure 8.84 A force acting directly in line and through the center of resistance will cause all points on the tooth to move the same amount in that same direction. This is termed translation (Photo by Dr. Robert Isaacson).

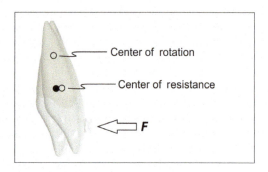

Figure 8.85 Tooth rotation from a kinematic perspective describes rotation from time 1 to time 2 as movement around a center of rotation. Note that the center or resistance moves in the direction that the force is acting (Photo by Dr. Robert Isaacson).

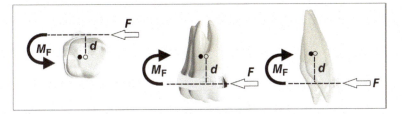

Figure 8.86 A tooth that receives a force not acting through the CRes feels a moment or tendency to rotate. The magnitude of this moment is measured as the magnitude of the force times the perpendicular distance from the line of the force to the CRes and is expressed in force × distance units, $MF = F \times d$. First-, second-, and third-order rotations are shown (Photo by Dr. Robert Isaacson).

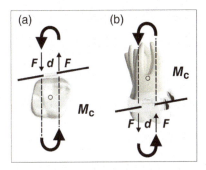

Figure 8.87 Moment of a couple (M_C) resulting in first-order (a) and second-order rotations (b). The two forces of the couple on each bracket are located equidistant from the CRes. The CRes and the center of rotation will be coincident. $M_C = F \times d$ (Photo by Dr. Robert Isaacson).

tooth movement. A couple can never move the center of resistance, and with a couple the center of rotation and the center of resistance will always be coincident. All tooth movement must be either translation and/or rotation as defined at the tooth's center of resistance.

The principles of physical science that control tooth movement are best applied to orthodontic procedures using basic well-established concepts.

8.39.1 Center of mass and center of resistance (Figures 8.84 and 8.85) [1–3]

Imagine a tooth as a motionless free body in space. Any force directed through the tooth's "center of mass" would cause the entire tooth to move in the direction of the applied force (Figure 8.84). A force acting through the center of mass results in a movement where all points on the tooth move the same amount in the same direction. This type of orthodontic tooth movement is termed **translation** or **bodily**

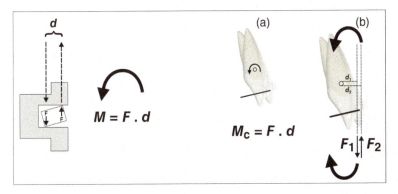

Figure 8.88 Moment of a couple (M_C) resulting in a third-order rotation where the two forces of the couple are not located equidistant from the CRes. No matter where the couple is located on the tooth, the CRes is always coincident with the center of rotation (Photo by Dr. Robert Isaacson).

movement. However, the *in vivo* tooth is not a free body because it is restrained from movement by its attachments to the supporting tissues. Therefore, the point at which all resistance to displacement may be thought of as concentrated is not at its center of mass but at its **center of resistance (CRes)** (Figure 8.84). The reality of *in vivo* tooth movement is that it is difficult to apply a force perfectly in line with the center of resistance. Therefore, we observe various tendencies for teeth to tip or rotate (various moments) around a center of rotation (Figure 8.85), and the center or resistance will move in the direction that the force is acting.

8.39.2 Orders of tooth movements and orthodontic terminology [1–3]

When an arch wire applies a force to displace a tooth, the tooth can respond with translation, rotation, or a combination of these two movements. The generic term "rotation" is used with more specific orthodontic applications as described below.

First-order rotation or rotation around a long axis of a tooth. In orthodontics, this is referred to as rotation of a tooth or of teeth (Figure 8.87a).

Second-order rotation or rotation around a facio-lingual axis of a tooth or teeth. This is referred to as **tip** in orthodontics (Figure 8.87b).

Third-order rotation or rotation around a mesiodistal axis of an anterior tooth, which is referred to as **torque** in orthodontics. Technically, the term torque refers to change along the long axis of a body. In orthodontics what we are actually doing is "torquing" the wire which causes a third-order tipping response of the tooth (Figure 8.88).

8.39.3 Force systems [1–3]

The force systems of arch wires are analyzed in terms of fundamental building blocks. These building blocks are either **single-point forces** or pairs of equal and opposite forces that are separated by a perpendicular distance (noncollinear). These noncollinear forces are called **couples**.

8.39.4 Single-point force and moment of force

A single-point force applied to a tooth has both a magnitude and a direction. If a single force could be directed perfectly through the CRes, the tooth feels a tendency to translate or to displace all points on the tooth the same amount in the same direction as the applied force (Figure 8.84). Only forces are capable of moving the CRes of a tooth. *In vivo*, it is difficult for a single-point force to be directly through the CRes. When a force does not act through the CRes of a tooth, the tooth rotates (Figure 8.85). The rotational tendency, or moment, produced by a force not acting through the CRes, is expressed as **moment of the force** (M_F Figure 8.85). The magnitude of the M_F is measured as the magnitude of the force (F) multiplied by the perpendicular distance (d) between the line of the force and the center of resistance ($M_F = F \times d$). In orthodontic applications, it is conventional to express the units of a M_F in terms of the force multiplied by a distance, that is, g·mm. Actually, the use of g·mm to express moments is an orthodontic convention. Grams are units of mass and not properly used to express forces. Forces are properly expressed as Newton. The conversion factors are: $1\,g = 0.00981\,N$ or $1\,N = 101.937\,g$.

8.39.5 Additive and subtractive couples [1–3]

An arch wire may also send a signal to the periodontium for tooth movement via a pair of equal and opposite forces which are separated by a perpendicular distance. This force system is termed a "couple." When a couple is applied to an object and the object responds by tipping or rotating the term we use "moment of the couple" or "moment from the couple"

(Figures 8.87 and 8.88). The force system of a couple is the sum of the force systems of the two equal and opposite single forces that comprise the couple. Alone, each force of a couple would move the CRes in the direction of the force as described for the single-point force. Because the two forces are equal and opposite, each force tends to move the CRes in an equal and opposite direction. *Therefore, no movement of the CRes can result from the application of a couple to a tooth, no matter where the couple is applied on the tooth.* When the lines of force of each of the two forces of the couple are located equidistant from the CRes both forces of the couple tend to rotate the tooth in the same direction around the CRes. These are termed "additive forces" (Figure 8.87). Even when the lines of force of the two forces of the couple are not located equidistant from the CRes, they still produce essentially the same tendency for rotation of the tooth.

In Figure 8.88b, a third-order couple is located at a bracket with the line of force of each of the forces of the couple acting at different distances from the CRes. The force nearest the CRes produces a smaller moment or tendency for rotation in a clockwise direction because the force is multiplied by a smaller perpendicular distance to the CRes. The force located further from the CRes produces a larger moment or tendency for rotation in an opposite counterclockwise direction because the force is multiplied by a larger perpendicular distance to the CRes. When the moment for clockwise rotation is **subtracted** from the moment for counterclockwise rotation, the remainder is a moment in a counterclockwise direction. This is essentially the same response as if the couple were positioned with the two forces equidistant from the CRes similar to those shown in Figure 8.88. Keep in mind that after subtraction of the forces, the remaining force is acting at a large distance from the CRes. Therefore, when a couple is applied to a bracket, *the resulting type of tooth rotation* is unaffected by the location of the bracket on the tooth or what torque is built into the bracket.

That is, the tooth can only respond to a couple with rotation around its CRes.

The rotational tendency produced by a couple is also referred to as a moment or the **moment of the couple**, M_C (Figures 8.87 and 8.88). The magnitude of the M_C is equal to the sum of the moments of the two equal and opposite single forces that comprise the couple. Therefore, the magnitude of the M_C equals the magnitude of one of the forces of the couple multiplied by the distance between the two forces of the couple. The uniqueness of the edgewise appliance arises from its ability to generate couples in three planes. No matter where a bracket is placed on a tooth, when a couple is applied at that bracket it can only cause the tooth to feel a tendency to rotate around its center of resistance. A couple alone will tend to not cause the center of resistance to move in any direction and the center of rotation and the center of resistance will always be coincident.

8.39.6 Equilibrium and tooth movement – Newton's third law [1–3]

Newton's third law requires that for every action there be **an equal and opposite reaction**. This is easy to visualize for single-point forces when a given wire is pressed against an identical wire and both wires deform equally in opposite directions. When the wires are of unequal resistance, the weaker wire will deform more, but both wires will still be pushing with equal and opposite magnitudes of force. **Equilibrium requires that the sum of the forces acting in any plane is equal to zero**. Equilibrium consists of a balance and requires that the sum of the moments in any plane equals zero. When an arch wire engages a bracket to create a couple at that bracket, the tooth feels a tendency for rotation around its CRes. The couple at the bracket is activated by bending or twisting the arch wire between the bracket and the next attachment of the arch wire. This creates strain in the wire to either move the bracket or the other end of the wire until the wire is again passive.

Although the couple created at the bracket results in a moment in one direction, the forces at the ends of the activated arch wire represent another couple with a moment in an opposite direction. The magnitude of the moment created by the couple at the bracket must be equal and opposite to the moment created by the associated equilibrium forces at the attached ends of the arch wire. This is equilibrium. Because the total force system present during equilibrium is difficult to visualize and is not intuitive, component parts can be overlooked and produce unexpected clinical tooth movements.

8.39.7 Force systems and tooth movements [1]

Arch wire bends, no matter how complex, send a message to the tooth consisting of a single force and/or a couple. The tooth can respond only with translatory and/or a combination of rotational movements. If it were possible to apply an isolated and single force acting exactly through the CRes, then tooth translation without rotation could occur (Figure 8.84).

Rotation occurs when a couple is applied to a bracket and the tooth feels the moment of a couple (M_C) (Figures 8.87 and 8.88). Atypical clinical example shown in Figure 8.89 is a single force directed at the bracket on a tooth attached to a continuous arch wire as shown. This force results in a moment of force (M_F) tending to move the CRes in the direction of the force and also to rotate the tooth around its CRes. To counteract this tendency of the tooth to tip in a clockwise direction, the edgewise bracket is designed to engage a second-order couple to rotate the tooth in the opposite, counterclockwise, direction. A perfect balance between the tendency of the M_F to rotate the tooth in a clockwise direction and the tendency of the M_C to rotate the tooth in a counterclockwise direction would produce tooth translation. In applied orthodontic terminology, this

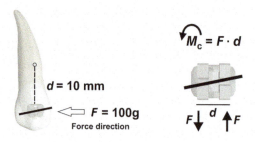

$M_F = F \cdot d = 100\,g \cdot 10\,mm = 1000\,g \cdot mm$

Figure 8.89 Canine retraction with 100-g force acting 10-mm coronal to the CRes creates a positive M_F of 1000 g mm. The edgewise appliance engages a second-order couple at the bracket that must create a negative 1000 g mm M_C to avoid distal crown tipping (Photo by Dr. Robert Isaacson).

relationship is expressed as a ratio of the M_C to the F that produces the M_F, or the moment-to-force ratio, M/F. For example, in Figure 8.89, canine translation is desired and a force of 100 g is applied 10-mm coronal to the center of resistance. This will tend to move the center of resistance in the direction of the force vector. Because the force is not acting through the center of resistance, a tendency for the crown to tip, or M_F, will also be present, and the crown will tip in the direction that the force is acting. The moment or tendency to rotate in this direction is quantified as 100 g × 10 mm = 1000 g·mm. The tooth will rotate to the degree that a couple is triggered in the edgewise bracket. Once the tooth tips enough to engage the couple, a tendency to rotate the tooth in the opposite direction of the single point force is provided by an M_C created by a second-order couple at the bracket. If the bracket is 4 mm long, an arch wire would have to exert 250 g at each end of the bracket to create the necessary M_C of 1000 g·mm of rotation in the opposite direction. If this could be achieved, all tendencies for rotation would be eliminated. Rather than a combination of a moment of force and moment of couple, the final results and net tooth movement (a combination of tipping and up righting) could then appear as translation in the direction of the applied force.

8.39.8 Mixed dentition example of one tube (bracket) and one couple system

(Figures 8.90–8.93)
A 0.018 slot with 0.016 stainless steel intrusion arch – base arch segment at the lower incisors is 16×16 stainless steel tied in the midline with 0.010 stainless steel ligature.

Consider a force system on **one side of the mouth only**. The simplest arrangement of an orthodontic force system involving a couple is an arch wire developing a single couple at one bracket. In a single-bracket system (the molar tube), one end of the arch wire is inserted into the tube with an activation bend located close to this attachment. This is shown in Figure 8.90, Patient 1 Time 1, where the activation bend is a "crown tip-back" bend at the lower second primary molar. The other end of the wire is displaced and tied with a stainless steel ligature between the lower central incisors. This is shown where the overlay wire is tied only in the midline between the central incisors. When the activated wire is tied at the point contact between the central incisors, the arch wire engages the molar tubes and two equal and opposite forces form the couple. One of the forces acts in the front of the tube and the equal and opposite force acts at the back of the tube. This couple produces an M_C or tendency to rotate the molar around its CRes. When a couple creates an M_C at a single tube, it is important to know the direction of the moment at that tube in order to know the direction of the forces of the associated equilibrium. With a one-tube, one-couple system, a useful clinical estimate of the direction of the moment created by the couple is possible by placing one end of an arch wire over, but not in, the tube where it is to be inserted. Place the other end of the wire at the location where it will be tied as a single-point contact (between the lower

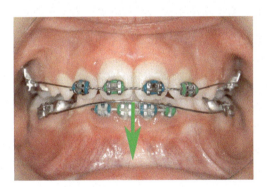

Figure 8.90   Patient 1 Time 1.

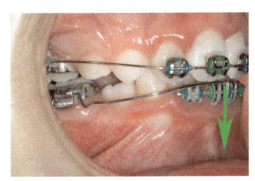

Figure 8.92   Patient 2 Time 1.

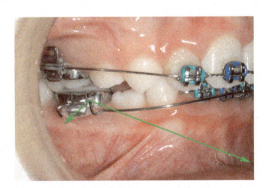

Figure 8.91   Patient 1 Time 2.

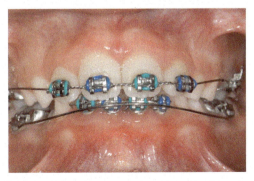

Figure 8.93   Patient 2 Time 2.

central incisors). At the molars, when the wire crosses the tube at an angle (Figure 8.90. Patient 1 Time 1), the tube may be visualized as rotating to the wire, and this is the direction of the moment that will be created. Knowing the direction of the moment at the tube permits identification of the direction of the forces in the associated equilibrium. The magnitude of the forces and moments in a one-couple system can be estimated clinically by measuring the force required to deform the wire for the tie at the anterior point contact. This force multiplied by the distance between the bracket and the point attachment of the arch wire equals a moment, which is equal and opposite in direction to the M_C at the bracket. To estimate the magnitude of each of the forces of the couple at the tube, divide the magnitude of this moment by the length of the tube.

The crown tip-back molar treatment response can be seen in Figure 8.91, Patient 1 Time 2, and incisor intrusion.

8.39.9 Mixed dentition: maxillary anterior root convergence

Comparing mixed to permanent dentition orthodontic treatment, when the maxillary permanent cuspids have not emerged, it is essential to converge rather than diverge roots of the maxillary lateral incisors. This is most predictably accomplished by "switching" the lateral incisor brackets by placing the maxillary left lateral bracket on the right lateral incisor and the maxillary right lateral bracket on the left incisor (Figures 8.94–8.99).

8.39.10 Orthodontic treatment of teeth with open apices

Fenn [4] analyzed orthodontic effects on maxillary incisors with open apices. Thirty patient with mean ages of 7.9 years were compared with a matched nontreated control group of 33 patients. The paired *t*-test indicated no significant differences in total root lengths of maxillary central and lateral incisors.

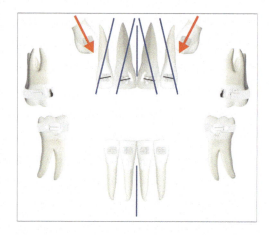

Figure 8.94 Mixed dentition root convergence. This is achieved by mesial gingival slot angulations of the maxillary anterior permanent incisors.

8.39.11 Two brackets – two equal and oppositely directed couples

Figure 8.100 [1–3]

When the M_C at each of two successive brackets are equal and opposite, their associated equilibrium forces at each bracket are also equal and opposite and function to cancel each other out and are subtractive in nature (Figure 8.95). This is sometimes referred to as a symmetrical V-bend, and it is assumed that it is placed equidistant between two collinear brackets. A symmetrical V is used when equal and opposite moments are desired at two successive teeth, and the forces of the equilibrium associated with each moment are not wanted. For a symmetrical V-bend to develop equal and opposite couples at two brackets, it is necessary that the brackets are collinear with the bracket slots in alignment with each other. Because malocclusions commonly show asymmetrically positioned or noncollinear brackets on the teeth, equal and opposite moments at two successive brackets often will not result from a V-bend placed equidistant between two brackets. The important point is not the location of the V-bend. Rather, it is the creation of equal and opposite moments at the two successive brackets. Equal and opposite moments are accomplished by adjusting the angle of entry

8.39 Definitions and terminology | **321**

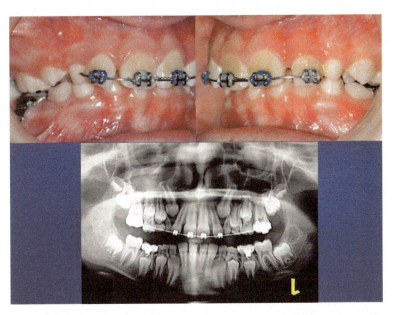

Figure 8.95 Mixed dentition root convergence. The maxillary centrals have "0" angulation. The maxillary laterals have been "switched" right to left and left to right, resulting in root convergence toward the midline.

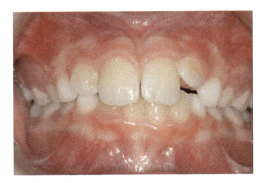

Figure 8.96 Time 1 mixed dentition anterior alignment.

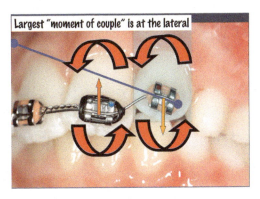

Figure 8.97 Time 1 mixed dentition anterior alignment using 0.012 nitinol wire anterior segment. Note additive moments of couples and reactive vertical forces.

of the arch wire until it is equal and opposite when the wire is placed over the two bracket slots before insertion (Figures 8.101–8.103).

8.39.12 Two brackets – two unequal oppositely directed couples

Figure 8.104 [1–3]

For clinical purposes, the effect of unequal and oppositely directed couples (subtractive) at two successive brackets may be thought of as the algebraic sum of the two single-bracket systems present. The relative magnitude of the moments at two successive teeth is approximated clinically by examining the wire passively placed over the two bracket slots. *The bracket with the larger angle of entry, and therefore the larger M_C, will have a greater tendency to rotate than the bracket with the smaller M_C. When the directions of M_C at two successive brackets are unequal and in opposite*

8.7 Section VII: Mixed dentition orthodontic mechanics

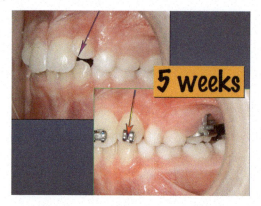

Figure 8.98 Time 1 and Time 2 mixed dentition anterior alignment using 0.012 nitinol wire anterior segment at 5 weeks.

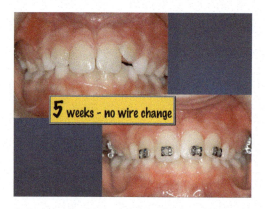

Figure 8.99 Time 1 and Time 2 mixed dentition anterior alignment using 0.012 nitinol anterior wire segment.

directions (subtractive), the larger of the two moments will determine the direction of the associated equilibrium forces. At each tooth, the magnitude of the equilibrium force associated with the larger M_C at each tooth will be modified by the equilibrium forces associated with the smaller M_C (subtractive). Each bracket will feel the net difference (Figure 8.104). This wire configuration is referred to as an asymmetrical V- or off-center bend, but it is not a question of where the V is located. The critical factor is the resulting orientation of the wire to each bracket slot. *This angle of entry determines the larger moment created and, therefore, the direction of the equilibrium forces present.*

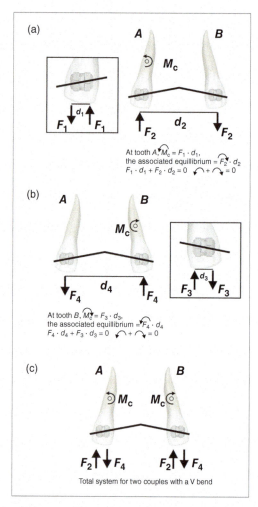

Figure 8.100 Forces and moments present in a two-bracket, two-couple system. (a) The M_C, $F_L \times d_1$ and its associated equilibrium, $F_2 \times d_2$, resulting from the engagement of the arch wire in tooth A. (b) The equal and opposite M_C, $F_3 \times d_3$, and the associated equilibrium, $F_4 \times d_4$, resulting from the engagement of the arch wire in tooth B. (c) The total system effect on the two teeth that is a combination of the separate effects shown in A and B (Photo by Dr. Robert Isaacson).

8.39.13 Two brackets – two "same direction, additive" couples including increased anterior incisor root torque

Figure 8.105 shows the equivalent of using an *extrusion* utility type arch plus torquing arch simultaneously. When the M_C at two

8.39 Definitions and terminology | 323

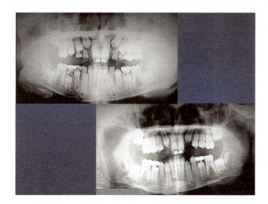

Figure 8.101 A case with congenitally missing permanent maxillary lateral incisors: clinical use of a centered gable bend segment used to converge roots of the central incisors away from developing permanent cuspids. Two adjustments at 6-week intervals.

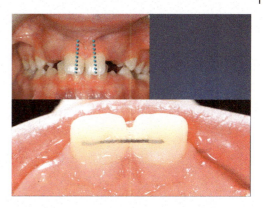

Figure 8.103 Overcorrected positions of the central incisors and bonded lingual wire retainer. Note the emerging maxillary right permanent cuspid.

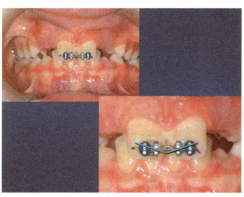

Figure 8.102 Clinical use of a centered gable bend 16 × 22 stainless steel segment with helical loop. This is used to converge the roots of the central incisors away from developing permanent cuspids with helical loop increases the range of wire dynamics. The blue lines represent the approximate angles of entry into the central incisor slots. The central incisor brackets have been tied together with stainless steel ligature. As the crowns begin to separate, the steel ligature creates a "new force" acting toward the midline causing the roots to upright and movement of the center of resistance of each central incisor toward the midline.

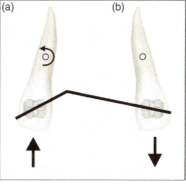
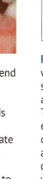

Figure 8.104 Two-bracket, two-couple system with an asymmetrical V-bend in the arch wire. This shows that the angle of entry is larger at Tooth a and creates a larger moment of couple at tooth a. This determines the direction of the associated equilibrium forces at a and b. The smaller oppositely directed moment at tooth b has smaller associated equilibrium forces that function to decrease the larger equilibrium forces associated with tooth a (subtractive force). Therefore, the overall response is for extrusion of tooth b, intrusion of Tooth a, large distal root rotation at tooth a, and slight distal root rotation at tooth b (Photo by Dr. Robert Isaacson).

successive brackets is in the same direction their associated equilibrium forces at both brackets are also in the same direction. Each tooth will feel the net result or the sum of the forces present. This configuration of a wire is sometimes referred to as a step bend and is basically two V-bends creating couples, moments, and resulting forces in the same directions (additive forces). When third-order couples for crown facial root lingual

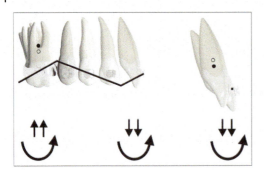

Figure 8.105 Two-bracket, two-couple system with additive force step bends in the wire. Both anterior and posterior couples act in the same (additive) directions. These are referred to as "additive couples." These couples generate associated equilibrium forces acting in the same vertical, additive directions (Photo by Dr Robert Isaacson).

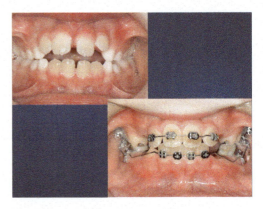

Figure 8.106 Mixed dentition lower incisor "additive force" extrusion utility arch using 16 × 22 stainless steel. In an attempt to decrease mesial crown rotation (tipping) of the second primary molars (E), resistance segments were placed, linking the first permanent molars into the system. Note the differences in rotational response at the lower right and left second primary molars.

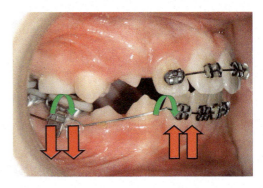

Figure 8.107 Additive system mechanics and approximate schematic vectors present in the system. In an attempt to decrease primary molar rotation and to enhance incisor extrusion 16 × 22 stainless steel "resistance segments" were placed from the second primary (E) to lower first permanent molars. This had some positive resistance effect at the lower right second primary. In addition, and as a result of incisor extrusion, subtractive forces (lingual crown rotations) are present at the lower incisors.

movement are applied to all of the incisor brackets, the facial crown movement appears clinically to manifest more rapidly than the lingual root movement. This is because the incisal edge is further away from the CRes than the root apex and, for any given number of degrees of rotation, the incisal edge will move a greater linear distance than the root apex. The apparent rapidity of incisor crown advancement with rotation around the CRes makes the torquing arch a valuable tool for anterior crossbite correction.

8.39.14 Clinical application – mixed dentition openbite, two "same direction, additive" couples including increased anterior incisor root torque

Figure 8.106 demonstrates the clinical application during the mixed dentition. The lower second primary (deciduous) molars are banded, and substantial mesial crown and distal root rotation of the molars are anticipated. In an attempt to decrease molar rotation and enhance incisor extrusion 16 × 22 stainless steel "resistance segments" were placed from the second primary to lower first permanent molars. Likely due to wire/tube interface "play" at the utility tube interface, this had some positive resistance effect at the lower right second primary molar (Figure 8.107). As shown in Figure 8.108, the lower left second primary molar showed substantial mesial crown and distal root rotations. This may have

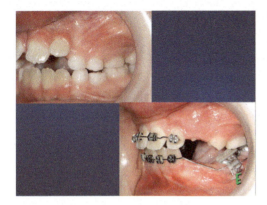

Figure 8.108 Mixed dentition lower incisor extrusion using 16 × 22 stainless steel. The lower left second primary molar (E) showed substantial mesial crown and distal root rotations. This may have been due to emergence of the lower left second bicuspid and subsequent root shrinkage of the primary molar (see Figure 8.109).

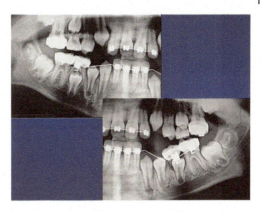

Figure 8.109 Emergence of the lower left second bicuspid and subsequent root resorption of the primary molar may have allowed more mesial crown rotation on the left side. No obvious negative effect on the vertical emergence path of the lower left second bicuspid is seen.

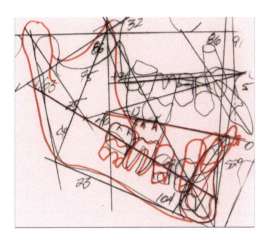

Figure 8.110 Superimposing on the corpus at PM point (Ricketts's method) reveals extrusion of the mandibular incisors. As desired by the clinician, the additive force extrusion utility arch can be adjusted for more or less lingual root/facial crown rotation (torque).

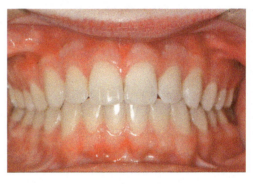

Figure 8.111 Two-year postorthodontic treatment. Using maxillary and mandibular fixed appliances, the patient received a short second phase of orthodontic detailing and finishing. This image was made 2-year posttreatment. The patient wears removable vacuum formed retainers two or three nights per week. No fixed lingual retention was used for this patient.

been due to the emergence of the lower left second bicuspid and subsequent root shrinkage of the primary tooth. Figure 8.109 shows no obvious effect on the vertical emergence path of the lower left second bicuspid. Figures 8.110 and 8.111 demonstrate cephalometric and dental alveolar changes, respectively. Figure 8.112 shows 2-year post-phase 2 facial balance.

The author would like to thank Dr. Robert Isaacson for allowing the use and modification of his excellent materials.

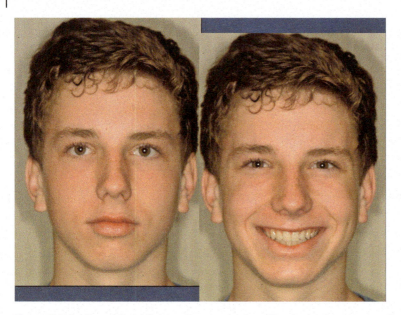

Figure 8.112 Dental facial balance 2-year postphase 2 orthodontic treatment. Smile arc is within acceptable limits.

References

1 Isaacson RJ. *Seminars in orthodontics journal, Vol 1, No 1*. Chicago, USA: Elsevier Publications, 1995 Mar.
2 Mulligan TF. *Common sense mechanics in everyday orthodontics II*. Phoenix, AZ: CSM Publishing, 2009.
3 Marcotte MR. *Biomechanics in orthodontics*. Philadelphia, PA: BC Decker, 1990.
4 Fenn KM. The effect of fixed orthodontic treatment on developing maxillary incisor root apices. *Am J Orthod* 1998;**114**(5):A1.

Index

a

achondroplasia 37
additive and subtractive couples 316–17
additive couples 322–6
adenoidectomies 122
adenoids 302–4
adenoids, enlarged 303–4
adenotonsillectomy 310
aesthetic concerns 109
  delayed eruption of maxillary incisors 241, 246
agenesis (congenitally missing teeth) 274, 278
airway interferences 121
alignment problems, anterior mandibular 60–3
allergic rhinitis 122
allergies and respiratory infections 304–5
altered eruption 44–6
altered tooth number 42–3
altered tooth structure 43–4
alveolar bone 279, 281–2
alveolus 258, 278
amelogenesis imperfecta (AI) 37, 43, 47
American Academy of Pediatric Dentistry 286
American Academy of Sleep Medicine (AASM) 310
American Association of Orthodontists (AAO) 7
American Association of Pediatric Dentistry 5
American Board of Orthodontics (ABO) 29–31
American Board of Orthodontics complexity index and outcome assessment 29–31
anesthesia 277, 303
Angle's Class II malocclusion 286
ankylosis 94, 240–1, 290
anodontia 42
anterior crossbite 15, 17, 19, 21, 23
anterior incisor root torque, increased 322–4
anterior mandibular malalignment 60–3
  contact displacements 62–3
  eruption problems 61–2
  predisposing factors 60–1
anterior maxilla transplantation 279
anterior open bite 29, 30, 32, 72, 225, 229
anterior root convergence, maxillary 320
anteroposterior (AP) categories/positions 107
apices, open, orthodontic treatment of teeth with 320
apnea-hypopnea index (AHI) 301
Araújo approach 227–9, 232
arch wire bends 318
arch wires and orthodontic mechanics 313–26
arch(es), dental
  dimensional changes
    deciduous teeth at stage 1 11
    deciduous teeth at stage 2 13–14
    deciduous teeth at stage 4 18–19
    lip bumper therapy 84
    serial extraction and 94–5
  length/size of
    crowding and 61
    serial extraction (in severe tooth size arch length discrepancy) and deficiency of 92–102
  size. *see* size
  recognizing and correcting deviations (changes of form) within 51–63
  skeletal relationships between, and class III malocclusion 51–63
autotransplantation of premolars. *see* premolar autotransplantation

axial inclination 62
AXIN2 mutation 42

b

backward rotators 118
banded expander 190
Baume
   type I occlusion 11
   type II occlusion 11
Berlin questionnaire 300–1
bilateral crossbite 142
biogenesis of deciduous
   teeth 9–11
bionator therapy 117
bite-jumping appliances 139
bodily movement 315–16
bodily movements (translation),
   mixed dentition 314
body mass index (BMI) 304
Bolton ratios/relationships
   class II malocclusions
   119, 120
   class III malocclusions 173
Bolton tooth-size
   discrepancy 119
bonded expander 190
B-point 111
bracket removal 293
brackets with mixed dentition
   one 319–20
   two 321–2
Brodie bite 148
Brodsky scale 302
bruxism 15
buccal crossbite 31, 72, 148
buccal hooks on maxillary
   expanders 191

c

canines 96
   deciduous 10, 13, 15, 17, 19,
   72, 93, 95, 219
   eruption 9
   serial extraction and
   premature loss of 93
   intercanine width changes
   (from 6 to 16 years
   of age) 55–6
   permanent, eruption
   17, 20–1, 94
CBFA1 mutation 38
cementum-enamel junction
   290
center of resistance (CRes)
   314, 316
center of rotation 314, 315, 317
central sleep apnea (CSA) 299
cephalometric changes 153
cephalometric data 76, 78,
   142, 150
cephalometric diagnosis 183
cephalometric film 142
cephalometry, class III
   malocclusion
   diagnosis 199
chincup orthopedics
   191–4
chincups 156
chondrocranium 119, 172
chromosomal abnormalities
   37
chromosomal anomalies 47
cleft lip ± palate 39
cleidocranial dysplasia
   (CCD) 37, 38
clinical examination 35–6
clinical stages, of occlusion
   development
   deciduous dentition
   12–17
   deciduous teeth,
   eruption of 9–11
   mandibular canines and first
   premolars 20–1
   maxillary canines and second
   molars 23–4
   permanent molars, eruption
   of 16–20
   second premolars,
   eruption of 21–3
Cochrane systematic
   review 287
cognitive functions 306
communication to family in
   class III malocclusion
   187–8
complexity of treatment,
   assessing 27–31
computed tomography
   (CT) 252
cone-beam computed
   tomography
   (CBCT) 273
contact displacements
   62–3
continuous positive airway
   pressure (CPAP)
   therapy 310
contract displacements 62–3
contralateral permanent
   maxillary central
   incisor 245
convergence, maxillary anterior
   root 320
corpus length (corpus
   LT) 113, 116
couples 314, 316
   additive and subtractive
   couples 316–17
   moment of 318, 323
   Newton's third law 317–18
   one-couple system 319–20
   second-order 318
   third-order 314
cranial base/CB 111, 116, 117,
   121, 163
craniofacial inheritance 187
craniofacial microsomia
   (CFM) 40, 42
craniosynostosis 40
crooked teeth 155
crossbite
   anterior 15, 17, 19, 21, 23
   buccal 72, 135
   elastics 148
   lingual 72
crowding 54–6
   and irregularities 61
   in mixed dentition. *see* mixed
   dentition
crowns, implant-
   supported 258, 259
cusp-to-cusp relationship
   17, 51, 70

d

deciduous dentition
  biogenesis 9–11
  normal characteristics of 12
deciduous mandibular cuspids 247
deciduous maxillary canines 95–6
deciduous maxillary incisors 246
decoronation technique 290–2, 294, 297
deep bite 155
Delaire chincup 191
delayed tooth eruption (DTE) 239–40
Dental Aesthetic Index (DAI) 28
dental diagnosis 183–4
dental eruption 38
dental follicle 279
dental imbalance 137
dental malocclusion 216
dental procumbency 137
dental protraction 137
dental protrusion 137
dental trauma
  decoronation approach 288, 290–7
  orthodontic treatment 286–9
  overview of 285–6
dental traumatic injuries (DTI) 285, 287, 288
dentinogenesis imperfecta (DGI) 43
dentoalveolar compensations 63
dentofacial orthopedics 2
diagnosis
  cephalometric diagnosis 183
  class III malocclusion 183–7
  dental diagnosis 183–4
  facial diagnosis 183
  functional diagnosis 184–5
  hereditary diagnosis 185–8
  OSA and SDB 300–2

diamond drill 290
diastema 4
discrepancy index (DI) 29, 139
Down syndrome 305
drug-induced sleep endoscopy (DISE) 302
dyslexia 142
dysmorphology 36–7

e

ectodermal dysplasia (ED) 42
ectopic eruption 239, 240
efficacy, defined 27
electric pulp testing (EPT) 279
endodontics 285, 295
enlarged tonsils 302–4
environmental factors 3, 23, 24, 38, 41, 43, 75, 121, 239
eruption deviations
  ankylosis 240–1
  delayed tooth eruption (DTE) 239–40
  ectopic eruption 239, 240
  and PIOM
    completion of deciduous dentition 241, 242
    mandibular canines and first premolars 242, 247–8
    maxillary canines 249–52
    maxillary first permanent molar ectopic eruption 242–4
    permanent incisors 244, 245
    second molars 249–52
    second premolars 247–9
  sequence, changes in 239, 240
  tooth ankylosis 239–41
E-space maintenance 21–2
exaggerated overjet 308
excessive daytime sleepiness 305
external apical root resorption (EARR) 47
extraction. see serial extraction

f

face mask 21, 191–4
facial analysis 148
facial convexity 286
facial diagnosis 183
familial microsomia 40
fibrous dysplasia (FD) 45, 46
first-order rotation 316
force 314
  moment of 314–16
  single point 316
force systems 316, 318
full orthodontics treatment 145
functional appliances 117, 136, 139, 167
functional defects 107, 161
functional diagnosis 184–5

g

general dentistry 295
genetic defects
  altered eruption 44–6
  altered tooth number 42–3
  altered tooth structure 43–4
  chromosomal abnormalities 37
  clinical examination 35–6
  dysmorphology 36–7
  multifactorial inheritance 38–42
  nonsyndromic malocclusion 40–1
  personalized medicine 35
  radiographic deviations 45–7
  single gene defects 38–9
gingival recession and alveolar destruction 93
gonial angle 114, 115, 118, 122, 166
gubernaculum dentis 239

h

Haas-type expander 190, 191
Hawley appliance 75, 193, 293
hemifacial microsomia (HFM) 42

hereditary diagnosis 185–8
Hickham chincup 191, 199
home sleep apnea testing (HSAT) 301
hybrid expanders 191
hyperdivergence 115, 122
hyperdivergent retrognathic phenotype 121
hypodontia 40, 42
hypohidrotic ectodermal dysplasia (HED) 42

i

imaging tests 302
implant-supported crowns 258, 259
incisor morphology 281
Index of Complexity, Outcome, and Need (ICON) 29
Index of Orthodontic Treatment Need (IOTN) 28
inferior mandibular displacement 58
informed consent 94, 187–8
interceptive treatment 3, 6, 23, 24, 27
intraoral radiographs 280
Iowa Growth Study 53

j

jaw
  abnormal jaw kinematic patterns 109
  growth and position 310
  lower 53, 115, 117, 174, 306, 308
  size 61–2
  upper 308
  vertical growth displacement 58
Johnston, Lysle 131
juvenile growth spurt 17
juvenile periodontitis 45

k

keratinized gingiva 278

l

Leeway spaces 55, 70–2, 194
lingual crossbite 30, 52, 72
lingual tonsil hypertrophy 303
lip
  bumper 59, 83, 84, 89
  cleft lip ± palate 39
local anaesthesia in premolar autotransplantation 277
long face syndrome 306, 308
loss
  of arch perimeter 118
  ectopic eruption of molars 94
  lip seal 183
  of upper incisor 274
lower holding lingual arches (LHLA) 21
lower incisor inclinations 114
lower lingual holding arches (LLHAs) 252
lowered mandibular posture 122

m

malalignment, anterior mandibular 60–3
  contact displacements 62–3
  eruption problems 61–2
  predisposing factors 60–1
malocclusion 5
  American Board of Orthodontics (ABO) 29–31
  class I malocclusion 31
    anterior mandibular malalignment 60–3
    crowding, in mixed dentition. *see* mixed dentition
    dental compensatory mechanism 58–9
    development of 52
    maxillary and mandibular malalignments 51
    mixed-dentition arch analysis 52
    prevalence 52–8
    tooth size arch length discrepancies (TSALD) 51, 67–8
  class II malocclusion 15–19, 21, 23, 31–2
    anteroposterior and vertical deviations. 137
    Brodie bite, buccal crossbite 135
    development of 108
    developmental changes 115–19
    distal step adaptation 136
    division 1 phenotype 111–15
    division 2 phenotype 110–11
    etiology 119–23
    extreme crowding and protrusion 133
    hyperdivergence, accentuated protrusion 134
    indications 131–2
    normal growth and development 134
    open bite, severe hyperdivergence, unilateral crossbite 135
    prevalence 109–10
    psychological problems 132
    severe deep bite, crowding 133
    traumatic injury 132
    treatment selection 137
  class III malocclusion 6, 16, 18, 19, 21, 23, 32–3
    cephalometric analysis 205
    cephalometry 199
    characterization of 163–7
    chincup for bed time 196
    communication 187–8
    CR/CO discrepancy 195–6
    dental crossbite 212

Index

detrimental facial esthetics 161
development of 162
diagnosis 183–7
early intervention 188–90
emotional well-being 182
etiology 170–4
face mask and/or chincup orthopedics 191–4
facemask therapy 214
finishing 194–5
functional diagnosis 202
growth reevaluation 196–220
habit, breakage of 227–9
induced cranium deformation 182
intraoral composite of 181
Leeway space control 194
mandibular premolars 200
masticatory function of 162
maxillary expansion and protraction 216
modified Hawley 207
nonsurgical approaches 179
nonsurgical procedure 199
normal occlusion 162
open bite with premature contact 219
orthodontic mechanics 194
orthopedic resources 182
overbite and overjet 208, 215
permanent occlusion 197
pretreatment records 207
prevalence of 163
protocols 183
protraction Hickham chincup 199
protrusive mandibles 161
retention 195–6
self-esteem evaluation 180
skeletal components of 161
tongue physiology 226–7
tongue thrusting and forward resting posture 227
treatment 229–35
untreated premature contacts 182
Wits appraisal 169–70
Dental Aesthetic Index (DAI) 28
Index of Complexity, Outcome, and Need (ICON) 29
Index of Orthodontic Treatment Need (IOTN) 28
Peer Assessment Rating (PAR) 28
Summers' occlusal index 28
mandibular arch 212, 247
mandibular canines 97
mandibular canines and first premolars 20–1
mandibular deciduous incisors 9
mandibular first premolars 96
mandibular incisors 122
mandibular irregularities 52
mandibular lip bumper 155
mandibular permanent incisors 18
mandibular plane angles (MPAs) 110, 114
mandibular posture 122
mandibular retrognathism 137
mandibular second molars 245
mandibular second premolars 249
Marfan syndrome 38
marked mesial inclination 247
Maryland bridge delivery 295
maxillary arch 21
maxillary canines
  permanent canines 251
  and second molars 23–4
  spontaneous eruption 251
maxillary crowding 54–6
maxillary cuspids 245
maxillary dental protraction 137
maxillary front teeth 4
maxillary incisors 246
maxillary lateral incisors 4
maxillary protrusion 112, 121
maxillary retrognathism 137
maxillomandibular differential 170
mesial migration 58
methotrexate 40
midface prognathism 137
midline shift 93
mini-screw implant (MSI) 132, 139
minor anomalies 35
mixed dentition
  additive and subtractive couples 316–17
  center of mass 315–16
  center of resistance 315–16
  clinical application 324–6
  dental arches
    arch dimensions changes 84
    arch length and mandibular incisors/MP 84, 85
    arch length and mandibular molar/MP 84
    leeway space/E space 70–2
    maxillary expansion and headgear 73–84
    maxillary transverse deficiency 72–3
    Schwarz appliance 86
    transverse changes 84, 85
    two-by-four fixed therapy 86
  equilibrium and tooth movement 317–18

mixed dentition (cont'd)
  force systems   316
  force systems and tooth movements   318
  maxillary anterior root convergence   320
  one tube (bracket) and one couple system   319–20
  orthodontic treatment   320
  serial extraction
    fundamentals of   92–3
    indications and contraindications for   93–6
  single-point force and moment of force   316
  Tanaka–Johnston analysis   68
  tooth movements and orthodontic terminology   316
  TSALD   69–70
  two brackets–two equal and oppositely directed couples   320–1
  two brackets–two unequal oppositely directed couples   321–2
  unilateral crossbite in   68
modified Mallampati score   302, 303
molar widths   115
moment   314
  of couple   314, 315, 317
  of force   314–16
multifactorial inheritance   38–42
muscular atrophy, spinal   122
myofunctional therapy   310

n

nasal endoscopy   302
nasal septum   172, 173
National Health and Nutrition Examination Survey, Third (NHANES III)   52
NCHS nationwide survey   52
Newton's third law   317–18
nonankylosed primary molars or a   277
nonrapid eye movement (NON-REM) sleep   299
nonsyndromic malocclusion   40–1
nutritional counseling   304
nutritive sucking habits   225–6

o

obesity   304
objective grading system (OGS)   29
obstructive sleep apnea (OSA)   299
  apps and devices for   310
  children, risk factors for   302–5
  classification of   301
  diagnosis and management   300–2
obstructive sleep apnea-18 (OSA-18) questionnaire   300
occlusion development
  deciduous dentition
    dental arches   13–14
    interdental spacing closure in   12
    management, of occlusal development   14–17
    mesiodistal measurements   13
    normal characteristics of   12
  deciduous teeth, eruption of
    biogenesis of deciduous dentition   9–11
    dental arches   11
    management, of occlusal development   11
  mandibular canines and first premolars   20–1
  maxillary canines and second molars   23–4
  permanent molars, eruption of
    dental arches   17–18
    first permanent molar   16–18
    management, of occlusal development   19–20
  second premolars, eruption of   21–3
Online Mendelian Inheritance in Man (OMIM)   35
open apices, orthodontic treatment of teeth with   320
open bite   308
oral habits   14–15, 17, 19, 21, 23
Orofacial clefts (OMIM #119530)   39
orthodontic treatment   247
  agreement and disagreement   2
  clinical decisions   3
  decision-making   1
  early treatment   1–2
    effectiveness and efficiency concepts   3, 6–7
    maturational stage of development   7
    psychological aspects   5
    severity of malocclusion   5–6
  emancipation of   1–2
  follow-up protocol   3
  key questions   2
  occlusal characteristics   3
  occlusal deviations, with indications   3–5
  PIOM program   3
  role of heredity   1
orthodontics   295
otodental dysplasia   47
overeruption   123

p

palatal cribs   309
parathormone   300
parathyroid receptor 1 (PTHR1)   44
patient self-esteem   289

pediatric sleep questionnaire (PSQ)   300
Peer Assessment Rating (PAR)   28
periodontal tissues   279
periodontics   295
permanent central incisor   250
permanent mandibular incisors   245
permanent maxillary lateral incisors   250
permanent maxillary left central incisor   245
personalized medicine   35
Petite chincup   191, 192
Pierre Robin anomaly   40
polysomnography (PSG)   301
postdecoronation   296
posterior bite blocks   156
posterior crossbite   15, 17, 19, 21, 23
premolar autotransplantation
  alveolar bone   281–2
  anterior maxilla transplantation   279
  class II malocclusion and congenitally missing lower second premolars   274
  dental follicle and adjacent gingiva   279
  follow-up   279–80
  labial cortical plate   277
  periodontal healing   281
  postoperative instructions   279
  pulp healing   280–1
  reshaping to incisor morphology   281
  root growth   281
  selection of anesthesia   277
  surgery   277
  surgical burs   278
  traumatic loss of upper incisor/s   274, 276–7
  uneven tooth distribution   274
premolars   96

preventive and interceptive orthodontic monitoring (PIOM)   9
primary failure of eruption (PFE)   43–4
prognathism   137
protrusion   133, 134, 137, 166
protrusive incisors   286
pulp healing   280–1
pulp necrosis   280

q
quality of life (QoL)   5

r
radiographic deviations   45–7
radiographs
  intraoral radiographs   273, 280
  panoramic radiographs   29
randomized clinical trials (RCT)   131
rapid eye movement (REM) sleep   299
resistance segments   324
retention   142
retention records   296–7
retroclination   123
retroclined maxillary central incisors   107
retrognathic mandible   309
retrusion   112
Ricketts's method   325
root formation   246
root growth   281
root malformations   43
rotation   318
rotation (with mixed dentition)
  center of (Crot)   314
  first/second/third-order   316
RUNX2   38

s
sagittal classification   13
Schwarz appliance   86
second deciduous molars   95, 97
second molars   249–52

second premolar teeth
  camouflage approach   262
  class I mixed dentition crowded malocclusion   263
  deciduous molar
    disk and buildup   258
    early permanent dentition   261
    mixed dentition and spaces/modified serial extraction   261–2
    space and restore   258–61
  extracted deciduous molars   257–8
  interproximal reduction   256
  longevity of
    infraocclusion   257
    resorption   256–7
  missing mandibular premolar socket   269
  molar class II relationship and midline discrepancy   265
  overall dental health and cost   258
  space closure   267
second premolars   247–9
second-order rotation   316
selective tooth agenesis (STHAG)
  hypodontia   42
self-esteem   5
sella–nasion–B point (SNB) angle   37
serial extraction
  fundamentals of   92–3
  indications and contraindications for alternative extraction sequences   95–7
  AL/tooth size deficiency   93
  ankylosis, of deciduous molars   94
  dental arches   94
  ectopic eruption of molars   94

serial extraction (cont'd)
　facial type and balance 93
　gingival recession and alveolar destruction 93
　impacted/ectopically displaced lateral incisors 93
　path of eruption 95
　premature loss, of deciduous canines and midline shift 93
　sequence of eruption 94, 95
　skeletal imbalance 93
　surgical skill in extractions 95
　timing of eruption 94–5
short root anomaly (SRA) 47
single bracket system 319
single gene defects 38–9
single nucleotide polymorphisms (SNPs) 37
single point force 316
size
　AL/tooth size deficiency 93
　arch 61
　Bolton tooth-size discrepancy 119
　jaw 61–2
　of deciduous vs. permanent incisors 13
　tooth size arch length discrepancies (TSALD) 51, 67–8
skeletal dysplasia 38
skeletal imbalance 93
sleep apnea 299
sleep needs 299
sleep-disordered breathing (SDB)
　apps and devices for 310
　consequences of 305–9

diagnosis and management 300–2
　treatment options 309–10
sleep-related breathing disorder (SRBD) scale 300
small gonial 110
SNB angle 122
soft tissue dehiscence 279
space creation 15, 17, 19, 21
space maintenance 15, 17, 19, 21, 23–4
space regain 15, 17, 19, 21, 23, 24
speech therapy 310
spinal muscular atrophy 122
square jaws 110
subtractive couples 316–17
sucking habit 225–6, 234
Summers' occlusal index 28
supernumerary permanent maxillary lateral incisor 245
supernumerary teeth 42
supraeruption 58
surgical burs 278

t
taurodontism (OMIM 27200) 45, 47
temporary anchorage devices 274
temporary skeletal devices (TADs) 229
third-order rotation 316
timing
　of early treatment 1–2
　effectiveness and efficiency concepts 6–7
　maturational stage of development 7
　psychological aspects 5
　severity of malocclusion 5–6
　of eruption 94–5

tongue
　spurs 231, 235
　tongue physiology 226–7
　tongue thrusting habit 227–9
tonsil hypertrophy 303
tooth agenesis 42
tooth ankylosis 239–41
tooth mobility 279
tooth movements 58, 315, 316, 318
tooth rotation 314
torque 314, 316
trabecular bone 279
transitional deviations 4
translation 314, 315
transplanted premolar 276
transseptal fibers 61
traumatized incisors 279
Treacher Collins syndrome 40
tricho-dentosseous (TDO) syndrome 47
Trisomy 21, Down syndrome (OMIM #190685) 37
true mandibular rotation 116
true rotation 116

u
uneven tooth distribution 274
upper anterior dentition 111

v
vertical chincups 156
vertical molar eruption 58

w
weight management 304, 305
Wits appraisal 169–70
World Health Organization 285

x
X-rays 302